Basic Steps in Planning Nursing Research

FIFTH EDITION

Basic Steps in Planning Nursing Research

From Question to Proposal

Pamela J. Brink, RN, PhD, FAAN

Marilynn J. Wood, RN, DrPH
Professor

Faculty of Nursing, University of Alberta
Edmonton, Alberta, Canada

JONES AND BARTLETT PUBLISHERS
Sudbury, Massachusetts
BOSTON • TORONTO • LONDON • SINGAPORE

World Headquarters
Jones and Bartlett Publishers
40 Tall Pine Drive
Sudbury, MA 01776
978-443-5000
info@jbpub.com
www.jbpub.com

Jones and Bartlett Publishers Canada
2406 Nikanna Road
Mississauga, Ontario L5C 2W6
CANADA

Jones and Bartlett Publishers International
Barb House, Barb Mews
London W6 7PA
UK

ISBN: 0-7637-1571-9

Library of Congress Cataloging-in-Publication-Data
Brink, Pamela J.
    Basic steps in planning nursing research: from question to proposal/Pamela J.
Brink, Marilynn J. Wood.—5th ed.
        p. ; cm.
    Includes bibliographical references and index.
    ISBN 0-7637-1571-9
        1. Nursing—Research—Planning. I. Wood, Marilynn J. II. Title.
    [DNLM: 1. Nursing Research—methods—Nurses' Instruction. 2. Research
Design—Nurses' Instruction. WY 20.5 B858b 2001]
    RT81.5 .B74 2001
    610.73'07'2—dc21
                                                                00-067145

Production Credits
Acquisitions Editor: Penny M. Glynn
Associate Editor: Christine Tridente
Production Editor: AnnMarie Lemoine
Editorial Assistant: Thomas Prindle
Manufacturing Buyer: Amy Duddridge
Cover Design: AnnMarie Lemoine
Interior Design: Nesbitt Graphics, Inc.
Composition: Nesbitt Graphics, Inc.
Printing and Binding: Malloy Lithographing, Inc.
Cover Photograph: © Photodisc

Printed in the United States of America
05 04 03 02 01   10 9 8 7 6 5 4 3 2 1

Contents

8   *Selecting the Sample*   *131*

9   *Selecting a Method to Answer the Question*   *149*

10   *Reliability and Validity of Measurement*   *173*

11   *Ethics in Nursing Research   199*

12   *Planning for Analysis of Data   217*

13 *Writing the Research Proposal* 241

Appendix: Sample Research Proposals 265

Index 399

Preface to the Fifth Edition

The essence of this book is that the way you ask a question will irrevocably determine the way you will answer the question. We thought we had made this point very clearly in chapter 1 and that every generation of nursing students who read our books had understood it. We were wrong. Not long ago, a teaching assistant who had read *Basic Steps* and had taken the course asked, "What is the difference between asking a 'Why' question and asking a question that begins with 'What is the effect? . . .' Everybody else asks, 'What is the effect ...' questions. I can't see the difference in the two questions. Why do you insist on having students write questions your way?" There was a moment of stunned silence and disbelief, then disappointment that somehow she had missed the point.

As teachers and authors of textbooks, all that any of us has to offer is our distinctive way of looking at the world. People come to study with us because of our uniqueness. Although numerous research texts are on the market, each text has a particular view of research and the research process. Some are entirely numerical and statistical, some are entirely qualitative, and others are oriented to clinical utilization. Some texts cover a broad range of material while others are specialized and limited in scope. Each text offers a special perspective that makes that text different from all others.

This text asserts that the way you think about the research process, the way you put all the parts of the process together into a plan, is the first step in conducting research. We believe that planning a research project is a problem-solving process. You need to know enough about the components of research to pick and choose those most appropriate to your study. A novice researcher who is given all the components at once can be overwhelmed by the possibilities and never accomplish a thing. However, when given the major components and how they interact with one another, a researcher has a better chance of solving problems successfully. None of it is particularly relevant if you don't know what to study.

Deciding what to study, considering all the options, is a serious and sometimes frustrating task. While this decision is the primary responsibility of the researcher, it requires discussion with others and reading what has been written about the subject. Perhaps the hardest task of all is deciding on one well-defined study on one well-defined topic. There is so much to do that it is hard not to want to do it all at once. We have found that the refocusing and redirecting process of deciding on the subject is assisted by learning a few simple rules about how to ask a researchable question. Just as learning to use a computer for word processing greatly assisted the person familiar with only a typewriter, these few simple rules for writing research questions will facilitate your thinking and planning process in research.

This book, then, offers what we believe are the basic steps in planning nursing research based on the first step: asking a researchable question.

Pamela J. Brink
Marilynn J. Wood
Edmonton, Alberta 2001

Preface

This book is written as an introduction to the research process and deals solely with the beginning phase of research—the research plan. The book begins with finding a research topic and ends with the written research proposal. This book cannot, and does not, claim to stand alone as an exhaustive treatment of all phases of the research process. It is a beginner's book and treats the planning process as an art in and of itself. All attempts at sophistication have been ruthlessly blue-penciled, replaced by simple words and terms that are easily understood.

The basic thesis of this book is that research is only as good as its plan and that a well-conceived plan is of immeasurable assistance throughout the rest of the process. But planning takes thought, library research, organization, and a lot of hard work. Showing the student where to find information, what kinds of organization are possible, what to look for in the literature, and how to ask a researchable question in the first place, should provide a clearer picture of what a research project entails and how to go about it.

Any research project begins with the planning phase. This involves finding one problem, and only one problem, for study; asking a question about that problem; intensively reviewing the literature on the problem; deciding how to solve the problem; planning how to collect the data; deciding which method of analysis best suits the data; deciding how to best protect the rights of those in the sample; and then writing a proposal that is clear to anyone not familiar with all the thinking that went into the plan.

Once the proposal is written and approved by a committee on the protection of human subjects, data collection can begin. Data collection is the actual legwork of research, done either by the researcher or a research assistant. If the proposal is clear and precise, anyone can collect the necessary data.

After data are collected, the researcher must try to make sense of it by analyzing, thinking about, and organizing the data into a reasonable and explainable package. The data analysis plan in the proposal is used as the basis for this phase but may be altered to allow for unanticipated results. Unless the research design is a very rigidly controlled experimental design, there will be data that do not fall within the analysis plan. This is the time for rethinking the entire research process.

The final step in research design is writing up the results. Although the research itself may have evolved in fits and starts, the written report needs to be an even statement of procedures, discoveries, and conclusions. The report should be logical, consistent, readable, intelligible, and carefully documented throughout. Clarity and completeness are critical to this report, because other researchers may want to replicate the research.

Although based on previous stages, each phase requires different skills, levels of information, and solutions to the problems that inevitably arise. No one research text can possibly do justice to each phase. If each phase were handled adequately, the size of the volume would look something like an unabridged dictionary, taking up enough space to require a desk of its own!

This book is intended specifically for the student who is taking an introductory course in research, whether at an undergraduate or graduate level. Most introductory research courses are based on the planning phase of research, but few introductory research texts devote adequate space to this portion of the research process. This text is designed to fill that gap. Recommended readings are listed at the end of each chapter to provide more in-depth treatment on that particular subject.

Pamela J. Brink
Marilynn J. Wood

CHAPTER 1

How to Write a Researchable Question

Ever since the first person said, "There must be a better way," human beings have been asking questions about the universe and trying to improve the quality of life. The invention of the wheel, the electric light, and the automobile all resulted from painstaking thought, trial and error, problem solving, and research to find that better way. The same is true of new surgical techniques and new drugs—both are products of a need to improve the human environment.

The human mind is always questioning. As children we asked, "Why is the grass green? What makes the sun go down? Why does my dog have fur? Why do I always fall down instead of up?" Most adults would answer the questions with "because," which satisfied us as a statement of fact. But if we found a different opinion in every answer, or if we heard "I don't know," we kept asking questions because, as human beings, we had to know.

The purpose of research is to answer questions, whether they arise from a practical need or simple curiosity. But not all questions can or need to be answered by research. Some questions already have answers. Others, by their very nature, can only elicit an opinion—for example, "How many angels can dance on the head of a pin?" Other questions can be satisfied with an immediate answer: "What's the fastest way of getting to your house?" Questions asking "What should I do?" or "Where should I go?" require opinions and, therefore, are not suitable for research.

What, then, is a research question?

A research question is an explicit query about a problem or issue that can be challenged, examined, and analyzed and that will yield useful new information.

Answers to research questions add to our general knowledge. They can be used by other people in other places because the answers are valid no matter who asked the question or where the answer was found. This is the critical feature of research findings—they must be facts, not opinions.

Identical duplication of research questions, while possible, is rare. Similar questions occur over and over again and give rise to replication studies that can be useful in themselves, but identical questions that are significant and usable are extremely unusual. If you have thought of a specific, clear research question, you can be assured that in all probability no one else has asked exactly that same question. Whether your question explores an entirely new avenue of thought or examines an area that has been explored before, the exact question is yours.

If you can support your position and document your procedure, you have done something unique: no one else has thought of your exact question.

The research question is a reflection of the opinions, past experience, and ideas of the researcher. The questions and the problems chosen for study are as varied as the people who choose them. Some people are interested in minute detail, others in the overall picture. Some are interested in people, others in mechanical objects. Some are interested in ideas, others in actions. All such topics are amenable to research. And they are all subjected to the research question.

In order to do research, the first step is to find a topic to research. Where can topics be found, and how do you know they are researchable?

RESEARCH TOPICS

Finding a research topic isn't as hard as it seems at first. Once you develop the ability of looking for researchable topics, they appear everywhere. Experienced researchers become so good at spotting research problems that they usually have at least a dozen ideas waiting to be investigated. But finding topics can be intimidating at first.

Where do you look for research topics? The most fruitful area for research topics is your own thoughts, observations, and experiences. What have you been reading lately? Who have you been talking to, and what did you talk about? Where have you been? When you read a book, you may find yourself disagreeing with the author, or you may feel that the author didn't prove the point to your satisfaction. You may think of several arguments to refute the author's position. You may find yourself annoyed with the author's bias. Whenever you disagree with something you have read, you have the beginning of a research topic. If you have experienced a similar reaction to a conversation or someone's behavior, you also have a potential research topic.

That research topics arise out of these areas is natural. You know something about the subject. You have some facts or opinions that contrast with another's point of view. You read something that contradicted the position you just heard. You were taught a slightly different approach. Your personal experiences did not agree with the generalizations being made. Or you found a flaw in the logical development of the argument. Whatever the source of your disagreement, you found yourself frustrated by the fact that you could not positively prove that the other person was wrong. This is the basis for the research question.

The second aspect of topic selection is that irritation or frustration indicates interest in the subject being discussed. Just how interested you are depends on how long your reactions linger. If you immediately forget your irritation, you aren't that interested. If it keeps nagging at you, you probably have an interest that will sustain you throughout the research. Because you need a subject that will interest you long enough to complete the research process, use this rule to gauge your interest level. Knowing enough about your topic and being interested in it are basic requirements for selection.

How do you know if your knowledge is extensive enough? Take stock of what you do know. Where did you learn it? If your entire stock of information is based on accidental, personal experience, you may find that this amount of knowledge is not enough to sustain you. If, on the other hand, you have talked to many people about this subject and have been reading in the area, and if your personal observations have reinforced what you have read and heard, you certainly know enough to begin.

If you want to do research on nursing supervisors and their leadership strategies, but your entire stock of information is based on being a staff nurse, you don't know enough to do a study of supervisors. What you do know about is being a staff nurse who is subjected to different administrative strategies. If you have talked to other nurses about different supervisors and have read about supervision and how it is best accomplished, you are well on your way to doing research on nurses' perceptions of various administrative strategies. But you would have some difficulty with administrators' perceptions and decisions on supervisory strategies because that's not where your real interest lies. You might, in fact, bias your research against the supervisor simply because your interest is in the staff nurses. Knowing enough about your subject means that you know what you are specifically interested in; that is, you must identify your point of view.

Judging the extent of your knowledge about a particular subject depends on how specific the problem is. The more general the problem, the more people share facts and opinions about the problem. Suppose your research problem was nursing and your research question was, "What is nursing?" You wouldn't be proving anything one way or another because a general description of nursing already exists. On the other hand, a question such as "What is primary care nursing, and how effective is it in health maintenance?" requires more specific information about primary care nursing. You would have to read about the subject, determine the arguments for and against this specialty, and use the information to formulate your opinion, which must be susceptible to testing with new facts.

Nursing research topics include studies of patient populations and potential patient populations, or studies of people's responses to health problems or potential health problems. A student once said about her research question, "I only chose this topic for my research because it is a nursing topic." When questioned further, she revealed that she was very interested in middle-aged women and their self-perceptions; in fact she had read everything published on the subject but had hesitated to write her proposal on that topic as she did not think it was a "nursing" subject. She was quickly disabused of that notion and she happily wrote an excellent proposal on "her topic." If you are particularly interested in a topic, as this woman was, and have read exhaustively in the area on your own, try to find something about the topic that you can research. You will be much happier if you do.

Fortunately, you have been studying nursing and command a wealth of information that you may not realize you have. This knowledge can provide sources for research problems. In the area of patient care, you know about a variety of pathologies and medical interventions. You also know that there are different nursing care strategies based on which health agency the patient comes to and for what health problem. Have you formed any opinion on how to improve patient care in any of these areas? Do you think you would be able to document it? If so, how? You may have noticed that certain patients within the same agency and with the same problems receive different care. You wonder if this is because of the patient or the staff. You have been reading about stereotyping and wonder if patients are being stereotyped and treated according to the label.

Theoretical issues provide an entire area of research topics. Role theory offers innumerable ideas, whether relating to singular roles, such as the sick role, or studies of roles in interaction, such as the patient role versus the nurse role. Concepts concerning the patient's psychological reactions, such as grief, loss, denial, alienation, and immobility, can be applied to almost any patient situation for testing.

Testing assessment and intervention strategies is another field for exploration. How these strategies are used and developed, and who uses them and for what, are areas open to divergent opinion and fact building. Behavior modification, crisis intervention, and implosive therapy are interventions that need to be tested on a variety of patients in a variety of settings.

No single theory, hunch, opinion, or even fact is ever totally researched. There is always room for further challenges and explorations. The less that is known about a particular subject, the more work needs to be done. The more work that has been done, the more refinement is necessary.

Now that you have a general idea about research topics and where to find them, the next step is to ask a question about the topic.

WHAT IS A RESEARCHABLE QUESTION?

A researchable question is one that yields hard facts to help solve a problem, produce new research, add to theory, or improve nursing practice. A question that yields opinion rather than facts can lead to an interesting article or essay but is not researchable. Research deals with facts—that is, with observable phenomena in the real world. A question that will provide answers that explain, describe, identify, substantiate, predict, or qualify is a researchable question.

For this reason nursing research must be *usable*. Because research deals with the real world, the findings should add to knowledge that can be used by other researchers, theorists, or practitioners. Whether the question deals with improving patient care, administration, services, or educational strategies, the answer should actually help to improve those areas. Whoever reads the published report with the intention of using the findings, relies on the researcher having been *ethical* in writing the report—that the facts as presented are true and based on a valid and reliable study. If findings are to be used, the study must be honest and reliable.

To be of use, nursing research questions should be *now* questions. No matter how good the research is, if the society does not need or want the research findings, they will be ignored. Therefore, questions should be relevant to the issues of the day. In nursing, clinical questions, in particular, are *now* questions. Nursing desperately needs answers to clinical questions that are practical and immediately usable.

Research questions need to be *clear*. Fuzzy questions yield fuzzy answers. A fuzzy answer is neither usable nor ethical. Therefore, the clearer the question, the clearer the answer and the more usable in clinical settings.

Finally, a researchable question lends direction to the rest of the research report. If the research question were about an event, directive questions would ask: What happened? When did it happen? In what way did it happen? To whom did it happen? What difference did it make, now that it has happened? These questions demand more of an answer than a simple "yes," "no," or "maybe." Without some movement in it, the question is just a "sitter," without impetus or direction. *Sitters* are questions that elicit answers such as, "Yes, that's interesting," or "And then what?" or even worse for the researcher, "Well, now, what are you going to do about it?"

Now is the time to examine the research question in more detail, to show how it is written, what the parts are, and what each part of the question does. Because many people find research a difficult process and feel overwhelmed before they are through, they stop before they have any sense of completion or accomplishment. One of the reasons for this is that either they did not have a clearly stated question to work with, or they chose a highly complex question as their first effort. Both are guaranteed to produce a sense of hopelessness before the plan is completed. As a research novice, starting with a simple, clearly stated question practically assures you of seeing the research plan through to the finished proposal. A simple question is less likely to lead to a complicated research design than a complex question, which assuredly will. As you progress through this book you will find that this statement is true, but for the moment, just accept the fact that the simpler the question, the greater the chance of satisfaction from this, your first effort.

Everything in your research plan depends on your question. It is the point you want to make, to explore, to describe, or to know, stripped clean of any superfluous verbiage. It is your research purpose stated in one simple, comprehensive sentence. To arrive at this point, you will have to eliminate all interesting but irrelevant distractions, seek out the essence of what you want to know, and move from a very broad subject to one specific point you want to make. Now let's build research questions and see how the process works.

ASKING RESEARCH QUESTIONS

Although there are no hard-and-fast rules for asking research questions, there are guidelines that you can follow that will simplify the process. The way research questions are worded can have a profound effect on the research process that follows, so the more you know about asking questions, the closer you become to being a skillful researcher.

There are two basic components to every question, the stem and the topic. "Who stole the cookies?" In this question, the stem is "who" and the topic is "stolen cookies." The question could as easily have been, "What nurses wear white uniforms?" in which case the stem is "what" and the topic, "nurses wear white uniforms." A simple question has one stem and one topic. You may recall in the last section we recommended that beginning researchers *start with a simple question* (our first rule of thumb) to keep from feeling overwhelmed by the research process. That means a question with one stem and one topic.

After simplicity, the next most important thing about research questions is that they be *action-oriented,* demanding some activity on your part to provide the answer (our second rule of thumb).

The type of question you ask about your topic is the basis for the design of your research plan. Whether you go to the library or into the community, whether you observe a group of children playing, or whether you work in a laboratory to find the answer, your particular activity is inherent in the question you have asked. For this reason, the next rule is to *ask an active question.*

You may have noticed in published reports of research that the author presented a statement or a hypothesis rather than a question. This is appropriate for a finished report or a published study, as you will see later, but at the beginning of the research plan you need something that will provide direction. Because you are concerned with the planning phase of the research project, you are dealing in future tense—what you will and won't do when you start to collect your data. A question, rather than a statement, is called for in this instance. Notice the difference in the following sentences:

Mastectomy has an effect on women.

What are the reactions of women to mastectomy?

In the first sentence, the statement is a declaration of fact requiring no action on anyone's part. The question, on the other hand, demands an answer. The following series of statements and questions illustrates the differences between a question and a statement:

Age has an effect on convalescence.
What is the relationship between age and convalescence?

Black women have smaller babies than white women.
What is the relationship between ethnicity and birth size of infants?

Ice water increases heart rate.
What is the relationship between temperature of ingested drinking water and heart rate?

As you can see, a statement of fact demands no action, whereas a question does.

You will find as you start to write questions that some do not require action. Any question that can be answered by a "yes" or "no" is not action-oriented. These questions are "stoppers." The question has been answered, obviating the need to do any research. Questions that begin with "should" or "could" are also stoppers; they elicit opinions, not facts. For example:

Should nurses wear white uniforms?

Should nurses allow patients to participate in care planning?

What should patients do about noisy roommates?

· Should patients bathe in the morning?

Everyone has an opinion on each of the above questions. If your question can be answered by a simple "yes," or "no," or "I don't know," then you don't need to do research to find the answer. Try rewriting each of your "should" questions into action questions that require some investigation to find the answer. You will notice a great difference between action and opinion questions.

As you write your initial questions, try to write questions that begin with "what," "what is the relationship," and "why." Avoid using inactive verbs such as "do" at the beginning of your question. Questions beginning with "do," like questions that begin with "should," can be answered by "yes," "no," "maybe," or "I don't know," and are considered stoppers. They elicit an opinion rather than some activity directed toward research. Notice how questions that begin with "do" look.

Do nurses neglect patients?

Do all patients respond to pain in the same way?

Do patients with coronary heart disease tend to keep their clinic appointments more regularly than other types of patients?

Look at each of these questions in relation to its basic components, the topic and the question. In the first example the topic is "nurses neglect patients," and the question is "do." "Do" doesn't imply much action, does it? Change "do" to "what," and the question becomes, "What nurses neglect patients?" If "what" were substituted for "do" in the second question, the same change would take place: "What patients respond to pain in the same way?" The answers can no longer be simple "yes" or "no" opinions; some form of action is needed to find an answer.

As you are trying to write your questions as simply as possible, don't be discouraged if you find yourself writing "yes" or "no" questions—even the most advanced researchers find themselves slipping into the habit of asking stoppers. Your first task is to try to write your question as simply as possible, which may entail writing a complex question first and breaking it down into its simple component questions. Once you have done that, you can look at the type of question you have asked.

Active questions require some form of observation or measurement for an answer. Active questions imply that the researcher will have to observe something, participate in something, or question someone to arrive at an answer. The way the question is worded determines how the researcher intends to measure the quantity or quality of the topic. Measurement, in the research sense, means examining an abstract idea to derive a concrete answer. Whether the answer is in numerical form or a description, it is observable and concrete.

An active question, then, provides some direction for the researcher to answer the question in a measurable (concrete) form.

As you begin working with your research questions, keep a workbook of your initial questions and your final, perfected questions. In addition, write working definitions of the major terms or ideas in your question. A *working definition* is your statement of what the term or word means to you in the context of your question; in other words, a working definition is a definition that is specific to your study. Working definitions, at the beginning of your study, are not dictionary definitions; they are your personal description of the term. Right or wrong, they are what *you* mean, not what *Webster's* means.

Keep your initial research questions and working definitions together so that you can refer to them as you develop your project. As you progress, you may change your mind on your project. Sometimes you change your mind because someone else did the study, sometimes because someone talked you out of what you wanted to do, and sometimes because you hadn't clearly formulated what you wanted to do initially. In any case, keep the workbook close by so you can refer to it as necessary.

EXAMINING COMPONENTS OF A RESEARCH QUESTION

Now that you have a general understanding of research questions, you can look at each component of your question in more detail. The two basic components, the stem and the topic, need to be examined separately to see what they do and how they will affect the rest of your plan.

Because all research requires some plan for collecting information to answer a question, the way you ask the question determines how you will answer it. A Chinese philosopher once said, "The answer is in the question." This statement is just as true in research as it is in philosophy.

The first step in phrasing a research question is to use an active stem. In the section on writing questions, changing the question from an opinion question to an active question required replacing words such as "should" or "do" with words such as "what" or "why." By altering the stem, we have changed the question from passive to active voice.

The second half of the research question, the topic, is simply what the question is about. The topic can be simple, embodying a single concept or idea; it can be complex, with multiple concepts; or it can be global theory. Asking research questions involves some narrowing of focus into a topic that can be attached to a stem to form a simple question. Let's look at some examples:

Stem	*Topic*
What	are the value orientations of the Annang of Nigeria?
What	are the characteristics of successful dieters?
What	are the health beliefs of the Amish?

In these examples, the topic is a fairly simple specific concept. In the first question, the topic is "value orientations of" something. The second topic examines "characteristics," and the third topic examines "health beliefs." Simple topics such as these are concerned with only one idea. As topics become more complex, they deal with two or more concepts in relationship to one another, and they require a different stem.

Stem	*Topic*
What is the relationship	between dietary intake and birth weight?
What is the relationship	between preoperative teaching and post-operative pain?
What is the relationship	between obesity and locus of control?

These topics contain two ideas or concepts. The stem asks if there is a relationship between them. These are still simple questions with one stem and one topic, even though the topic has become more complex. The stem is adjusted to fit the topic and vice versa. You can ask "what is dietary intake" or "what is birth weight," but if you want to put them together in one question, you must change your stem to "what is the relationship" to fit the change in your topic from a single idea to two such ideas or concepts.

The topic is even more complex when you ask a question beginning with a "why" stem. "Why" questions start with a set of relationships that have already been established through research, and the theoretical explanation for the relationship is being questioned. For example:

Stem	*Topic*
Why	do Japanese-Americans have a lower suicide rate than any other ethnic group?
Why	does preoperative teaching decrease postoperative anxiety?
Why	does increased assertiveness in nurses lead to lower nosocomial infection rates?

These questions are still simple from the standpoint that they have one stem and one topic; however, a topic developed for a "why" stem becomes quite complex because it shows that a cause-and-effect relationship has been established between the two concepts.

Levels of Questions

Research falls into one of three major levels, each level based on the amount of knowledge or theory about the topic under study. At the first level, there is little to no literature available on either the topic or on the population and the purpose is to describe what is found as it exists naturally. At the second level, there is knowledge about the topic and about the population, but the intent of the researcher is to do a statistical description of the relationship among the variables. At the third level, there is a great deal of knowledge and theory about the topic and the purpose of the study is to test the theory through direct manipulation of the variables. Each level of knowledge limits the type of study that can be done.

Questions at Level I are designed to elicit descriptions of a single topic or a single population previously ignored in the literature. There may be literature about the topic but not in relation to a specific population, or there may be no literature at all that you can find anywhere on the topic. On the other hand, the topic may have been studied before, but you want to take a fresh look at it, perhaps from an entirely different viewpoint. Other Level I questions are based on some piece of missing data that other studies have overlooked. Level I studies are exploratory by their very nature (their intent is to explore all facets of a topic or a population) and their intent is to describe what is found. Level I studies take place in natural settings to describe what exists, as it exists. Answers to these questions provide a complete description of the topic.

If your topic has already been described and you have found a description in research literature, then you know too much for a Level I question and you move to the second level. Second-level questions focus on the relationships between two or more variables previously described but never before studied together. (A *variable,* in research, is defined as anything that varies, that has two or more properties, or two or more qualities. Age, sex, height, and weight are all examples of variables.) At this level, you have considerably more knowledge about the topic than you did at the first level, but you don't yet know enough to predict the relationship between your variables. You can, however, develop a good rationale for why they *should* be related. If, when you read about your topic, you find that you can predict that one variable influences the other in a certain way, then you know too much for a Level II question and you should move on to the third level.

Questions at the third level require considerable knowledge of the topic. These studies test predictive hypotheses about the variables. The knowledge required for the development of hypotheses is based on the results of Level II studies; therefore, the action of all variables can be predicted.

Finding the appropriate level for your question determines your subsequent course of action. Because this is such a critical step, we will give you detailed guidelines to follow. These guidelines will save time and energy and, at the same time, will help you focus on what you want to study. Now let's look at each level in detail.

LEVEL I QUESTIONS. At this level there is little or no prior knowledge of the topic. The stem question is always "what is" or "what are," and the topic is a single entity or concept. Level I questions are asked in such a way that they lead to exploration (by the researcher) and result in a complete description of the topic. Here are some examples:

Stem	*Topic*
What are	the eating problems of retarded children?
What are	the characteristics of suicidal patients?
What are	the spiritual needs of transplant patients?

All these questions have the same stem and address a single topic: "eating problems," "characteristics," and "spiritual needs." Each contains a reference to the population that the researcher wants to study: "retarded children," "suicidal patients," and "transplant patients." Most research questions refer to the study population in some way so that they focus on the researcher's interest. When the topic is broad, such as "problems," "needs," or "characteristics," it will need further clarification so that the question really asks what you plan to examine. Thus, you specify "eating problems," "spiritual needs," and "characteristics of suicidal patients" so that there is no doubt about your meaning. Each question spells out both the concept to be studied and the population in which it will be studied. These are the components of a good Level I question. In addition, these questions require that some type of activity, such as observing, questioning, or listening, be undertaken by the researcher to describe the topic completely.

The most important characteristic about Level I questions is that they are based on topics that either have not been studied before or have not been studied in that particular population. If you look at the examples above, you can see the idea. In the first question the topic is "eating problems" and the subjects are retarded children. There may be a great deal of literature on eating problems but little or no literature on the eating problems that are specific to retarded children. The second question refers to population characteristics. In sociology, an entire field of demography is devoted exclusively to studying population characteristics, but at the time this question was asked no study had described characteristics of suicidal patients. The third question deals with the needs of patients. There may be many studies in nursing literature on patient needs, but at the time this question was asked there was little information on the specific topic of "spiritual needs." There may be studies on spiritual needs of other populations such as soldiers, the dying, or children, but little literature specific to the spiritual needs of patients. These questions ask about *one concept only*. No reference to "relationships," "causes," or "effects" should be included in a Level I question.

Whenever you write a question at the first level, go back over that question and read it critically to see if it has the following characteristics: *one* variable, concept, or topic, and a reference to the population in which that variable, concept, or topic will be found.

A question such as, "What causes nurses to avoid suicidal patients?" has two variables. One is "nurses' avoidance," and the other is the "cause," which is unspecified but implied. Even if you don't know the cause, you have assumed that there is one and that the nurses' behavior is the effect. When you review your question and find that you have assumed a cause-and-effect relationship, try the second level. The same is true of questions that include words such as "influences" or "effects" or "results from." These are red flags. Whenever you see these words in a Level I question you know you will need to rethink and rewrite the question. All of these words *assume* a second variable, and at Level I we are doing research on only one variable.

LEVEL II QUESTIONS. Second-level research questions build on the results of studies at the first level. When a topic has been thoroughly described, it is possible to identify measurable variables. The next step is to look for relationships between these variables. At Level II, the stem question asks, "What is the relationship?" and the topic contains two or more variables. The answer to the question at the second level is determined by the statistical significance of the relationship between the variables.

Because Level II questions are built on existing knowledge, some research literature will always be available on all of the variables in the question. You know something about the variables even though they have not been examined together before. When you study variables together, you need to have a rationale to explain their proposed relationship. You need to discuss the concepts behind the variables and propose that a relationship may exist between (or among) them. The answer to the question will verify whether such a relationship exists.

Now, let's look at some Level II questions:

Stem	*Topic*
What is the relationship	between relaxation and pain in postoperative patients?
What is the relationship	between pain and length of convalescence from hysterectomy?
What is the relationship	between the educational level of nurses and their membership in professional organizations?
What is the relationship	between preoperative teaching and postoperative anxiety?
What is the relationship	among prenatal nutrition, birthweight of newborns, and age of the mother?

Each of these questions begins with the stem "What is the relationship?" and has a topic with at least two variables. For each question, a rationale is developed to explain why the variables might be related. Be sure that you can identify a minimum of two separate variables in your question.

When we say that each variable must vary, we are referring to the fact that there is no sense in doing research on something that does not change or has only one characteristic. It (whatever *it* is) simply exists, and we don't have to do research on it. We do research on phenomena that have more than one property so that we can describe or measure that property and look at its relationship to other phenomena. When we are studying an attribute of a person, such as an attitude, there must be at least two categories of that attribute in order to say that it varies. Attitudes, for example, may be measured as positive, negative, and neutral. The minimum measurement of an attribute is to say that it is present or absent—two categories of measurement. If we specify that the variable is always present, it is no longer a variable and becomes a fixed entity. For example, in the question "What is the relationship between the LeBoyer method of childbirth and the weight gain of infants during the first month?" the "LeBoyer method" is the only method that will be looked at in relation to weight gain so there is no variation. Each variable must be written so that it can have at least two categories. In this example, the first variable should have been "method of childbirth," allowing for more than one method to occur. By specifying the LeBoyer method, no variation was allowed. The second variable "weight gain during the first month" is written properly because it does not restrict itself to any one amount of weight gain but rather allows for variable weight gains to be measured. This is an easy mistake to make, especially when you have something in mind that you are hoping to prove, such as that LeBoyer's method is better than any other method of childbirth. Just remember that you must measure the others, too, or you have nothing to relate to the amount of weight gain in your sample. Later on in the planning of your study, you will discover that you will be collecting data only on the variables in your question and, if something is not in your question, it won't be measured. This may help you to see the importance of writing the variables so they can vary.

When writing questions at Level II, examine them critically. Each question must have a minimum of two variables, written in such a way that they both vary.

A question that asks "What is the relationship between nurses' positive and negative attitudes toward alcoholics?" has only one variable, "nurses' attitudes." Positive and negative are merely two categories of attitudes. When a Level II question is written properly, it will ask about the relationship between _____ and _____. If you look carefully, it is easy to spot a missing variable.

The process of writing research questions involves deciding the appropriate level of your question. After this has been done, the rest of the research process follows easily in a series of steps, all of which depend on the level of the question. So, when you are analyzing your Level II question, there are a couple of "red flags" to watch for that will help you decide if you are at the right level. If you find that you can predict the exact relationship between your variables (that is, you know which one influences the other and what direction the influence will take), this is a red flag. Try a Level III question. Also, if you cannot study your variables without testing a cause-and-effect relationship between them, you have run into another red flag. These questions may belong at Level III.

Although you may know one variable comes first in time (for example, pain), you really don't know if pain, in fact, is related to convalescence. If there were to be a relationship, you would not be able to predict the direction of the relationship.

LEVEL III QUESTIONS. The third level of research builds on the results of previous research. Research at this level begins at a significant relationship between variables. At Level III, the question asks *why* this relationship exists, and you must provide the answer, which always begins with "because . . ." and ends with an explanation. Assume that at Level II you had asked the question, "What is the relationship between sensory stimulation and weight gain in premature infants in the nursery?" You found that, of the four types of sensory stimuli examined, two of them were more effective in increasing weight gain than the other two. You are now in a position to ask the Level III question, "Why are these two more effective than the other two?" You will have to check the research and theory literature on sensory stimulation, breaking it down into its component parts regarding weight gain until you find something that provides an explanation. You can then safely design a study that begins, "If I manipulate this variable, then that particular result will occur." Now you have the basis for a predictive hypothesis and an experimental design. **All Level III questions lead to experimental designs.** The questions look like this:

Stem	*Topic*
Why	does patient satisfaction increase with positive attitudes toward self-care?
Why	is a decrease in dietary iodine associated with goiter development?
Why	does increased vitamin C in the diet decrease skin fragility in elderly people?

Each of these "why" questions has two variables, and each question specifies that one variable either causes or influences the action of the other variable in a certain way. The "why" question is answered by you, the researcher, who searches the literature for the theory necessary to explain the relationship. The study resulting from a Level III question will test the theory. The process of asking a Level III question is more complex than either of the other levels because much more information is needed to begin. You must answer the initial "why" question before you can propose to test the exact relationship between your variables. Here is an example:

Stem	Topic
Why	is urinary tract infection lower among spinal cord injury patients who drink cranberry juice?[1]

The information used in this study to explain the relationship between urinary tract infection and cranberry juice was developed from other research findings and began with:

> Because the metabolism of cranberry juice results in acidic urine. This lowered urinary pH may be providing a bacteriostatic medium within the urinary tract.

This question is based on both actual observations in a clinical setting and research findings. Patients who drink cranberry juice were noted to have fewer urinary tract infections than those who don't drink cranberry juice. The researcher wondered "why." The answer came from physiological literature as well as through research and theory. The researcher, after reviewing the literature, proceeds with any one of several new "why" questions: Why does cranberry juice metabolism result in acidic urine? Why does a bacteriostatic medium result in decreased urinary tract infections? Why does lowered urinary pH provide a bacteriostatic medium? If each of these questions can be answered through the literature, then the researcher can test the assumptions in the original question and set up an experimental design to show, beyond question, that increased cranberry juice ingestion decreases incidence of urinary tract infection. Level III questions require thinking through the answer as well as reviewing the literature to prove that the researcher's "educated guess" was on the right track. Here is another example:

Stem	Topic
Why	does structured communication decrease anxieties in families of surgical patients?[2]

> Because, using Festinger's theory of cognitive dissonance, the human organism strives for internal harmony among its cognitions. When this harmony does not exist, the organism experiences dissonance, which the individual seeks to reduce by seeking new cognitive elements that are consistent with existing cognitions. Structured communication can reduce dissonance by facilitating cognitive restructuring, thereby decreasing preoperative anxieties.

At Level III, you can predict what will happen and provide a theory based on previous research findings to explain it. At Level II, you propose that two

---

1. Kinney, A. B., and Blount, M., Effect of cranberry juice on urinary pH, *Nursing Research,* September/October 1979, *28*(5), 287–290.

2. Silva, M. C., Effects of orientation information on spouses' anxieties and attitudes toward hospitalization and surgery, *Research in Nursing and Health,* September 1979, 2(3), 127–136.

variables might be related, based on what you know about each one individually, but you cannot predict how or even if they are related. If you find a significant relationship at Level II, you move on to Level III because you will want to explain the "why" and document the precise nature of the relationship.

Remember that at Level III you must be able to design an experiment to test the action of your variables. Some questions, however, simply are not amenable to Level III studies. These are the "why" questions that require studies of variables that we have no ethical right to manipulate on human subjects or that are impossible to manipulate. Look at these examples:

Stem	*Topic*
Why	does age increase convalescence time for postsurgical patients?
Why	does gender influence the number of postoperative medications a patient takes?
Why	does smoking increase the probability of lung cancer?

In the first two examples, the causes, or influencing variables, are age and gender. Neither of these can be altered or manipulated by the researcher. You can, however, study them as they occur naturally in a Level II study. In the third question, the causal variable is "smoking." A study manipulating smoking with human subjects to see if lung cancer could be increased would be unethical. With questions such as these, rewrite them at Level II and see how they fit:

Stem	*Topic*
What is the relationship	between age and length of convalescence?
What is the relationship	between gender and amount of postoperative medication?
What is the relationship	between smoking and incidence of lung cancer?

In each case, the study can be done quite easily at Level II by finding a sample where these conditions occur naturally—that is, patients who have lung cancer already and whose smoking habits can be documented, or who are convalescing from surgery and whose age can be related to the length of time they take to convalesce.

At Level III, you can (and must) specify the direction of each variable in relation to the other, and *the causative variable must be amenable to manipulation by you.* Many studies can be done on the same two variables but at different levels. For example, you might ask the Level II question, "What is the relationship between preoperative teaching and patients' postoperative anxiety levels?" To answer this question at Level II, you would need to find comparable patients in areas where some nurses did preoperative teaching and others did not so that you could compare the patients' anxiety levels. The same two variables could be studied based on a "why" question asking, "Why does structured preoperative teaching significantly decrease the patients' postoperative level of anxiety?" In this study, you would design an experiment to test different kinds of structured preoperative teaching strategies and determine which one was more effective in reducing the anxiety. To do this study, however, you would first develop a theoretical explanation for why the particular teaching strategy was more successful at decreasing anxiety.

Rewriting Your Question

Many people who begin research feel that their written questions are perfectly clear; yet, not everyone will be able to understand what they mean. We have found that practicing the writing of research questions greatly improves their clarity. Table 1.1 presents examples of questions that were written by nurses of various backgrounds and, following group discussion, were rewritten more clearly. You may find these examples useful.

As you read these questions and their revisions, several common problems become apparent: Level I questions can have only one variable. Words like "effect," "cause," "factors," "reasons for," all refer to an assumed variable that the author failed to include. If you don't know enough to specify what those variables are, rewrite the question at Level I. If you know what the variables are, rewrite the question at Level II. If you know what the variables are but cannot specify the cause and effect (or if it would be unethical to manipulate the causal variable), rewrite the question at Level II. If you know the cause and effect and want to test the relationship experimentally, write a "why" question at Level III. Many of the examples in Table 1.1 were written by people who knew too much about their topics but still tried to use Level I questions. When rewritten at Level II or III, the questions suddenly made sense.

When two or more variables exist in the topic, write the question at Level II before trying to write it at Level III to be sure you have the answer before proceeding. Remember, Level III questions are based on the answers to Level II questions.

In attempting to write a Level II question, you may be writing about one variable with two extremes (such as the high and low incidence of medication errors) rather than writing about two variables. Questions such as this one need to be rewritten at Level I.

The following simple rules summarize the problems you may encounter and will help you write more effective research questions.

1. At Level I, have only one variable and one population in the topic.

2. If you have a cause or effect in your question, write the question at Level II or III.

3. If the words "cause," "effect," or any of their synonyms appear in your question, either eliminate those words or specify what they are and how they vary.

4. At Level II you need a minimum of two variables.

TABLE 1-1	*Examples of Rewritten Questions*

Original Question	Rewritten Question	
What are the effects of a child's admission to a psychiatric unit on the siblings?	Level I:	What are the feelings of children who have had a sibling admitted to a psychiatric unit?
What is the clinical significance of oliguria in the postoperative patient?	Level I:	What are the characteristics of patients who have oliguria postoperatively?
What is the level of pain relief in pediatric postoperative patients having received TENS (transcutaneous electric nerve stimulation) instruction?	Level I:	What methods of pain relief are available to pediatric surgery patients?
	Level II:	What is the relationship between level of pain and type of pain relief instruction (including TENS) among pediatric postoperative patients?
	Level III:	Why does preoperative TENS instruction significantly decrease postoperative pain levels in pediatric patients?
What is the relationship between medication nurses with low error incidence and high error incidence?	Level I:	What are the characteristics of medication nurses with high error incidence?
	Level II:	What is the relationship between error incidence and education level among medication nurses?
What is the relationship between administrative and staff nurses?	Level I:	What are the administrative characteristics of nurses?
	Level II:	What is the relationship between interpersonal skills of nursing staff and their job titles?
What happens to quality of nursing care with nursing registries?	Level II:	What is the relationship between quality of nursing care and type of nursing personnel (registry vs. hospital-based)?
What is the reason for hip fractures being more prevalent in women than men?	Level I:	What are the characteristics of patients with hip fractures?
	Level II:	What is the relationship between gender and hip fractures in elderly people?
What effect does discharge planning have on post-MI patient?	Level II:	What is the relationship between discharge planning and course of recovery at home for the post-MI patient?
What are the effects of relaxation/imagery techniques on asthmatic patients?	Level III:	Why do relaxation/imagery techniques decrease the number of asthmatic attacks in chronic asthmatic patients?

5. All variables must be written so that they vary.

6. At Level III there must be two variables that specify a cause and an effect.

7. If you have written a Level III "why" question, make sure it is both ethical and possible to manipulate the causal variable. (If not, rewrite the question at Level II.)

BE INTERESTED IN YOUR IDEA

A solid research topic is always worth doing and doing well, but research is only as good as the time and effort put into it. Don't choose a research topic because it looks easy. All research requires painstaking thought, writing, and reading before the proposal is finished. You might get by with a minimal effort, but you will have lost an opportunity to explore something meaningful to you. On the other hand, don't choose a topic that is so grandiose or complex that it can't possibly be done effectively. You may attract the attention of your instructor or supervisor, but that isn't a solid basis for learning research.

Choose a topic that truly interests you and will keep you going back again and again to search the literature, your notes, or your own thoughts. You need not necessarily retain the first thoughts you had when you began to write your question. On the contrary, you may focus on one small aspect of the larger problem that you had never thought of before. But this will not occur without your being intimately involved in the larger topic to begin with. This involvement is necessary if your research project is to be successful.

RECOMMENDED READINGS

American Nurses' Association Commission of Nursing Research, *Guidelines for the investigative functions of nurses,* Code D–693M, Kansas City, Mo: ANA, 1981.

Artinian, B.M., and Anderson, N., Guidelines for the identification of researchable problems, *Journal of Nursing Education,* 1980, *19*(14), 54–58.

Diers, D., *Research in nursing practice,* New York: Lippincott, 1979, Chap. 1,2.

Ellis, R., Asking the research question, *Issues in research: Social, professional and methodological.* Selected papers from the American Nurses' Association Council of Nurse Researchers Program Meeting, 1973, 31–35.

Fawcett, J. and Downs, F. S., *The relationship of theory and research* (3rd ed.), Philadelphia: F. A. Davis, 1999.

Johnson, B. K., How to ask research questions in clinical practice, *American Journal of Nursing,* 1991, *91*(3), 64–65.

Moody, L., Vera, H., Blanks, C., and Visscher, M., Developing questions of substance for nursing science, *Western Journal of Nursing Research,* 1989, *11*(4), 393–404.

Rempusheski, V. F., Ask an expert . . . Formulating research questions, *Applied Nursing Research,* 1990, *3*(1), 44–46.

Rempusheski, V. F., From where do nursing research questions emerge? *Applied Nursing Research,* 1990, *3*(1), 44–46.

From Question to Problem

Throughout the first chapter, the words "research topic," "research problem," and "research subject" were used interchangeably. This was done quite deliberately. In research, the research problem stands by itself as the moving force behind the research plan. It is developed from the research question and is the final and complete synthesis of everything you have thought, read, argued over, and written. It substantiates what you propose to do and why. Before this point, however, you have been talking about problems that occur in real life, situations that need solutions, topics or ideas that interest you, and subject areas that you want to explore. As they were used in the first chapter, the terms "subjects," "topics," and "problems" referred to a less sophisticated order of thinking than the research problem for your proposal.

In research, the research problem is the full exposition of your idea that you want to study. The problem statement or the problem definition—however you prefer to think of it—is a logical progression of ideas and arguments about your research idea. The problem introduces your topic, explains its importance, condenses facts and theories about the topic, and then in a final, decisive section justifies conclusively your choice of topic. The full problem answers all of the possible "who," "what," "where," "when," and "why" questions that anyone not involved in your project would ever dream of asking.

And those answers are firm, so definitive that there are no loose ends, no gaps, and no fuzziness in the reader's mind.

In essence, the research problem is an essay about your research topic. An essay is a statement of opinion, substantiated by facts, that proves the position taken on a subject. A good essay offers an orderly progression of ideas that carries the reader through to the logical conclusion. Research problems should be written in the same way as good essays.

Because many research reports begin with the research problem, you may wonder why this book began by asking a question. The question serves the same purpose in research as the thesis serves for an essay. In an essay, the thesis is "the author's opinion boiled down to one arguable statement."[1] The research question does the same thing—it is the entire research design boiled down to one measurable question. Just as the entire essay is built on the thesis statement, the entire research proposal is built from the research question. Explaining how to build a research plan from your research question is the sole object of this book.

In the previous chapter, you were introduced to some of the functions of the research question and pinning down your subject. In this section, you will be refining your question into its clearest, most concise form and moving into the development of the research problem.

FINDING THE LEVEL OF KNOWLEDGE ABOUT A TOPIC

Now that you have written your question, your next step is critical analysis of your question with the ultimate aim of using it to search the literature on your topic. In Chapter 1 you were introduced to the idea of three levels of research based on three levels of knowledge and theory development. Take a moment right now, if you have not already done so, to write out your topic at all three levels. Remember that:

Level I questions have one variable in one population

Level II questions have two or more variables in one population

Level III questions have cause and effect

Suppose you find that you have one variable in two populations, or two or more variables in two or more populations, and cause and effect that cannot be manipulated by the researcher. What do you do?

When you have one variable in two populations, write two simple Level I questions, each with one variable in one population. In this case, for example, "What are the characteristics of patients in a 'typical' nursing home in

---

1. Payne, L. V., *The lively art of writing*, New York: Mentor Books, 1965, 25.

Scotland versus the United States?" you will do two Level I studies, one in each population, and then compare the results of each complete study. You still have a Level I study—you simply have two of them to compare. This type of study is the basis for the Human Relations Area Files at Harvard University. These files are collections of anthropological field studies or single case studies of cultural groups that have been collected into one vast resource for secondary analysis. For the most part they are all Level I studies of single variables in single populations or descriptions of population characteristics. Anyone wishing to use the files can take two or more cultural groups to compare and contrast but the initial studies were all at Level I.

Suppose you had written a question such as, "What is the relationship between ethnicity and post-hysterectomy convalescence?"[2] How would you know whether this was a Level II question or two Level I questions? The difference lies in (1) the amount of knowledge about the variables and (2) the intent of the investigation. In the case of the single variable in two populations, the purpose would be to do a thorough verbal description of a single variable within the context of its population. The intent of the second-level question is to take selected portions of a previously studied variable (convalescence) and selected ethnic groups (Anglo and Mexican-American) and see if they relate to one another in a statistically significant way. In the first type of question the answer is a simple description of a variable in two different groups. In the second, the answer is a statistical relationship in which two or more ethnic groups are considered to be different categories of one variable.

Suppose you know enough about your variables to write a cause-and-effect statement, based on fact rather than hunch, but you know that there is no ethical way you as the researcher can change the independent variable as required for a third-level study. What do you do? Rewrite the question at Level II but use the theory as the base for your study. Or, if you have access to a laboratory setting, you may leave the question at Level III and use the theory base to answer the question and test the theory on animals, cells, cultures, or other appropriate subjects.

The way you write your question is the way you will answer it, so be perfectly clear at the very beginning about your level of knowledge about the topic. It is your level of knowledge that takes you to the library to discover the level of knowledge available there. Based on your literature review, you may change your question to a different level.

One way of finding out your level of knowledge about the topic you have chosen to study is to try to write questions at all three levels. You will immediately recognize your level of knowledge about the topic. If you cannot write a Level III question, it may be because you don't know the answer to the Level

2. Williams, M.A., A comparative study of postsurgical convalescence among women of two ethnic groups: Anglo and Mexican-American, *Communicating Nursing Research*, Boulder, Co.: Western Interstate Commission for Higher Education, 1972, *5*, 59–73.

II question. This is what happened to Ginnette Miles, a graduate student at the University of Iowa. Here are her questions and her working definitions of terms:

Level I Question "What are the craniofacial features of preterm infants with postnatal cranial molding?"

Craniofacial features—the physical traits of the upper skull and fore-head including head shape and curvature, measurements and anterio–posterior diameter, biparietal diameter, forehead length and width.

Preterm infants—infants who were born before or during the 37th week of gestation.

Postnatal cranial molding—symmetrical flattening of the lateral aspects of the cranium and forehead which develops in preterm infants as the head is repositioned from one side to the other on a mattress.

Level II Question "What is the relationship between the craniofacial features of preterm infants and their physical attractiveness as perceived by adults?"

On the other hand, you may know a great deal about your topic right away and will have no difficulty in writing your topic at all three levels. In this case, you need to decide which question you prefer as well as which question has already been answered before you proceed with your research proposal.

The following questions were written by Deborah Sholz when she was a graduate student at the University of Iowa. Notice the amount of knowledge needed to write these questions.

Level I. What are the body positions into which nurses place low-birth-weight intubated infants?

Body position: a configuration of the body which describes whether prone, supine, side-lying toward right or left; whether head is turned 90°, 60°, 45°, 30°, or 0° from midline either to the right or left; whether chest is rotated right or left; whether hips are rotated right or left; whether extremities are extended, flexed, medially or laterally rotated, including hips, knees, ankles, shoulder, elbows, wrists; whether head is in alignment or tilted backward or forward.

Intubated low-birthweight infants: infants with an ET tube in trachea weighing less than 1500 grams.

Level II. What is the relationship between body positions and heart rate in the intubated low-birthweight infant?

> Heart Rate: beats per minutes as detected by cardiac monitor.

Level III. Why does supine body positioning decrease heart rate in the intubated low-birthweight infant?

> Supine body position: infant's scapulae and buttocks are flat against bed mattress.

Although there are any number of ideas that you could have chosen to research, most research topics can be grouped into a few primary categories: theory, concepts, observed situations, prior research, and tool development. Each category has different requirements for solution and different end products. Each has its practical aspects, drawbacks, literature, and logic. Each has its supporters and its detractors. But all are valid. No one is better than another; it's simply a matter of what interests you the most. Some people always start with questioning a theory, some always start by questioning an observed situation. It's really a matter of "goodness of fit" between the researcher and the topic. If you want to question a clinical situation that has been bothering you, don't drop the idea because it's not a theory question. On the other hand, don't just attach any old theory to your question; your question will direct you to the appropriate one. Conversely, if you are a theorist at heart, your question will direct you to the appropriate situation to study; not every situation will suit your theory. The point is, your question will tell you where you are going and what you are going to do. Remember that it's your question and no one else's; how you develop it is your responsibility.

Now let's take some research topics and divide them into groupings:

Observations
Some patients refuse medications.

Some patients are called demanding.

Some call lights aren't answered.

Mastectomy seems to affect some women more than others.

Detoxification programs don't always work on addicts.

Behaviors
Listening

Eating

Touching

Distancing

Avoiding

Talking

Concepts
Addiction

Dependency

Hopelessness

Independence

Nausea

Privacy

Theories
Loss theory

Role theory

Alienation theory

Theories of aggression

Psychopathological theories

Theories of change

Learning theory

Germ theory

Biorhythmical theory

Ethological theory

Systems theory

Each category of topic classifies a different order of phenomena. Observations arise from real-life situations that can be seen, smelled, touched, tasted, or heard by any individual. Often an observation is stated as a generalization about a repeating occurrence. It is the generalization that is usually tested in the research project.

Behaviors are specific types of observations that can be seen and thought about. In nursing, research frequently is based on observed behaviors of patients or nurses. Because behavior is frequently seen as purposive or goal-directed, however, analysis of behavioral intent is more abstract and more removed from reality than a direct personal observation. Therefore, research on behavior is more abstract than research on observations and should be treated as a different level of abstraction.

Kim defines a concept as: "[a procedure for labeling or naming] a symbolic statement for describing a phenomena or class of phenomena."[3] Concepts are single abstract ideas, often expressed in a single word, that represent two or more interrelated ideas. A concept can represent a single group of observations or facts that are closely linked to one another in a distinguishable pattern. Research can be done on one concept and its component parts, but the interconnections between the ideas, which form the basis for the study, must be discussed.

You have been exposed to concepts all your life, so when you see one, you will recognize it immediately. Concepts are simply terms that trigger a set of ideas. Isolation is a concept; so are privacy, assertiveness, burnout, patient care, ethnicity, and pain. Each word, as you think about it, stimulates ideas about your past experiences with the concept. Perhaps you have experienced burnout yourself or have known someone who did. Can you describe the experience, what triggered the phenomenon, what helped to alleviate the feelings, what were the behaviors that contributed to the diagnosis of burnout? Think about pain. What does pain mean to you? Have you had patients who reacted differently to a similar type of pain? Is there a difference between pain threshold and pain tolerance? Is pain physiological or psychological?

When you look at a concept for your study, you will want to answer all of the questions that need answering about the concept as you plan to use it in your study. You will want to determine just what it is you want to know about the concept and write it down before you begin your study.

"A theory is a statement that purports to account for or characterize some phenomenon" according to Stevens.[4] Fawcett defines a theory as: "A theory may be a description of a particular phenomenon, an explanation of the relationship among phenomena, or the prediction of the effects of one phenomenon on another."[5] Theories are explanations of two or more interrelated concepts; as such, they are the farthest removed from reality or direct observations. Theories are abstractions of processes, interactions, and observations.

As you can see, each successive category moves farther and farther away from the requirements of being observable and measurable because the level of abstraction increases. Because research deals with observable phenomena

---

3. Kim, H., *The nature of theoretical thinking in nursing*, Norwalk, Ct.: Appleton-Century-Crofts. 1983, 8.

4. Stevens, B. J., *Nursing theory. Analysis, application, evaluation.* (2nd ed.) Boston: Little, Brown, 1984, 1.

5. Fawcett, J., *Analysis and evaluation of conceptual models of nursing*, Philadelphia: F. A. Davis, 1984, 19.

that can be described, classified, or explained, the closer the research topic is to observable fact, the easier it will be to pin down the elements in the research question. Not only are observations easier to pin down, but you also are more familiar with them since you have made one or more of these observations for yourself.

At the opposite extreme, theories are the most difficult to pin down as they are the farthest removed from observable facts. You may be familiar with the general idea of the theory and some of the work that has been done on it, but you are not as familiar or knowledgeable about theory as you are with observations. If you can refine a theory into measurable, observable terms, you should be able to pin down concepts and behaviors even more easily.

Because research requires explanation as well as observation, it will always involve some level of abstraction or theory. Whether you build your problem essay from an observation to a theory or begin with a theory and reduce it to measurable terms, you must relate theory to facts.

HOW TO SEARCH THE LITERATURE ON YOUR TOPIC

Whether you are a staff nurse, student, or faculty member, the library search of the literature will be limited by the library resources available to you. If your library does not have access to a computer search system in nursing or does not have up-to-date nursing literature sources, you are hampered in your search for recent studies. You are not, however, excused from searching the literature available to you. Begin your search on your topic by the easiest method. After isolating the key ideas from your topic, write synonymous concepts from *Roget's Thesaurus* or from your dictionary. With these synonyms in hand, turn to the book catalog in your library and see if there are any books listed under the themes you have listed. Ask your reference librarian for assistance. If there are many books on the topic, you may be at Level III and need to do some reading of the literature before proceeding with your search.

One of the most troublesome aspects of good research is a thorough review of the literature. You need to be as exhaustive as possible on your topic. One way of doing this is to examine everything available to you. Another way is to go beyond your own library resources and ask your librarian to assist you in obtaining references on interlibrary loan or to write to authors for reprints of their materials. A third method is to talk to those who know something about your topic. Each of these methods of "consulting the experts" or of reviewing the literature can and should be used, when appropriate. For your initial review you want to know if anyone has done your particular study before. As you go further, you need to find out what has been done that is central to, as well as peripheral to, your topic. And, finally, you need to know just what data-collection techniques have been developed that will be useful to you in your study.

The actual mechanics of a literature review require legwork on your part. Go to the library and look in the journals and books. Talk to the librarian and state precisely what you have read and examined. Direct the computer search of the literature based on what you have done. Because many computer searches are based on recent literature, you will need an additional search for your topic among earlier sources. Remember that there are many other sources. Computer searches are convenient, but they certainly are not exhaustive. You will find that many journals are missing from computer searches, and you will have to search those journals yourself.

Take your time at this stage of your proposal development. Read everything you can on your topic. Learn who the major authors are on your work. Get to know everything they wrote. Whether your question is at Level I, II, or III, you need to be as exhaustive in your search as possible. The more you know about your topic, the better your final project will be. It is certainly worth that effort at the beginning.

If you find few books (or none) on your topic, turn to your library's periodical holding list to find out which journals are on file in your library. Make a list of the nursing journals your library has on hand, so that, as you find a reference, you can check your list to see if you have that journal available to you. From the serials list turn to your major nursing indexes, *Cumulative Index to Nursing and Allied Health Literature* and the *International Nursing Index.* Other indexes will also be of use, such as the *Hospital Literature Index* and *Index Medicus.* Once you have located these sources, look up their major headings and subheadings for your topic and its synonyms. If you find your topic, check to make sure your library has the journal before writing down the reference. Start with the most recent year and go back a minimum of five years on your topic. At Level I, search broadly; at Level III, search narrowly.

When we get busy or pressured, we tend to forget the resources available to us in our research. Use your reference librarian as much as you need to—that's what a librarian is for. Don't hesitate simply because you aren't sure you know what to look for—ask for help.

LEVEL OF THEORY AND LEVEL OF QUESTION

As you saw in Chapter 1, there are three basic levels of research questions. The first level of question deals with a single topic or a population about which you know very little. Your knowledge was limited either about the topic of the question or about the people you wanted to study. Sometimes Level I questions are derived from observations of human or animal behavior that have never been questioned before. If you were interested in how children respond to pain after a burn,[6] you might want to do a Level I study. You may find a great deal of literature on pain, but most of it related to adults rather than children. In a recent study by one of the authors,[7] the research question was, "What are the variations in value orientations of the Annang of Nigeria?" Although there had been research done on value orientations in other groups, no one had done this basic study of the Annang. Therefore, the literature review on the topic consisted of reviewing all of the studies that had been done on value orientations, the theory on values and value orientations specifically, and the Annang. Because no study had been done on the value orientations of the Annang and very little literature existed on the Annang themselves, the study had to remain at Level I.

At Level II, studies have usually been done on the two or three variables that are being correlated. However, you will not find studies that have previously correlated the variables (unless you have found one study you wish to replicate and the purpose of your study is to replicate this particular study).

At Level II, you will usually find some previous research on which to base your rationale for attempting to study these variables together. At this level of research, you will also find concepts derived from Level I studies that are worth exploring or testing further. Sometimes you develop Level II studies from the findings of a Level I study. If, for example, you had read a study about privacy and the hospitalized patient,[8] and you enjoyed the concept that was developed from that study, you may wish to develop your study from that concept. There are many concepts at Level II that need to be developed further than the original paper. Bereavement, pain, privacy, burnout, helplessness are all concepts that deserve further study. Some of the studies will never go beyond Level II. If you are looking at behavioral variables, you are more likely to stop at Level II studies. If, however, you are looking at physiological variables, you are more likely to go directly to Level III studies.

At Level III, you will be dealing with theories or developing your own theoretical framework. At the third level, you must begin with theory, so you go through the process of outlining a theory to make it operational, as described in this chapter. Without the theoretical base, you simply don't have a third-level study. At Level III, however, you trace the linkages between each aspect of the theory. The linkages trace the logical steps from one point of an argu-

---

6. Kueffner, M., Passage through hospitalization of severely burned, isolated school-age children. In M. V. Batey (ed.), *Communicating nursing research,* Boulder, Colo.: Western Council for Higher Education, 1975, 181–199.

7. Brink, P.J., Value orientations as an assessment tool in cultural diversity: Theory, methods and examples, *Nursing Research,* 1984, *33*(4), 198–203.

8. Schuster, E.A., Privacy and the hospitalization experience. In M. V. Batey (ed.), *Communicating nursing research.* Boulder, Colo.: Western Council for Higher Education, 1975, 153–171.

ment to another. When you ask a "why" question you answer that question with a "because . . ." explanation. The explanation has a series of statements that are linked to one another logically and sequentially. This series of explanations can be diagrammed in a conceptual map[9] of the problem.

At Level III you are testing theory—that is the whole purpose of Level III studies. Your problem will be to find a theoretical framework for your study. You have asked a "Why . . . ?" question based on a good deal of knowledge. You asked, "Why does this particular variable change this other variable in this specific way?" You answer your own question by building an explanation for the relationships between those specific variables based on other people's research findings. You would not have been able to ask the question first if you did not know a lot about the way the variables impact on each other. The step-by-step explanation of the linkages between these variables, the impact of other variables on them, and how those other variables influence their actions, all form the basis for this theoretical framework. How to form those linkages is exemplified in Chapter 5 on how to write hypotheses.

You begin with your theory and you substantiate each point in the theory with the research that has been done by others. If you are right, and you hope you are, your explanation of how and why these variables interact in a particular way can be demonstrated through your project. Your literature review, therefore, is on those two variables and how they have been studied before. You are looking for the flaws in design that you will rectify in your proposal; you will look for proven tests that everyone uses because they work, you will look for all possible exceptions to the rule, and you will take notes on each study because you do not want to duplicate mistakes (but you do want to be sure to include all the correct maneuvers). Use your 5 × 8 cards, make photocopies of the critical articles, read extensively.

Physiological studies have the greatest literature base; support for your argument will be found in that literature easily. Behavioral studies are the most limited, as the conditions under which behaviors will differ are the least known and understood. Studies of human behavior are often culture specific, and to find behaviors that are cross-culturally valid for given circumstances is rare.

The level of theory is dictated by the level of question, but not all questions lead to theory since there is not enough research data on which to build theory. Much basic research needs to be done to advance nursing theory, and, for this reason, we advocate the use of all levels of research design in order to advance nursing knowledge rapidly. The level of question is based on the level of knowledge about a topic, and the level of knowledge dictates the level of theory. If, after having thoroughly reviewed the literature on your question,

9. Artinian, B., Conceptual mapping: Development of a strategy, *Western Journal of Nursing Research*, 1982, 4(4), 379–394.

you have found little or no data on either the topic or the sample, you remain at a Level I study. If you have found previous research on your variables but no linkage of the two together, you provide that explanation and test your conceptual framework at Level II. If your study shows a significant relationship, then you may proceed to ask "why" and test your theory at Level III. (A more detailed explanation of how to develop a conceptual or theoretical framework will be found in Chapter 3.)

DEVELOPING THE RESEARCH PROBLEM FROM THE LITERATURE REVIEW

The process of putting theory into an observable, measurable research question involves a thorough inventory of your knowledge about the theory: deciding which concepts within the theory most interest you; asking yourself which behaviors best exemplify the concept you have chosen; and, finally, choosing those observations that best represent those behaviors. Because you are narrowing down from abstraction to observation, you are moving from a generalization to a specific. Pinning down theory is a process of identifying what you want to know and filtering out all unnecessary material until you have narrowed your subject to its purest, most refined point. Let's see how it works.

Find Out What You Know

Let's say that your research question involves the concept of the patient role. You know that the term "role" stands for major concepts and theories, and you must decide which aspect of the word interests you. At the same time, you need to find out just how much you know about role to have a starting point for your literature search; you don't want to waste time going over familiar ground.

So you begin with your working definitions of your terms. Simply defined, working definitions refer to what *you* mean by the terms you are using *in context of the research question*. A working definition is *not* the definition of the term found in a dictionary. Nor is it a definition found in an English translation of a foreign language dictionary. A working definition refers to the meaning that you, the researcher, have in your head when you are talking about your research topic and its attendant variables. These are the definitions that get you to the literature, but they are probably not going to be the final definitions you will use in your proposal.

You define "role" as that group of behaviors commonly found among ill persons in a hospital setting. Suddenly you are uncomfortably aware of how far away you are from an observable, measurable definition of the term. As you look at your definition, you can see you need to define just what you mean by "that group of behaviors," since that phrase is very vague. You also see that you need to define "ill person" more specifically, and "hospital setting" isn't exactly the clearest term, either.

Role represents a series of concepts tied together into one word. And you should have a working (measurable) definition of each concept. Each concept must be divided into its component parts, each of which must also be defined in relation to some observable, measurable behavior. So you turn to the dictionary for help. You find that the dictionary defines role in terms of acting a part in a drama. This is not helpful as you attempt to clarify your idea.

Return to your original definition. You are interested in three major inter-related concepts in role theory: ill persons, hospital settings, and grouped behaviors. You have three areas in which to search the literature, look up definitions, plan a computer search, or seek out the reference librarian. On the other hand, you wrote working definitions of each area to narrow down, still further, just which aspects of the theories interest you and how much you know about each.

Ask Questions about the Theory

According to your question, you are most interested in how patients learn their role. Therefore, you ask:

Who teaches the role and how is it taught?

Are there different types of patient roles to be learned?

Is the patient role easy or difficult to learn?

Are patients satisfied or dissatisfied with their roles?

What kind of a role is the patient role?

What other roles interact with the patient role?

Is terminal illness a role situation?

Does the diagnosis of cancer change the patient role?

How does type of hospital affect the patient role?

All of these questions, as well as others you may think of, will need to be answered by some aspect of role theory. As you ask your questions and read what other people have thought or observed, take notes on the answers and opinions that you encounter. You can use index cards for your notes, making sure that you accurately cite the references to avoid having to look them up again.

Head each card with a question and, as you read, jot down notes on the answers, citing the author, title, publication date, and page number. When you are finished, group your cards under the appropriate questions. Examine each set of answer cards and decide which answers you agree with—or feel most comfortable with—and separate them from the other cards. You now have a beginning outline of those aspects of role theory in relation to ill patients that most interest you.

Look Up Interrelated Ideas

Since a concept is made up of at least two ideas, and a theory is made up of at least two concepts, there is always the possibility that at least one of the ideas will lead to an entirely different concept or even a different theory. Therefore, as you search the literature, look up all revelant, related concepts and ideas. You may find a fruitful new line of thought that leads you away from your original idea or reinforces your approach to your question. Look carefully at these ideas. Accept or reject them on the basis of knowledge, not hunch.

This search will also tell you whether you have eliminated too many ideas in the initial development of your question. Use this aspect of the literature review to clarify your topic, making sure you have left out nothing important and are not including anything irrelevant or superfluous.

Outline

Starting with the major heading, break down your theory into the component parts that address your question. (Remember that each major heading has at least two distinct subheadings.) This outlining process helps you become more specific about what aspect of the theory interests you and helps you identify relationships.

As you outline, include only those aspects of the theory that you agree with and exclude those areas that you consider to be irrelevant or unimportant. From this will emerge your specific point of view. Don't throw away the other arguments; keep them handy where you can refer to them when you are developing your full and final problem.

Role
    I. Role types
        A. Patient roles
            1. Inpatient
            2. Outpatient
            3. Convalescent
            4. Terminal
                a. patient doesn't know diagnosis

      b. patient knows diagnosis
        (1) recently told
        (2) has known for some time
     5. Short-term
     6. Long-term
     7. Emergency
   B. Staff roles
   C. Family roles
   D. Sick roles
  II. Role learning
 III. Achieved versus ascribed roles
 IV. Role distance
  V. Role behaviors
 VI. Role sets
VII. Roles in interaction

Convert Your Topic Outline to a Sentence Outline

For each heading in your outline, write one sentence or one definition that expresses your point of view. As you write your definitions, you may have to revise your outline because you may be moving farther away rather than closer to your original topic. As a handy reminder of your original thinking, you may include an example with your definition. If the definition does not follow from your example, try to rephrase it so that it does.

Role is the set of behaviors attached to a particular social position or status within a society.

   I. Role types are the specific roles attached to a particular position within a social position.
   A. Patient role is the set of behaviors expected of individuals who are receiving health-care services.
    1. Terminal patient roles are those behaviors expected of patients who are dying.
     a. Those behaviors expected of patients who are dying but don't know it.
     b. Those behaviors associated with patients who do know they are dying.
      (1) Terminal patients who have just been told may react with anger, crying, withdrawal, or a request to see their spiritual advisor.
      (2) Terminal patients who have known about their diagnosis for some time may be used to the idea, may refuse

to talk about it, may talk about their death freely, may be clearing up their personal affairs, or may want to be with their families as much as possible.

c. Those behaviors associated with patients who know they are dying but pretend not to know.

Relate the Theory to the Question

By outlining your theory and writing definitions about each relevant aspect, you now have some new working definitions for each term in your question. Not only do you have your terms defined, you have also added some new qualifying words to your research question. After your thorough review of role theory, your topic may have changed. In fact, you may have a whole new series of topics based on your review of theory. But remember, one topic is all you need for your research; more than one makes an overly complicated study.

Now that you have asked questions of your theory, defined each term in your question, outlined the relevant aspects of the theory, clarified exactly what you want to observe about each aspect and why, and, finally, substantiated each part of your outline with literature, you have the basic framework of your ideas and your literature review. This outline alone, when written in the form of an essay, constitutes your theoretical framework for the study. (If you had done the same work on one or more concepts, you would have the underpinnings for a conceptual framework.) If you are dealing with more than one theory or concept, your framework must show their relationship to one another as well as to your question.

BEGINNING WITH AN OBSERVATION

Remember that we began this discussion with the comment that starting with a theory and reducing it to specific, observable phenomena was more difficult than starting with an observation and relating it to specific situations. The latter instance requires proceeding from your personal experience and your familiarity with the subject.

You discover how much you know about your topic when you try to write questions at all three levels. If you find you haven't the vaguest idea how to write a cause-and-effect question on your topic but you can write questions at both Level I and Level II, you are already aware of how much you know about your topic. Begin your literature review with your question. For example:

What are the characteristics of successful dieters?

This is a Level I question about the variable "characteristics" on a population of "successful dieters." You can assume that there have been a number of studies of characteristics of various populations, but have there been any studies on "successful dieters"? First write working definitions of both characteristics and successful dieters. For example:

> Characteristics: The qualities or traits that distinguish individuals or groups of individuals from one another. These qualities or traits may be demographic such as age, sex, and socioeconomic status; or specific to my population such as prior dieting history, family history of obesity, onset of obesity, amount of body fat at the time of last diet, and so on.[10]

> Successful Dieters: Individuals who have deliberately lost at least 15 percent of their overall body weight and have kept it off for at least one year without gaining back more than five pounds.

With these two definitions in hand, the literature can be searched very carefully to see if there is any study at all that fits this description. Let us say that one or two studies were identified that looked similar to this one or were at least in the same general area of interest. Find those studies and read them. Do they answer the specific question you asked? Do they answer the entire question or do they leave things out?

Start by looking up the terms in your working definitions: successful dieters, diet history, family obesity, and so on. Let us say you found a study on successful dieters, but "successful" was defined differently. "Successful" was an individual who had kept the weight off for more than two years.[11] Or not all parts of your definition of "characteristics" were included. You can still proceed to a Level I study. The population in your study may have different characteristics from the other study's. You may find another study on successful dieters in which the authors defined successful as "having been overweight as an adult but not now overweight." In this case, the definition of successful is far more vague than yours so the findings of the study do not prevent you from pursuing a Level I study. You will take notes on these studies and write up the findings in your literature review. These two studies will help you isolate some other characteristics you did not think of, or may provide you with useful measures. They provide ideas for your study so you need to refer to them.

Suppose you found only studies of the characteristics of unsuccessful dieters. Look at these studies to see what kinds of characteristics they examined and which ones look promising to you for your study. Be sure to take notes on these studies and refer to them in your proposal, particularly when

---

10. All materials on successful dieters paraphrased from the grant proposal titled *Characteristics of successful dieters* submitted to the Division of Nursing by Pamela J. Brink in 1984, 1986.

11. Colvin, R. H., and Olson, S. B., A descriptive analysis of men and women who have lost significant weight and are highly successful at maintaining the loss, *Addictive Behaviors*, 1983, *8*, 287–295.

you develop your method of data collection. (Other studies can provide you with ideas on how to collect data.)

For a Level I study on successful dieters you will probably find studies on the relationship between obesity and many diseases, studies on different dieting programs, and studies on different explanations for the causes of obesity. None of these are directly relevant to your study but are essential reading to give you a general review of your topic. In your final literature review you will probably group many of these studies into summary statements or paragraphs. Tornquist has a very good section on how to write this type of summary paragraph.[12]

Let's take another example. Suppose you had started with an observation that certain patients reacted differently when learning that they had terminal cancer. Some reacted with anger, shouting, crying, and moroseness; others didn't react at all. Your original question might have been: "What are the reactions of oncology patients when they are told they are terminally ill?"

This question is already observable and measurable. It relates a particular situation to an abstract explanation. You may end up explaining the differences by using role theory, or you may find an entirely different theory, such as stimulus/response or loss theory. This type of question is easier to write about simply because, as a nurse, you are familiar with the subject. You have experienced these behaviors for yourself. You know what you are looking for and why. And, as a nurse, you can probably use the answer in your practice.

Just because you are familiar with your subject and begin with readily observable terms does not mean that you are free from the responsibility of reviewing the literature on your question. On the contrary, because your question is so specific, it may have already been answered by someone else. Your first task, then, is not to look up the theory but to examine the research literature.

Where Do You Start Your Literature Search?

Just as with the theory question, you begin with each specific idea in your question. In this instance, you may decide to begin with the words, "oncology patients." Card catalogs, the nursing index, and the *Index Medicus* will have a section on oncology but may not have anything specific on oncology patients. Just as in the theory question, you must then look up "patients" in the literature. But you are interested in specific patients, those with terminal illnesses. To adequately review the literature on this subject, each aspect of your question needs to be investigated for research that relates specifically or remotely.

Certain researchers discuss their findings in relation to new ideas and theories. As you read, take note of these interrelated ideas. One or more of them will strike you as being the *one* concept or theory that truly fits your question.

---

12. Tornquist, E. M., *From Proposal to Publication: An Informal Guide to Writing about Nursing Research*. Menlo Park, Calif.: Addison-Wesley Publishing Company, 1986, 25–30.

Just as with the theory question, keep your bibliography cards organized and properly annotated. You will probably want to head each card with the aspect of the question referred to, such as "oncology patients." From these cards, an outline will emerge.

Your outline practically writes itself. Your question is the major heading; your minor headings come from the individual words or specific ideas within the question. This outline takes the reverse of the theory outline format. You will move from your specific definitions to an idea or a concept. For example:

I. Oncology patients are inpatients of an oncology unit who were admitted with a tentative diagnosis of a carcinogenic process.
   A. Diagnostic studies have been completed, diagnosis has been confirmed, and the patient has been informed of the diagnosis of lung cancer. According to the chart the patient reacted with:
      1. Anger—explosive and abusive language to the staff and family.
         a. Anger can be a defense mechanism to protect an individual from an intolerable fact.
         b. Anger can be a normal expression for any disagreeable fact, opinion. Cultural behavior?
         c. Anger can be a usual response for some people. Stimulus/response?
      2. No response. After the patient received the diagnosis, chart states that the patient began to make pleasant conversation with the physician, changed the subject, or otherwise gave no indication of having heard or cared about the diagnosis.
         a. Heard partially. Higher levels of anxiety cause fragmented (spotty) perceptions.
         b. Denied the meaning of what was heard.
         c. May not wish to discuss the issue until given time to think about it. Motivation?
         d. May have the behavioral patterns of not discussing intimate details with strangers. Cultural beliefs?
         e. Explanation given may be so vague and technical, patient did not understand.
   B. Diagnostic studies have been completed as in A. Patient has been informed of diagnosis of leukemia.
   C. Diagnostics as in A and B. Patient informed of diagnosis of metastatic cancer from prior surgery.

You established your outline through ideas and reading, but because you began with a behavioral observation, your initial definitions are more specific and observable. Your review of research and theory is easier because you knew what you were looking for at the beginning.

When you are developing the literature review for a Level II question you proceed in exactly the same way. You write working definitions for each of the major variables in your study and begin your outline with your definitions. The following outline was developed by a graduate student during a beginning research course.[13]

"Question: What is the relationship between burnout in the NICU and type of coping mechanisms used among nurses?"

Coping is the cognitive and behavioral efforts used to manage specific internal/external demands that are appraised as taxing or exceeding the resources of the person.

I. Coping mechanisms are specific methods used to decrease stress.
 A. The types of coping mechanisms utilized in the ICU and NICU vary with each individual.
  1. Personal (reactive) strategies are informal methods of communication.
   a. Talking to people outside the unit.
   b. Talking with fellow nurses.
   c. Withdrawing self from the unit.
  2. Management strategies are professionally mediated therapy sessions.
   (1) Attending psychotherapy sessions for discussion.
   (2) Participating in neonatologist-attended meetings.
   b. Personal (proactive) strategies are behaviors initiated by the person.
   (1) Knowledge about the stress-producing situation.
   (2) The amount of control the individual perceives to have over the stressor.
   (3) The ability to laugh.
   (4) Confrontation of the situation.
II. Various stresses within the NICU produce a need for coping mechanisms.
 A. Interpersonal communication problems exist between staff and: physicians, nursing office, other departments in the hospital, and other staff members.
 B. The nurse's need for an extensive knowledge base in: patient teaching, cardiac arrest, pathophysiology of a neonate, and making many rapid decisions.
 C. Environmental stressors include: numerous pieces of equipment and failure, physical injury to nurse, physical set-up, and noise level of the unit.

---

13. By permission of Karen Goebel, University of Iowa, College of Nursing.

    D. The components of patient care include: work load and amount of physical work required, meeting the psychological needs of the patient, meeting the needs of the family and death of the patient.

III. Coping mechanisms are effective when there is a release of stressful emotions.

IV. Burnout is the loss of motivation for creative involvement resulting from stresses of the NICU.

    A. Characteristics of burnout manifest themselves in various ways.

        1. Physical manifestations are described.

            a. Feelings of chronic fatigue and exhaustion after adequate sleep and rest.

            b. Minor ailments such as colds, headaches, and stomach upsets occur frequently.

                (1) Emotions are altered by burnout. Symptoms of depression.

                (2) Hostility and negativism directed toward fellow workers, the unit, or patients and their families.

                (3) Guilt for having negative feelings.

        2. Burnout affects behavior.

            a. Detachment is expressed by avoidance and the use of diagnosis rather than name to identify patient.

            b. Overinvolvement is demonstrated by declining to take vacations and the inability to delegate responsibility.

    B. The causes of burnout are multivariate.

        1. The constant threat of imminent death with resulting guilt.

        2. Ethical dilemma about life and death issues.

        3. The demands of dealing with and supporting families of NICU patients.

        4. New and changing technology which must be learned.

        5. Understaffing which leads to exhaustion and frustration.

        6. Interdisciplinary conflicts due to roles not clearly defined.

        7. Intradisciplinary conflicts where strong leadership is required to maintain cohesiveness.

        8. Chronic patients who become a source of frustration and strain.

Starting with a problem close to home gives you the advantage of having more information about your question to start with, which, in turn, enables you to direct your reading and outline more specifically and to form working definitions.

The second aspect of starting with a problem close to home is that you are usually involved with the question you select. You either are working with the question on a daily basis or have had a recent experience with it that is likely to occur again. For this reason, the work you do on your problem—your thinking, your reading, and your attempts at clarification—is immediately applicable in your daily life and is not just an isolated incident. The more removed your research question is from you personally, the more removed you will be in the rest of your project. The more intimately involved you are with your question, the more interest you will generate, the more likely you are to sustain your interest, and the more practical your work will be.

On the other hand, if working with theory excites you, don't select a problem just because it's practical. Remember, this is your research project and no one else's—so whatever *you* want to know is the question you need to ask.

RECOMMENDED READINGS

Barnum, B. S., *Nursing theory. Analysis, application, evaluation* (5th ed.), Philadelphia: Lippincott, 1998.

Binger, J. L., and Jensen, L. M., *Lippincott's guide to nursing literature: A handbook for students, writers and researchers*, Philadelphia: Lippincott, 1982.

Chinn, P. L. (ed.), *Advances in nursing theory development*, Rockville, Md.: Aspen Systems, 1983.

Cooper, H. M., Scientific guidelines for conducting integrative research reviews, *Review of Educational Research*, 1982, *52*: 291–302.

Cooper, H. M., *The integrative research review*, Newbury Park, Ca.: Sage, 1984.

Cooper, H. M., *Integrating research: A guide for literature reviews* (2nd ed.), Newbury Park, Ca.: Sage, 1989.

Fawcett, J., *Analysis and evaluation of conceptual models of nursing* (3rd ed.), Philadelphia: F. A. Davis, 1995.

Fox, R. N. and Ventura, M. R., Efficiency of automated literature search mechanisms, *Nursing Research*, 1984, *33*:174–177.

Ganong, L. H., Integrative reviews of nursing research. *Research in Nursing and Health*, 1987, *10*: 1–11.

Gunter, L., Literature review. In Sydney D. Krampitz and Natalie Pavlovich (eds.), *Readings for nursing research*, St. Louis: Mosby, 1981, 11–16.

Kim, H. S., *The nature of theoretical thinking in nursing*, Norwalk, Ct.: Appleton-Century-Crofts, 1983, 8.

Lefort, S. M., The statistical clinical significance debate. *IMAGE: Journal of Nursing Scholarship*, 1993, *25(1)*: 57–62.

Light, R. J. and Pillemer, D., Summing up: *The science of reviewing research*, Cambridge: Harvard University Press, 1984.

Meleis, A. I., *Theoretical nursing: Development and progress* (3rd ed.), Philadelphia: J. B. Lippincott, 1997.

Nicoll, L. H. (ed.), *Perspectives on nursing theory*, Boston: Little, Brown, 1986.

Oxman, A. D. and Guyatt, G. H., Guidelines for reading literature reviews. *Canadian Medical Aassociation Journal*, 1988, *138*: 697–703.

Powers, B. A., and Knapp, T. R., *A dictionary of nursing theory and research*. Newbury Park, Ca.: Sage, 1990.

Silva, M. C., Selection of a theoretical framework. In Sydney D. Krampitz and Natalie Pavlovich (eds.), *Readings for nursing research*, St. Louis: Mosby, 1981, 17–28.

Strauch, K. and Brundage, D., *Guide to library resources for nursing*, New York: Appleton-Century-Crofts, 1980.

CHAPTER 3

The Full and Final Research Problem

In learning how to arrive at your full research problem, you developed all the necessary elements for the entire research plan—your question, your theories, your terms defined, and the type of measurement that you intend to use. Your next step is to put all these components together into a complete package, the research problem. This is very much like putting together a bicycle that you ordered from a catalog. If any of the parts was missing, or if you attached the pedals where the wheels belong, you wouldn't have a workable bicycle. Like the bicycle, the full problem should have a sense of completeness about it; all the parts should operate together, and the problem as a whole should work properly and be aesthetically pleasing. A poorly designed research plan is as useless as a box of parts and bolts.

To extend the analogy: putting a bicycle together is much easier, less time-consuming, and less frustrating if you know the relationship between the parts and the whole. If you know the "what" and "why" of the parts of a bicycle, then you know if you are putting things together properly and if you have achieved the full and final bicycle. A well-constructed bicycle is achieved because you know how it works, why it works, and what it needs to work.

A well-constructed research problem is achieved in the same way, because you know how and why it works, and what it needs to work. But before you can build your research problem, you need to understand the basic elements of the problem.

ELEMENTS OF A RESEARCH PROBLEM

Although some research texts and published research papers include all of the introductory matter (problem, rationale, purpose, literature review, and terms) under the heading, "Problem," it's best to know the elements of the problem itself and how it is developed as a separate and distinct section of the research plan. The elements are:

1. Review of the literature
2. The rationale for developing the question
3. The theoretical or conceptual framework

Each element, for its fullest development, requires a lot of thinking, reorganizing of ideas, and a logical progression of concepts and facts that leads the reader to your statement of purpose. Although research problems can be written in a variety of ways (see the research proposals in the Appendix), the same basic elements are present in all problems.

The problem is your frame of reference for the entire research project, your rationale for choice of literature, your point of view on your subject—all of which are substantiated by facts, theories, and arguments gleaned from your reading. The problem is your statement of what you are doing and why. If you are hesitant about your idea, your problem will be hesitant. If you are uninterested in your study, your problem will be dull. If you haven't done your reading, your problem will be merely a bucket of bolts. Whether you know it or not, your problem is the expression of your personality.

Review of the Literature

The rationale for the development of your question came from somewhere—ideas do not develop in a vacuum. Ideas often come from an outside source, either in written form or in an interview. Your review of the literature simply documents the source of your idea and substantiates the rationale behind your question.

The rationale for incorporating the review of literature in the problem essay is that when you substantiate what you say, you usually substantiate it through the literature you have read or through direct personal quotes. Therefore, since you must document your source for your rationale and your theoretical/conceptual framework, why separate your review of literature from the two other elements in the problem definition? You simply waste paper by repeating your sources in a different way.

The literature review is a series of references. It is not a bibliography. Only the literature that you have used to substantiate your problem is included in your literature review and in your subsequent list of references. Not everything that you have read about your problem is relevant to your research and therefore should not be included in the review. In high school you included your entire bibliography to prove to your teacher that you did extensive reading. But this is research, and only relevant literature is required in the literature review.

The Rationale for Developing the Question

The amount of space devoted to the rationale will vary, depending on the type of question you have chosen to answer. If there is no literature to support a given question at the exploratory level, more attention should be given to developing the rationale.

The rationale for asking the question is your statement of why you believe it is an important question to study, why you want the answer, and of what use the answer will be to nursing. What made you think of the question in the first place? You certainly had a series of ideas or questions that led you to this final research question. This is your rationale for the development of the question, and if not explicitly stated, it must be clear by the time the reader has finished reading the problem argument. This is your logic, your reasoning, your point of view—and the reader has the right to know what it is.

The Theoretical or Conceptual Framework

Although these words are frightening to the new researcher, they are not as formidable as they sound. The framework for your study is simply an explanation, based on the literature you have read, of how the variables in your study are expected to relate to each other and why. In this book, we put the framework in the form of an essay, and the structure of a good essay is in the form of an argument. The essay supports your rationale for developing the question; it is your explanation of how the theories you have found relate to your study; it provides the justification for your study; and it will give the reader a feeling for the value of the proposed research to nursing, not only in its contribution to the development of theory but also in its relationship to other research on the topic.

The framework is called a *conceptual framework* when your explanation is based on literature and research about the variables, or when the literature does not contain a particular theory that explains the relationship among your variables. The explanation, therefore, will be your expectation, based on the literature, about the action of your variables. You will evaluate this explanation after you have done the study and, depending on your results, you may or may not find that it actually provides a useful explanation for the action of the variable. Regardless, it will provide the central theme for the discussion of your results.

The framework is called a *theoretical framework* when the variables have been studied before and have been found to be related to one another. You have available to you either a theory that provides an explanation for the action of your variables, or a proposed explanation given by another author to explain the findings of his or her study of the same variables. In either case, the result would be a theoretical framework for your study. This framework will then be tested by you and will either be supported or refuted by your results. You, therefore, will add to the literature on the theory you are using.

Once you have read the literature and have established the existing level of knowledge about your topic, you are ready to develop the framework for your study. We already know that each level of research has its appropriate level of knowledge reflected in the literature, thus it makes sense that the framework also will be based on the level of knowledge about the topic and will differ for each level of research.

At Level I there may be no framework based on existing literature as there may be no prior research on the topic you have chosen. In this case, a rationale for the study customarily is developed to support the need for exploratory research on the topic, and to discuss the potential usefulness of the findings. Sometimes, however, Level I studies are based on theories or concepts that have been studied in other populations. For example, you might decide to explore the sick role in another culture. Since the theory of sick role was based on research done with the white U.S. population, its applicability to other cultures is not known. Your study, therefore, would explore the concept of sick role in another culture, using the existing theory as a starting point for the study, keeping in mind that it may not fit, and therefore allowing for flexibility in the design of the study. In this case, the framework for the study would include a discussion of sick-role theory as it would be used for your study and would provide a summary of the previous research on sick-role theory from the standpoint of the cultural or ethnic background of the subjects. In the discussion of your findings, you would be able to contrast your subjects with those of previous studies and might come up with some tentative ideas about the reasons for any differences that you found. These ideas could then provide the basis for further research on sick role.

At Level II, you must provide a conceptual framework for the study in your proposal. From the literature on the variables you plan to study, you will develop a probable explanation for the action that might occur among the variables. For example, in a study of the relationship among health beliefs, health values, and health promotion behavior, Brown et al. attempted to explain the potential relationships among these three variables using health locus of control as an example of a health belief system and utilizing what is known about values as predictors of behavior, to state that a strong internal locus of control along with placing a high value on health should be related to health-promotion behaviors in individual subjects.[1] The authors explain that this relationship might be expected to occur because the way individuals perceive the environment will determine their behavior in a particular situation. Persons with an internal locus of control perceive themselves as fully responsible for their own health, and if a high value is placed on health, a person should respond with health-promotion behaviors. Because not enough was known about these variables in relation to one another (they had not been previously studied together), this framework is conceptual rather than theoretical and represents the authors' "best guess" about what the findings might mean. Clearly, at Level II, the study is not exploratory but is looking for relationships among specific, predetermined variables to answer questions about these variables. The findings might lead to the development of a theory that could then be tested in further research.

Level III studies always have theoretical frameworks to explain what the researcher expects to find. Because these studies are always based on the results of Level II studies, you will always know the relationship between the variables in advance and can predict the direction of the relationship. Your prediction can be supported by a theoretical framework that explains why the variables affect one another the way they do. For example, in an experimental design, Rice et al. studied the effects of relaxation training on patients' responses to cardiac catheterizations.[2] In this case, previous research had already established that relaxation training reduces state anxiety in cardiac patients; therefore the authors knew that a significant relationship existed between those two variables and the direction of the relationship (anxiety is reduced). In fact, this relationship had not only been found in Level II studies, but also had been tested in other Level III studies using cardiac patients in a variety of situations (from postoperative to rehabilitation), but not with patients undergoing cardiac catheterization. The theoretical explanation for the effect of relaxation therapy is that it produces "an integrated hypothalamic response which results in generalized decreased sympathetic nervous system activity, and perhaps, also increased parasympathetic activity,"[3] and that positive somatic and cognitive changes occur during relaxation. The authors

---

1. Brown, N., Muhlenkamp, A., Fox, L., and Osborn, M., The relationship among health beliefs, health values, and health promotion activity, *Western Journal of Nursing Research*, 1983, 5(2), 155–163.

2. Rice, V. H., Caldwell, M., Butler, S., and Robinson, J., Relaxation training and response to cardiac catheterization: a pilot study, *Nursing Research*, 1986, 35(1), 39–43.

3. Benson, H., Beary, J.F., and Carol, M. P., The relaxation response, *Psychiatry*, 1974, 37, 37–46.

believed, therefore, that given the sympathetic and parasympathetic responses above, relaxation would provide both a distraction for the patient in a lengthy and difficult-to-understand procedure and a positive treatment for a situation involving high tension and anxiety. This study provided a further test of the theory by utilizing relaxation therapy in a situation that had not been studied before (the cardiac catheterization), and thus extended the use of this treatment with cardiac patients to include a major diagnostic procedure. As you can see, testing of theory at Level III is done in small increments, all of which eventually contribute to the overall understanding of the topic.

When you develop your problem essay, be sure that you are consistent with the level of your question, and use this as an opportunity to cross-check all the parts of the problem for consistency.

When you write your problem essay, you will be incorporating your rationale for the development of the question, your theoretical or conceptual framework, and your literature review into one (not three) definitive statement of what you are studying and why, and its relevance to you and your reader.

Remember, at this point you are the expert on your research. Now all you have to do is prove your expertise in an essay.

When you are looking up your topic initially, don't hesitate to look in theory, history, or even fictional literature for material on your idea. Sometimes there is not much available in the research literature but a great deal in other sources. Use any source available on your topic and check it for accuracy.

Be sure to check sources both in and out of the nursing field. Sometimes, the literature in the area is found only in history books or books on sociology. Check the various professional indexes for sources, look up synonyms and antonyms and check those out, talk to people, and ask them to help you think of sources for your search. Don't hesitate to use any source you can find that substantiates your topic. Nursing is an eclectic field and has built its knowledge on an amalgam of ideas outside its major areas of interest; the breadth of reading possible for any topic is enormous.

Remember that good research is ethical research. If you say that there is no prior research in an area, then you will be believed. Your word of honor is accepted until proven otherwise. Your statements are accepted at face value. If you say you have done your literature review, you will be believed.

A major problem that crops up over and over again is losing references. Be sure to keep a record of everything you have read about your topic and put it where you can find it until after you have finished the research project in its entirety. Don't throw away your bibliography cards—you never know when you will need them. Your can be absolutely sure that if you lose, misplace, or throw away one bibliography card, that is the one you will desperately need when you write your proposal.

THE PSYCHOLOGY OF ARGUMENT

Each element in your research problem is absolutely necessary to persuade the reader that your research project is sound, well though out, and well documented from observations or reading. This is the essence of argument—to persuade another person that your logic is correct and that your position is thought through.

To argue your point successfully, you will need to know your opposition as well as you know your position. For many of us, that's not an easy thing to do. We are so enamored with our own position we cannot think of any possible argument against it. But notice the technique in successful debates, successful salesmanship, successful books—they had all taken into account the opposition's point of view and had an answer for it. They were prepared to answer any question that required clarification, explanation, or further data. Whether you are trying to entice people to support your organization or accept your research plan, you need to plan ahead to win the argument.

The crux of the matter is that you have stimulated the argument and you are interested in winning. Winning just doesn't happen by itself. So if you are going to start an argument, be prepared to win it. You have the edge, because the opposition is not prepared for an argument, nor does it have a vested interest in its outcome.

Let's say that you have already experienced losing your research argument, which went something like this: "I want to study children's reactions to injections." Your instructor looks at you and says, "Well, that sounds like a reasonable enough topic, but why do you want to study it?" Somewhat taken back by being questioned at all, you respond with, "I'm in pediatrics, and I think it would be good to know." A pained expression comes over your instructor's face, perhaps even a sigh, and all of a sudden you feel pretty inadequate.

Suppose you had said, instead, "I'm on a peds ward, and I've noticed differences in children's reactions to injections. I have a hunch that there is a difference in boys' and girls' reactions after, say, about the age of 5 because of the way children are socialized into sex-stereotyped role reactions to painful experiences. I'm not sure just when—what age, I mean—these differences begin to be noticed, nor am I sure if it has anything to do with previous experiences with injections. But it seems to me that if we could find out when those differences occur—if they do—and if there is any relationship between prior experience, age, and sex, we as nurses could then change our approach to giving children medications on the basis of these findings."

Result? Full approval and a go-ahead.

Why? Because you thought out your rationale for why you want to do your study, you gave a personal observation to back up your idea, you suggested a theory to explain your observation, and you pointed out a use for the information that you might gather from your study. You won your argument simply because you answered all the questions. Your position was logical, sound, and thoughtful. Perhaps without knowing it, you incorporated all of the elements on problem selection. You spoke with authority.

Your argument also had a basic structure. You began with the general problem area that you wanted to study. Then you conceded that you didn't know all the answers ("I have a hunch. . . ."), and, third, you pointed out the practicality of the project. This was your punch line, which you shrewdly left for the end. Strong arguments always include (1) central points, (2) concessions, and (3) the points in favor of the position.

The basic elements of the full problem follow the requirements for an argument. Your rationale for developing the question uses the style of arguments—the central issue you are dealing with, the many and diverse ideas or situations that could be explored through research, and your reason for settling on this particular project. Your argument is strengthened by your literature review. Each point you make in a concession, or in your favor, should have relevant, documented facts to substantiate your statements.

The conceptual or theoretical framework also follows the logic of argument, whether you integrate your framework into your rationale for developing the question or write it as a separate section. You will begin with your central point, make concessions to other relevant theories or concepts, and then point out exactly which theory or concept is most applicable to your study and why. Here, again, your literature review substantiates your basic framework.

Whether you are doing research on a theory, an observation, or a particular tool, use the psychology of argument in the development of your problem.

STRONGEST ARGUMENT LAST

Imagine for a moment that you are the teacher of a research course, and all your students have handed in their problems for you to read. Which of the following problems would you make the student rewrite and which would convince you?

Problem 1

Recently bereaved widows have greater difficulties adjusting to the social problems of daily living than the literature on bereavement suggests. Most of the research and theory on bereavement deals with the phenomena of psychological adjustments to loss. Nurses need to know more about loss and grief. This study will add to the body of knowledge on loss and grief in widows.

Problem 2

Nurses are constantly interacting with patients who have suffered some form of loss—the death of a spouse or child, loss of a job, or loss of a limb. Most theories on loss are psychological explanations relating to grief or bereavement. Few studies have explored the relationship between a particular loss and the resulting daily social adjustments that must be made. Yet, a major area of nursing care is to assist the patient with problems of daily living and adjustment to the loss—not just to assist patients to cope psychologically without the lost object. Therefore, a study that focuses on the social adjustments to loss should provide nurses with some ways to assist the patient in adjusting to the social changes resulting from the loss. For this reason, this study will focus on the social adjustments of daily living that newly bereaved widows must make.

If you agree that Problem 2 makes the stronger statement, look at the structure of the problem again. Notice that it begins with a generalization and ends with a specific, from "loss" to "widows' daily adjustments to a loss." Then it builds to a climax, "Therefore, a study that focuses on . . ." and presents the final, irrefutable argument supporting the focus of this study. Finally, the problem deals with the usefulness of the data to be learned. The structure of the argument is maintained by listing concessions first and points in favor later. The movement in Problem 2 is from the problem area to the purpose of the study. In one paragraph, the skeletal outline for the entire research problem has been presented.

On the other hand, Problem 1 starts with the specific and ends with a generality; it makes the major point first and ends on a weak note. The same argument presented in Problem 1 is presented in Problem 2, but the ordering of the problem is different. Putting the strongest argument last leaves a stronger impression in the mind of the reader, who will have forgotten the first sentence by the end of the paragraph. The last sentence is the one the reader will remember, therefore, it should be the strongest.

Notice that Problem 2 is longer than Problem 1, even though both are single paragraphs. This result is due to the logic of the argument. When you begin your argument with your major point, it is difficult to create concessions and defenses afterward. If you start with the general problem, make concessions, and then build your defense from minor to major points, your argument is necessarily longer. But, because of its structure, you can easily check it to see that you haven't left anything out.

Read a good essay, article, or research report, and notice the way the author leads you from the general to the specific, from minor to major points, from concessions to defense. Remember that the advantage is always to the person who has the final, definitive argument.

SUBSTANTIATE WHAT YOU SAY

By now, you should have your research question; a topic outline of your theories, concepts, or observations; working definitions of every major term in your question; and a one-paragraph statement of your entire problem area. In other words, you should have the skeleton of the final research problem for your written proposal. Before you proceed to write the full and final problem as an essay, however, you have one final area to check—your review of the literature. It is this step that substantiates your argument.

Look at Problem 2 again. Notice the sentences that begin: "Most theories on loss . . ." and "Few studies . . ." In your full and final problem, you can't get away with those statements just as they are. You have to justify those statements with facts. Here is where your review of literature comes in.

To be at this stage in your project where you have the skeleton for your final problem, you need to have done some reading. If you have bibliography cards or annotated references on everything you have read, you are now ready to build a case for your project.

Begin the process with your research question, which, after all, is the central point you are trying to make. Put it up somewhere in front of you so that you can refer to it frequently. Now reread your question. Which is the most central point you are trying to make in your question? Which is the topic of the question, the fulcrum around which all the rest of the question revolves? Underline that portion of the question. Take every other word or phrase and rank them under the central point in descending order of importance. Do your outline and definitions agree with this order? If not, look at your question again. Does it include your strongest argument? If not, you need to rewrite it. Your question must contain your strongest argument.

Now take your outline and arrange each point under the headings you made from your question. You are now restructuring your outline from the most relevant issues to the least relevant. You also have a reference for each point in your outline. Separate the pros and cons under each heading. Make sure that for each heading you have references both in favor of and against that point.

As you work with your question and your outline, you will begin to notice two things happening to your notes. One, you will find interesting, but irrelevant, pieces of information. Set those aside. You may need them later, but right now you are building your argument and don't need them. Second, you may find that some of your notes fit under more than one topic heading. That always happens. Cross-reference your topic headings so that you can easily find your notes. Sometimes a reading will give both the pros and cons for the subject. Don't throw them out. You can always use the same author or even the same reading in several different places.

You now have a topic outline of your problem from the strongest to weakest argument, with concessions and defense. And for each topic heading, you have a list of readings. Recheck your outline to see if there are any gaps in your argument. Does every heading in your outline have at least two contrasting subcategories? Does your argument include both pros and cons? Do you feel you are an authority? Are you confident that you can defend your position from any point of view?

If you feel that you are being overwhelmed by reams and reams of paper, there is another way of developing the outline for your problem. Outline the central and substantiating areas of your question. Then arrange your annotated cards under the appropriate outline headings. Now arrange each group of cards according to the major and minor points. Then divide the cards under each heading according to pros and cons. Instead of a written outline, you now have your reference cards sorted into an outline. This is the advantage of writing references on 5 × 8 cards. They are easier to sort and hold up better than paper.

You might want to use a shoe box or a card file and make dividers under each content heading to keep your cards sorted. That way, as you begin your problem essay, all you have to do is pull out the appropriate cards and write directly from them. This method saves wear and tear on your nerves and prevents the loss of that one significant point you want to make.

The critical objective in this discussion is that you have ready references for every point you are making in your problem. You can quickly and easily substantiate your position with a quote, paraphrase, or reference to authors who have said essentially the same thing. Because you have done your homework, you can prove your point—you have become an authority.

RECOMMENDED READINGS

Chater, S., Search of research? The teaching of selecting and stating the problem, *Nursing Outlook*, 1965, *13*, 65.

Diers, D., Finding clinical problems for study, *Journal of Nursing Administration*, November/ December 1971, 15–18.

Donely, Sister R., Why has nursing been slow in developing a theoretical base? *Image*, 1980, *12*(1).

Flaskerud, J. H., Nursing models as conceptual frameworks for research, *Western Journal of Nursing Research,* 1984, *6*: 153–155.

Flaskerud, J. H., and Halloran, E. J., Areas of agreement in nursing theory development, *Advances in Nursing Science,* 1980, *3*: 1–7.

Hunter, J. E., and Schmidt, F. L., *Methods of meta-analysis: Correcting error and bias in research findings,* Newbury Park, Ca.: Sage, 1990.

Hurley, B., Why a theoretical framework in nursing research? *Western Journal of Nursing Research,* 1978, *1*(1), 28–41.

Jacox, A., Theory construction in nursing: An overview, *Nursing Research,* 1974, *23*(1), 4–13.

Moody, L. E., *Advancing nursing science through research* (vols. 1 and 2), Newbury Park, Ca.: Sage, 1990.

Myers, S., The search for assumptions, *Western Journal of Nursing Research,* 1982, *4*(1), 91–98.

Polit, D. F. and Hungler, B. P., *Nursing research: Principles and methods,* (6th ed.), Philadelphia: Lippincott, 1999.

Smith, M. C., and Stullenbarger, E., A prototype for integrative review and meta-analysis of nursing research, *Journal of Advanced Nursing,* 1991, *16*(11), 1272–1283.

Wandelt, M., *Guide for the beginning researcher,* New York: Appleton-Century-Crofts, 1970.

CHAPTER 4

Critical Review of the Literature

Whether you have been reading extensively or not, the nature of the material determines if a simple reading will suffice or if a critical review is necessary. A critical review does not imply criticism, although that can occur. A critical review means taking an analytical approach to your reading.

An analytical approach to any literature review implies purposive reading. You read the literature for a particular purpose. So the first criterion for the critical review is *usability*, just as with research itself. Whether you plan to use the material for general background information or as a reference in your proposal, whether it is a research report or a theoretical one, it must be practical.

Many people have less trouble determining the usability of theory than of research. The theory "feels right" or explains something not fully understood. The usability of a research report is not as readily perceived. The findings may support your hypothesis, but whether or not you can use the report depends on your ability to understand the report and its conclusions.

Some people feel immediately defeated when asked to read research. "I just don't understand statistics," they say. But look again at the structure of the research plan. How much of the plan is statistical? Very little. The structure of the research report is exactly the same as that of the research plan, except that the report is written in the past tense. The statistics are only one part of research, and you can get help with statistics if you understand the rest of the report.

Someone else will sigh and say, "But I just don't have a logical mind, so there's no point in my reading research." Nonsense. You may think differently from other people, but this doesn't make you illogical. Did it ever occur to you that perhaps the reason you couldn't understand the report was because the report was illogical? Just because research is published doesn't mean that it's well done or even well written. So don't decide you can't understand research until you've had a chance to evaluate the report.

Evaluating a research report for its usability is a simple matter of asking a series of questions. Research is usable only when the person who reads it knows its strengths and weaknesses on the basis of the critical review. The reader is also the person who will apply the findings. Applicability means more than use in further research. When reading research reports, look at your own professional practice—can this information be used in clinical practice, in educational settings, or in administrative functions?

When we know the side effects of a particular level of medication dosage, then we can reduce the amount if we wish to decrease the side effects. If we know that increased age affects length of convalescence, we can plan for longer periods of convalescence. If we know that certain types of patients adversely affect the nursing staff, we can alter nurses' attitudes, patient type, or simply make everyone aware of the situation.

Finally, applicability means the use of research to further our knowledge base. Pure and applied research are both usable in nursing. Simply because research is usable does not make it applied; pure research is also usable.

The second criterion for any research critique is *completeness*. The report must be comprehensive, addressing all your questions about the problem, the sample, the data collection technique, and the method of evaluating the data. As you read, are you still left with questions? Do you feel you don't quite understand the point being made? If so, the author probably left something out.

A good way to check for completeness is to see if you can replicate the study. If you have to ask the author for more information, the report is incomplete.

Incomplete studies are easy to spot. Look for the key words: purpose, problem, hypotheses, definitions, sample, methods, analysis. Does the author give you complete information on each? Or, are there omissions such as who forms the sample? Does the author mention only who is excluded? Does the author forget to tell you about the interview, if one was used? These and other gaps mean you cannot use the report as the basis for a similar research project, so its usability index goes down.

The third criterion of a critical review is *consistency*. Every area of the report must proceed logically. Can you follow the logical progression of ideas from problem to purpose, sample, data collection, analysis, and, finally, to the conclusions? Does the sample section follow from the problem? Is the data analysis consistent with the sample? Or, were some of the research subjects thrown out without explanations? Whether you start with the conclusions and recommendations and read back or begin with the introductory matter, the relationship between each component of the research process needs to be clear and logical. If the report is inconsistent, it is incomplete and therefore not usable.

Your critique of the literature, therefore, is your analysis of its usability, completeness, and consistency. In your best judgment, and according to your own logic, *you* decide if what you have read will serve your purpose.

A final point needs to be made. Don't expect perfection! Not everyone is perfect—not even published researchers. So don't "throw the baby out with the bathwater" when you are reading research. Evaluate the report with a critical eye. Look for ideas you can use—even a poor report might offer something useful. Look for ways of improving on the research.

CONTENT OF A CRITIQUE

Despite everything you may have heard, read, or thought before, the purpose of a research critique is to determine whether the findings are usable for you. Because you are the person doing the reading, you decide whether you can use the research.

You may have noticed in your reading that some journals regularly publish a critical review or a critique along with the published research. These critiques are done by professionals who know research forward and backward. They bring up points and issues that other people may not have thought of; their critique is as thorough and as detailed as time and space allow. These critiques have specific purposes: (1) they raise points that should be considered in further research on the problem; (2) they provide an analysis of the entire research process for people who don't know how to critique; and (3) they add information about one or more aspects of the research process that can be used by other researchers.

As a beginner, you are not expected to do such an extensive critique. But if you look over these critiques, you will observe that the same general questions are asked, and in the same order, as those discussed in the following pages. Only the detail is missing.

WHAT TO CRITIQUE

Unless a critique already has been presented in conjunction with a research report, you will be expected to critique every piece of research literature you read. Remember that you must be able to supply reasons for your choice of material and the way you use it in your proposal. Your critique should supply you with these reasons. No matter which aspect of your project you are attempting to substantiate with the literature, you will need a rationale for inclusion or exclusion of the relevant material. And your rationale is always based on your analysis of the literature.

Remember, all research is subject to a critique, including yours. The best research has been critiqued from the inception of the idea all the way through to the published report. But until you, the reader, have critiqued the report yourself, you have no way of knowing if it is, in fact, good research. Much of the information you need can be found in computer databases, such as CINAHL. Abstracts found in the database provide enough information to decide whether or not the article is usable.

With this in mind, let's move on to the actual technique of doing a research critique.

HOW TO DO A CRITIQUE

There are several methods of doing a critique. Which one you choose depends on your background and experience. The more experienced you become in critiquing and the more you know about research, the more detailed you will become in your analysis. But when you are starting out, you simply need some basic guidelines to follow. You will be surprised at how adept you become at critiquing.

Before you critique an article, even before you read the paper all the way through, scan the conclusions and recommendations. Using your usability index, decide if you want to read the rest of the paper. If you can't use the findings or recommendations, you probably won't want to use the rest of the report either. If you are looking for a particular research instrument, scan the section on methods or design to see if it is there. If you can't use the material, you will not be interested enough in the full report to critically analyze its contents. So before you commit yourself to an article, scan it for usability and interest. A major failing in reported literature is the separation of the theoretical framework from the rest of the problem statement. It should be an integral part of the problem. When you see this format, separating the two, it is quite likely the theoretical framework will prove to be meaningless for the study.

Another problem you may run into is the use of secondary sources in a literature review. If the secondary sources are inaccurate, so will be the current review. Always check original sources as the basis for a project.

After selecting an article to critique, scan the entire article from beginning to end. Look for the key terms: problem, framework, purpose, design, sample, methods, findings, analysis, protection of human rights, and conclusions. They should be in approximately this order. Is each area of the report given a sub-heading that corresponds with each step in the research process? They usually aren't, in which case you should reread the report and underline each of the major topic headings. (Of course, you do this on your own copy of the article, not in the journal itself.) If you cannot find a title to underline, then jot your own key term in the margin. This gives you an easy reference guide to all of the steps in the process.

Now scan the order of the headings. Do they follow the ordering you have learned? For example, can you find the introductory matter in the headings, or is it somewhere else? Whether you had to label the content yourself or the author provided the appropriate headings, you are looking for the logical progression of the material in the report.

You now have a basic outline of the report's content. Now look for gaps. Has any area been left out? Make a note of that to yourself. You may have missed it in your scan, or it may not be there. In either case, you will be looking for gaps and misplaced material as you continue your critique.

Now go back to the article and look at the section you have labeled as either "Introduction" or "The Problem." Read that section carefully and watch for three things: clarity, significance, and documentation. You will decide on the basis of these three items if the report is defective, substandard, or adequate.

A defective problem lacks clarity, significance, and documentation of earlier work. The writing style is ambiguous, unclear (you don't know the point being made), and inconsistent. The research itself is meaningless, unsolvable, or trivial. Either the documentation is missing entirely or the references are incorrect.

A substandard problem is either incomplete/unclear, of limited interest, or not fully documented.

An adequate or standard problem, on the other hand, covers all the major research objectives. The writing style is clear. You know and understand what the research is about, and the progression of ideas is logical. The documentation of the problem seems to be reasonably complete and is used correctly. Finally, its significance is clear in that the problem needed solving or the results are unquestionable.

To make this evaluation of the problem, you must first identify it. If the author doesn't clearly label it, you must find it on your own, which means reading the report thoroughly. Use your outline of the article as your guide. If you find yourself reading about the sample or data collection, you have read beyond the problem. Go back to the introduction and look for the problem there. It might be stated as a question, a statement, or a hypothesis. You decide how well or how poorly it is stated—but first you have to determine what it is.

As you read this book, you are given certain rules of conduct about the research process and the writing of a proposal not found in previously published reports. In fact, some of the research articles you read will directly violate some of the principles you read here. Try to keep in mind the function of this book—you are learning how to *write* a research proposal and how to *plan* a research project. The plan for the project and the final, written report do not always look the same.

A difference you will find between this book and final, written research reports is the way in which the purpose of the study is written (see Chapter 5). Most published nursing research reports have hypotheses rather than purposes. You can find research reports with hypotheses at all levels of research design—some even write null hypotheses as the purpose of the study. Regardless of the method used by the researcher to state the purpose of the study, you need to determine whether or not the statement accurately reflects what *you* believe the research purpose to be.

The purpose of a study tells us the (1) aim of the study; (2) objective of the study, (3) intention of the study, (4) plan of the study, and (5) the design of the study. Without a stated "purpose" for doing the study we cannot know, for certain, what the study is about. We must "guess," or assume. The purpose of a study directs the researcher's and the reader's attention to what the study is about, in one succinct statement.

The purpose of a study follows the problem essay and is, in essence, the culmination of the problem essay. After you have read the problem, the purpose should not be a surprise. It tells you precisely what the study is about. In some research reports, the researcher will write both hypotheses and questions. This gives you a more specific idea of exactly what they are looking for in their research.

The conclusions and discussion in a research report must answer all the questions asked, tell you whether the hypothesis was supported or rejected and why, and tell you if the statement of fact was indeed a fact. If there is no relationship between the stated purpose of a study and the conclusions, you have a faulty study. The purpose of the study tells the reader what the variables are and who the population is, and indicates the methods or design used. If these three pieces of information cannot be extracted from a statement of purpose, it will be difficult for you, the reader, to critique the rest of the research report. For example, sometimes you will see a predictive hypothesis given as the basis for a descriptive study. We don't know if the hypothesis was really written before the study was conducted or if the hypothesis was written for the article after the researcher found some interesting things in a descriptive.

When you read research studies with predictive hypotheses, look at the hypothesis and see if it is a direct cause-and-effect relationship or a more remote cause-and-effect statement. If it is remote, then the assumptions linking one part to the other must be in the problem essay. Remember, predictive hypotheses are stated positively. A predictive hypothesis is also called the *research hypothesis.* A null hypothesis is negative in tone, stating that there is no relationship. You learned about null hypothesis in statistics. People write a null hypothesis at the beginning of a research study either because they are ignorant of the difference between a research hypothesis and a statistical or null hypothesis, or because they do not want to find a relationship. You need to figure out for yourself what the researcher is trying to say.

The purpose of the study should be stated before description of the study design is given. If you find the purpose hidden among the conclusions, the report is defective. If, on the other hand, the purpose is where it should be but not as clearly expressed as it should be, the report is merely substandard. An adequate statement of purpose can be written as a question, a statement of relationships, or a hypothesis, but it must clearly describe what the study is all about.

Research designs are specific labels used by an author to designate a precise form of research process. The parts of the research design are the method of sampling; the process of data collection; and the method of data analysis. When the author of a research article labels the design, you can expect to see certain things in the research report. If you know what the author thinks is the design, then you can critique the study according to the author's statement. Sometimes the author is wrong and the editor of the journal and the reviewers are also wrong. The worst errors in design labels are in qualitative research approaches. Many authors and their reviewers mislabel their designs. The design of a study has a purpose and a direction. A research design is chosen because of the type of question the researcher asks and the level of knowledge about the topic to be studied. Design choices should make logical sense. If you want to find out how people feel about things, an experiment is an illogical choice. If you want to find out what people *do* under certain circumstances, an interview or questionnaire is an illogical choice (they will tell you what they *think* they do—which is not the same thing at all). If you want to find out about the health of Albertans, or even what most Albertans think about health care cuts, interviewing a few nursing students at one school does not make sense. So the purpose of the study dictates the design and the design dictates the sample, the methods of data collection, and the data analysis. Research makes logical sense.

Just as with the problem, you will evaluate the research design as either defective, substandard, or adequate. You will be looking at the sample, the methods of data collection, and the analysis.

What do you need to know about sampling when you are reading a research report? First, you need to know the purpose of the sample. The general purpose of sampling is to represent the population as closely as possible. Samples are small portions of a population. A population is the group of people the researcher wanted to study. A *total population* is everyone in the world who meets the criteria wanted. No researcher can possibly study a total population unless it is extremely small. A *target population* is the "theoretically available" group to whom the researcher wanted to generalize the results. Researchers usually sample from a theoretically available population to which they have access. This means that populations are (1) geographically available; (2) available by phone; (3) available through some address list; or (4) available through some secondary source. Usually, the researcher will report the way in which the sample represented the population from which it was drawn.

Next you need to ask, what is the size of the sample and what is its proportion of the population? Samples can range in size from one to thousands. They should be as large as possible given the time and resources of the researcher; given the amount of error the researcher is willing to accept (stated in the research report), and given the research design, which includes the number of variables being measured, the number of times each variable is measured, the type of variable being measured, and the type of measurement of each variable. How samples are selected will affect the sample size. The criteria for sample selection reflect the decisions made by the researcher on who will be included and who will be excluded from the study. Only those included in the study are said to "represent" the target population. The stated criteria, therefore, "limit" the generalizability of the findings to people having the same characteristics as the sample. If the purpose of the sample is not meant to statistically represent the population, then what is it meant to reflect? Next, you need to ask yourself, "How was the sample selected?" What were the criteria used for sample selection and what was the sampling procedure? Was it a probability or non-probability sample?

Does the sample "make sense" in light of the research purpose? Samples should make sense in relation to the purpose of the study. Note the following:

1. If there is no complete list of a population, a random sample is not possible.
2. If each variable is measured many times, the sample can be smaller.
3. If each member of the sample is measured only once, the sample should be larger.
4. If the sample is measured with numerical measures, the sample should be larger.
5. If the sample is measured with qualitative measures, the sample should be small.

Finally, as you review the research report, you will note the sampling procedure—whether the sample selection was through probability or nonprobability sampling. Probability sampling is recognized by terms such as:

Simple random sampling: which means every member of the target population has a known probability of being included in the sample either through (1) a percentage of the population or (2) a predetermined number of subjects.

Stratified random sampling: which refers to the target population being stratified (divided) on some characteristic or variable. Equal numbers or percentages of subjects are drawn from each strata or group.

Cluster sampling: refers to geographic stratification of the population.

Random assignment to groups in which there are a preplanned number of subjects in each group; the method of assignment to groups is pre-established and, depending on the number of groups and the number of subjects in a group, can be established by computer assignment.

The second major sampling procedure is called *Nonprobability sampling,* which includes *convenience or accidental* sampling (whoever is available and willing to be studied); *network samples* in which friends recruit friends into the sample; *quota samples* (also known as non-probability stratified samples); and *systematic samples* in which every nth person/object is included. Systematic samples may have a random or a nonrandom start. All these terms are discussed further in Chapter 8.

A defective sample does not represent the population in a logical manner. The sample may have nothing to do with the population. Or, the sample may not be fully described. You may feel that the author selected a biased sample from the population. If the sample is meaningless, inconsistent with the problem, or biased, it is defective.

In a substandard sample, the author is unclear regarding either the population or the sample. The sample may be meaningful to the problem but not to the population. Or, you may simply have a hunch that something is wrong within the sample.

An adequate sample is clearly specified, defined, and related to the particular population and problem being studied. It is representative.

Data collection methods are based on the problem and the sample. Again, look for the clarity, significance, and documentation of the methods in relation to the adequacy of the report.

If the data collection methods have no relationship to the problem or the sample, or if they simply are not presented, they are defective. Phrases like "an interview was conducted," "a questionnaire was constructed," and "available data were used" are insufficient in themselves. Sometimes authors will actually use a method of data collection that is inappropriate to the labeled research design. This means either the author does not know the design or has simply failed to be clear. Remember, if you cannot use the information—if you cannot replicate the research on the basis of the information given—the report is defective.

Substandard methods give only partial information. You may have a general idea of what the author has done, but not enough detail to use the information. If the author used a reference for the method, look that reference up. If the reference is unavailable from the usual sources and you have to write to the author, the report is inadequate. On the other hand, you may have full and complete information on the methods used, but you decide on the basis of your readings that only a partial or tentative solution can be achieved through this method.

An adequate or standard report on methods will tell you what, why, and how it was done in sufficient detail that you can make an informed decision about it.

The method must be logically consistent with the problem and the sample. Look at the age of the report you are reading. Is it an old piece of research? Was any work done in that area prior to this research? If not, the relationship between problem, sample, and method is critical. If the work is new, does the author rely on prior literature to establish the relationship between problem, sample, and methods? Or does the article deviate completely from established sequences? When the methods are irrelevant to the problem, the research is illogical and defective.

At this point in your critiquing, your analysis of data is rough and somewhat skimpy. Unless you understand statistics, you will have some difficulty with this part of the critique. Nevertheless, you should look at the clarity of the reporting style, the documentation of method, and the relationship between analysis and method.

Most research reports have tables of information, charts, and graphs. Can you find the sample adequately represented in the table? What about the methods—are they exemplified anywhere? If you were to develop an answer to the question based on the methods and sample, what would you include? See if the author has included this critical information.

A defective analysis does not answer the question that was asked. Such an analysis is unclear, ambiguous, unrelated to the data, or inconsistent with the rest of the research. A substandard analysis shows bias toward one aspect of the data over another, or does not fully present an analytical tool. The adequate analysis, on the other hand, is comprehensible, responsive to the data, and congruent with all preceding material in the article.

Finally, you are ready to examine that aspect of the report that discusses the findings, conclusions, and usability of the research. You have read the report quite thoroughly to this point and can form an impression of the findings or conclusions. Are they clear? Relevant? Usable?

The findings and conclusions have to be generated from the research. If the researcher makes some assumptions or conclusions that have not been adequately substantiated elsewhere in the report, you may suspect bias. One small research project, as you know, will not solve global problems. So look for the type of generalizations made by the author. If they go too far beyond the research, the author probably is too egocentric. Or, the conclusions might be too narrow or too specific. You are, after all, looking for some creativity from the researcher.

Defective conclusions are either too broad, too specific, or nonexistent. Substandard conclusions lack completeness. The adequate conclusion has a sense of finality and closure and is derived directly from the problem, and accurately reflects the findings.

You now know this article backward and forward. You have an opinion on its value by the end of the report. Now let's see how objective that opinion is.

Go back to the beginning of the report. Get out a pencil and paper. Start at the top left-hand side of the paper and list each of the major portions of the research report: *problem, sample, methods, analysis, findings/conclusions.* Across the top of the paper, list your headings: *defective, substandard,* and *adequate.* Now check off under which heading each section of the article falls. Add up the number of checks you have made in the *defective* column and multiply by 1. Add the checks in the *substandard* column and multiply by 2. Multiply the sum in the *adequate* column by 3. Total the scores. If you gave the report at least 12 points, it is adequate. If the report scored from 8 to 11, it is substandard. If the score fell below 8, you have a defective study.

Check your score against the impression you had after you had thoroughly analyzed the article. Do they agree, or is the score totally inconsistent with your impression? If similar, you have just verified the reliability of your perception. But, because feelings and impressions are not always reliable indicators of how good each aspect of the report is, use your objective scoring method until your feelings and the scores agree consistently.

GUIDELINES FOR CRITIQUE OF PUBLISHED RESEARCH

Another method of critiquing a published research report is to evaluate the study based on the following questions:

1. What is the research question on which the problem for this study is based? (Restate according to Level of Design.) Is the problem clear and logically stated? Is it *appropriately* supported by the literature?

2. Research design:

   a. *Sample:* What is the target population? What are the criteria for inclusion? How is the sample selected? What is the sample size? Are these four elements of sample appropriate to this design? Was an *appropriate* power analysis provided?

    b. *Methods:* What are the variables under study? What methods were used to collect data for the study? Where issues of *reliability and validity of measurement* adequately addressed? Are the procedures adequately explained? Are the methods the most appropriate ones that could have been selected?

    c. *Data analysis:* Did the data analysis provide an answer to the research question? Is there sufficient power to support statements made about the relationship(s) between/among independent and dependent variables? Are the analysis techniques appropriate and properly conducted?

    d. *Internal validity:* Could there be an alternative explanation for the relationships observed (or not observed) among the variables? If so, what might these be?

    e. *External validity:* Would the findings be applicable to other settings, times, people, places?

3. How can the findings of this study be applied to nursing practice, nursing education, or nursing administration without further research? [Acknowledging that all studies are flawed, and assuming that this study is no more flawed than most, how could you see the results in practice? Remember that if we refuse to use the study findings without further research, we can probably make the statement about most published nursing research.] Be specific.

4. What is the next logical research question that arises from this study? [Remember that all research raises more questions than it answers, and assume that the researcher will do replication studies.]

WHERE DOES THE CRITIQUE BELONG?

It may surprise you to find out after all this work that the critique doesn't belong anywhere. The critique is a basic part of your development as an authority in this area of research. You won't find critiques at the end of research proposals as appendixes. You won't include your critique as part of your proposal. But you will use the results of your critiques throughout your research plan, data collection, analysis of data, and final written report. As specific entities, they don't belong anywhere. As a process critical to your development as a researcher, they belong everywhere all the time.

The process and the end result are different. Your critiques are a part of the process of building your proposal. Thus, you will cite either in your bibliography or in your list of references every adequate piece of research you have actually used to develop your proposal. You will reference inadequate or substandard reports only when they are all that is available, specifying how they were inadequate and why you used them anyway. In order to do all this with reasonable veracity, you must have critiqued what you read.

No one can, or will, do this for you; it is your responsibility. The results, however, are worth it.

RECOMMENDED READINGS

Avis, M., Reading research critically. II. An introduction to appraisal: Assessing the evidence. *Journal of Clinical Nursing*, 1994, *3*, 271–277.

Beyea, S. C., and Nicoll, L. H., Qualitative and quantitative approaches to nursing research, *AORN Journal*, 1997, *66*(2), 323–325.

Carr, L. T., The strengths and weaknesses of quantitative and qualitative research: What method for nursing? *Journal of Advanced Nursing*, 1994, *20*, 716–721.

Donely, Sister R., Why has nursing been slow in developing a theoretical base? *Image*, 1980, *12*(1).

Dyer, I., The significance of statistical significance, *Intensive and Critical Care Nursing*, 1997, *13*, 259–265.

Fleming, J. W., and Hayter, J., Reading research reports critically, *Nursing Outlook*, 1974, *22* 172–176.

Giuffre, M., Reading research critically: Threats to internal validity, *Journal of Post Anesthesia Nursing*, 1994, *9*(5), 303–307.

Giuffre, M., Reading research critically: Assessing the validity and reliability of research instrumentation—Part 1, *Journal of Post Anesthesia Nursing*, 1995, *10*(1), 33–37.

Giuffre, M., Reading research critically: Assessing the validity and reliability of research instrumentation—Part 2, *Journal of Post Anesthesia Nursing*, 1995, *10*(2), 107–112.

Harrell, J. A., Reading research reports: Should I apply the findings to my practice? *Tar Heel Nurse*, 1995, *57*(2), 26–27.

Hek, G., Guidelines on conducting a critical research evaluation, *Nursing Standard*, 1996, *11*(6), 40–43.

Hinshaw, A. S., and Schepp, K., Problems in doing nursing research: How to recognize garbage when you see it!, *Western Journal of Nursing Research*, 1984, *6*(1), 126–130.

Jacox, A., and Prescot, P., Determining a study's relevance for clinical practice, *American Journal of Nursing*, 1978, *7*(11), 1882–1889.

Leininger, M. M., The research critique: Nature, function and art, *Communicating nursing research: The research critique*, Boulder, Co.: Western Interstate Commission for Higher Education, July 1968, 21–23.

LoBiondo-Wood, G., and Haber, J., *Nursing research: Critical appraisal and utilization* (4th ed.), St. Louis: Mosby, 1998.

Morse, J.M., Evaluating qualitative research, *Qualitative Health Research*, 1991, *1*(3), 283–286.

NLN Research and Studies Service, Search or research: Criteria for a research report, *Nursing Outlook*, August 1964, *12*, 60.

Norbeck, J., The research critique: A theoretical approach to skill development and consolidation, *Western Journal of Nursing Research*, 1978, *1*(4), 296–306.

Stetler, C. B., and Marram, G., Evaluating research findings for applicability in practice, *Nursing Outlook*, September 1976, *24*, 559–563.

Summers, S., Defining components of the research process needed to conduct and critique studies, *Journal of Post Anesthesia Nursing*, 1991, *6*(1), 50–55.

Tanner, C. A., Imle, M. and Stewart, B., *Guidelines for evaluation of research for use in practice*, New York: NLN Publication, May 1989, (15–2232), 35–60.

CHAPTER 5

Stating the Purpose of the Study

You might wonder, "Why state the purpose of the study when the question has already been developed into the problem and supported by a logical argument? Of what use is a statement of purpose?"

The main benefit of the statement of purpose is that it says exactly what you intend to do to answer your question. The purpose includes what you will do to collect data (for example, observe and describe, listen and describe) or what variable you will observe or measure (for example, age, occupation, self-image). Second, include some information about where the data will be collected (the setting of the study). Third, the purpose should include who the subjects of the study will be. The stated purpose of a study comes after the written research problem and is a one-sentence encapsulation of the study you propose to do. The question you wrote initially included what you were going to study (your study variables), and who you were going to study (your population). The statement of the purpose of the study expands on the question to include where, when, and sometimes how.

The statement of purpose, therefore, includes what and who you plan to study; *plus* where, when, and how you plan to do the study. The "what," "where," "when," and "who" of the purpose are stated in such a way that the research design follows logically.

The three ways of stating the purpose of a study are (1) a declarative statement, (2) a question, and (3) a hypothesis.[1] The appropriate method depends on the level of the question and the extent of the existing knowledge about the problem.

LEVEL I: THE PURPOSE WRITTEN AS A DECLARATIVE STATEMENT

When your knowledge about the research topic is limited because little or no research has been done, your study will focus on a search for information. At the simplest and most basic level, your initial question begins with "what." These questions are exploratory. For example:

> What are the behaviors exhibited by mothers and infants during the first week of the infant's life?

> What are the characteristics of nursing students who fail state board examinations?

Because these questions have a "what" stem, we can assume there is either no literature available that answers the specific question, no theory to explain it, or no previous research on which to base a study. Therefore, these questions lead to an exploration of the topic in great depth and detail. Instead of starting with concepts and a conceptual framework, you will develop concepts as your end product. Now, how does the statement of purpose differ from the original question?

The statement of purpose states exactly *what* you intend to do, *where* and *when* you intend to do it, and with *whom,* in order to answer the question. Purposes written as declarative statements *always* result in description.

The question, "What are the behaviors exhibited by mothers and infants during the infant's first week of life?" exemplifies the type of Level I question that had to be explored and described prior to the development of the theory on maternal/infant bonding. If you are familiar with the theory, you will have difficulty thinking back to that basic question, but the question had to be

---

1. The idea of stating the purpose depending on the level of the study was adapted from Wandelt, M., *Guide for the beginning researcher,* New York: Appleton-Century-Crofts, 1970. Wandelt related these differences to the level of knowledge and available theory about the topic.

answered before the theory could be tested. At the initial phase, someone had to examine thoroughly mothers' and infants' behaviors in order to describe and classify those behaviors into some meaningful taxonomy. The statement of purpose of that original study would have been written as follows:

> The purpose of this study is to explore (as observed) and describe the behavioral interactions that occur between mothers and their infants during the first week of life in the hospital and in the home.

In exploring behavioral interactions (as expressed by observable behaviors), new concepts may emerge. No predictions are possible from this kind of data, only descriptions and classifications. Therefore, the purpose states what the study will describe, including what will be done, where, when, and with whom.

The next question, "What are the characteristics of nursing students who fail state board examinations?" came from a nurse educator who had been puzzled about why some students fail and others do not. She, the teacher, did not know enough about the characteristics of those students to ask a Level III "why" question. Although theories existed to explain failure among students, the nursing students did not seem to fit those theories. No description could be found of students who failed state boards. The appropriate purpose of this study, therefore, is to explore and describe. The purpose would be stated as follows:

> The purpose of this study is to describe the characteristics of generic nursing students at X School of Nursing who failed state board examinations between 1980 and 1985.

The setting and the sample are described briefly in general terms; specifics are given later in the proposal. All Level I statements of purpose are written exactly the same way because they always intend to provide description.

Sometimes, Level I studies are explorations of a single process or single-process variables with the express intent of exploring the variable in depth and describing the process as completely as possible. These studies all begin with a "what" question on one variable or one concept and are obviously based on no known literature on the topic. Examples of such studies are usually found in reports using qualitative research methods.

> The purpose of this study is to identify and describe the social-psychological processes nurses use in a Level III Neonatal Intensive Care Unit.[2]

2. From Hutchinson, S.A., Creating meaning: Grounded theory of NICU nurses. In W.C. Chenitz and J. M. Swanson (eds.), *From practice to grounded theory: Qualitative research in nursing,* Menlo Park, Ca.: Addison-Wesley, 1986, 192.

Other studies at this level will look at a single concrete variable in a population under two different circumstances. First, the variable may have been studied before in other populations but not in the present one. Second, the population may be well known, but the variable has been unexplored. Studies of single variables in single populations are also Level I.

LEVEL II: THE PURPOSE WRITTEN AS A QUESTION

When you know what you will be observing but cannot predict the findings, your purpose is stated as a question. How much knowledge is enough but not too much? How can you tell if your study should be at this level? Let's look at some sample questions:

What is the relationship between age and rate of learning in autotutorial settings?

What is the relationship between ethnicity and suicide rate?

These questions start with concepts about which the researcher obviously has some knowledge, because the question asks about relationships between concepts or among ideas within a concept. The immediate difference between these questions and the exploratory kinds is that these begin with a concept.

The concepts from which the first question emerges are maturation and learning. These concepts have to be discussed during the development of the problem to clarify the frame of reference. You know that the concept of maturation was based on Erikson's stages of development and the concept of learning stemmed from stimulus/response theory. However, nothing in the literature gives any basis for predicting the effect of maturation on learning; therefore, the question asks, "What is the relationship?"

This question raises another point. Maturation was described in such a way that the age of the individual represents the level of maturation. Other aspects of maturation that might be measured by psychological or physiological variables are not considered in this study.

One of the effects of the statement of purpose is that it limits the study. This prevents you from being sidetracked. Therefore, the statement of purpose should be as specific as possible to make the rest of the proposal easier to develop.

The purpose of the study derived from a Level II question would look like this:

The purpose of this study is to answer the question, "Is there a significant relationship between age and rate of learning pharmacology among staff nurses in an autotutorial program at the Queens Hospital in 1990?"

The difference between this purpose, written as a question, and the initial research question is that the answer will be "yes" or "no" as determined by the data. Because the significance of the findings will also be determined, the answer to this level of question always requires statistical analysis. This level of purpose leads to a descriptive design, but it is not exploring the unknown as was the declarative statement.

Let's look at another example of purpose stated as a question.

What is the relationship between ethnicity and suicide rate?

This question deals with two concepts: ethnicity and suicide. Both may be studied alone or in combination with other variables. In this case, they are being examined together to determine if they vary together. The question is a simple one, asking if ethnic groups differ with regard to suicide rate. The literature tells you that in traditional Japanese society, *harakiri* or *seppuku* was practiced as an honorable form of death for a warrior. You might speculate, therefore, that the Japanese-American would have a higher suicide rate than other groups *if* traditional values about suicide were retained. Other ethnic groups might have different values that would affect suicide rates. This is an appropriate question for Level II, and the purpose would be stated as follows:

> The purpose of this study is to answer the question, "Is there a significant relationship between ethnicity and rate of suicide among adults between the ages of thirty and sixty years in X community in 2000?"

The answer will be that there is, or is not, a statistically significant difference in the suicide rates among ethnic groups in X community.

As a statement of purpose at Level II, your question changes from "What is the relationship?" to "Is there a significant relationship?" Why couldn't you have written your question this way in the first place? The reason is a matter of emphasis. First, notice the difference between the three levels of questions: (1) "what?" (2) "what is the relationship?" and (3) "why?" Questions 1 and 2 begin with "what" because they are descriptive studies. When the purpose of the study is stated, however, it is written differently because it evokes a different answer. As a final example of the difference between the original question and the final statement of purpose, notice the difference in the complexity of the two.

Level II Question
What is the relationship between a patient's length of stay and the immediate needs of the patient's significant others?

Level II Statement of Purpose
The purpose of this study is to answer the question: Is there a statistically significant relationship between a critical care patient's length of stay in an

adult medical, surgical, coronary, or combined intensive care unit and the perceived immediate needs of significant others, at the University of Iowa Hospitals and clinics, VAMC, and Mercy Hospital in Iowa City from May, 1986, to October, 1986?[3]

At Level I, you cannot predict the answer because you will explore a new area of research. At Level II, however, you know exactly what the content of the answer will be as the purpose has limited the scope of the study. The statement of purpose at Level II specifically excludes everything except the variables to be studied. The description provided by the answer will be narrow in focus and will describe the statistical relationship between the variables. When you originally asked the question at Level II, you were not sure whether this relationship was already known. Asking "what is the relationship?" question emphasizes the descriptive nature of Level II studies and facilitates searching the literature for related studies. It leaves the issue of prediction for Level III.

Look back at the questions and purposes on page 73. Notice that two of the variables are age and ethnicity. Both variables are mentioned first in their individual questions and both can be assumed to come first in time; we may even be able to predict that as age increases, rate of learning will also increase. So why are we maintaining that these are Level II questions? Why not Level III? The reason is very simple. All Level II studies are descriptive studies—they are designed to describe the relationship among variables—while all Level III studies are experimental studies in which the investigator manipulates the independent variable. Neither age nor ethnicity can be directly manipulated by the investigator. You can create a sample based on different age groups or different ethnic groups, but this is not "manipulation"—actually changing something. You can change the temperature of water, you can show different movies, you can teach different content using different techniques, but you can only observe the effects of age and observe the effects of ethnicity as they occur naturally. You cannot age a person and you cannot change his or her ethnic identity—these are inherent human qualities not amenable to experimental manipulation. It is equally impossible to do Level III studies when manipulation of the independent variable might cause harm to the subject. Even if you know a great deal about a disease process, you cannot (ethically) cause that disease in humans in order to have a Level III study. The best you can do at Level III is a laboratory experiment using tissue cultures or animal subjects. These studies are difficult to generalize to human subjects. Although you may

---

3. Margo Halm, Research proposal, December, 1985.

know a great deal about the variable and its effects, you cannot write the question or study it at Level III with humans.

LEVEL III: THE PURPOSE WRITTEN AS A HYPOTHESIS

When you have enough information to predict the outcome of your study and you intend to test the significance of your prediction, your question is stated at Level III as a hypothesis.

A hypothesis is simply an assertion of a specific relationship between two or more variables. Hypotheses are possible only in studies based on conceptual or theoretical frameworks; they are supported by an argument developed during the definition of the problem. Although hypotheses are sometimes referred to as "hunches," in reality they are calculated guesses that can be supported by theory and previous research.

The term *hypothesis* in this text is used interchangeably with *predictive hypothesis,* in which the exact relationship between two variables is predicted. A predictive hypothesis specifies which variable is the cause and which is the effect, or which is independent and which is dependent. We believe the predictive hypothesis is preferable to the simple statement of a relationship between two variables found in some literature, such as, "There is a relationship between gender and successful weight loss among dieters." The latter sounds like a statement of fact and may lead the researcher to feel that the point has been proved before the study has been done. We believe that predictive hypotheses are precise statements of relationships that should not be made unless they can be supported through the literature. If you cannot predict the direction of the relationship, go back to Level II to identify and describe it first.

Hypotheses are predictions of causal relationships between variables that must be tested. At this level of study, your focus becomes quite narrow. At Level III, the independent variable or cause is the one that you, the researcher, manipulate. You are fully responsible for this variable as it is under your full control. Without a good idea of what the result will be, it is unethical to inflict your independent variable on people. The result is the dependent variable. That is why predictive hypotheses must be developed from previous research findings and from the theoretical answer to the "why" question. There is always a great deal of information available about the variables in Level III studies. Without sufficient data, it would be impossible to predict cause-and-effect relationships. Consider the following Level II question:

What is the relationship between ethnicity and suicide rate in Los Angeles County in the year 2000?

The answer was that Japanese-Americans had a significantly lower incidence of suicide in Los Angeles than any other ethnic group.

A search of the literature, however, did not reveal a theory to explain this finding; therefore there is not enough information to write an ethical predictive hypothesis. In addition, you could not ethically manipulate ethnicity and suicide in an experimental design.

Here is another finding from a Level II study:

> Nurses who work for ten years or more in long-term psychiatric facilities are significantly more authoritarian (as measured on an authoritarianism scale) than are medical/surgical nurses working for the same length of time.

Think about the two variables in this study. If you asked why the relationship exists, you would not be able to predict a cause or effect from the answer. Which is the independent variable? Does the psychiatric setting foster authoritarianism, or does authoritarianism influence the choice of nursing specialty? When your knowledge is still too general to predict exactly how one variable influences another, you are not ready to write a predictive hypothesis.

Extensive research and theory on teaching and learning by nurses have been effectively used in the clinical setting. You can predict, for example, that any structured teaching program is more effective than an unstructured teaching program for all patient populations and for all types of knowledge. Because there has been extensive research on these theories, they can be safely tested on patient populations. There are different levels of prediction, however, based on the level of knowledge of patient/teaching studies. For example, take the following hypothesis:

> Diabetic patients who receive structured group teaching about their diabetes will have a significantly lower readmission rate than will diabetic patients who receive the usual ward teaching.

In this situation, you are trying to prove that there is a direct relationship between structured teaching and readmission rates on the basis of a series of assumptions: structured teaching improves knowledge, which improves understanding, which improves adherence, which improves health, which decreases the need for hospitalization. The predictive hypothesis was written to indicate that the investigator knew about teaching/learning theory and was applying it to a specific patient population. You can see from the hypothesis that only structured versus unstructured teaching and readmission rates will be measured on the diabetic studies. The assumptions themselves are not being tested in this study. They are accepted as true. If you cannot support these assumptions through research literature, you go back and test each one before measuring the effect of teaching on readmission rates. When you write a predictive hypothesis, you need to be able to list the assumptions underlying the prediction you have made regarding your independent and dependent variables. These assumptions are then supported in your theoretical framework.

Because research studies build on previous results, each subsequent patient teaching study should become more precise than the previous study. "Precision," in this case, means a narrower focus on patient teaching. Once you have established that structured teaching affects other variables such as readmission rate, you refine structured teaching into narrower units, such as contrasting group teaching with individual teaching or comparing multimedia instruction with a lecture format. The hypothesis would be written like this:

> Patients who receive structured group teaching will have a significantly higher level of knowledge than patients taught by any other method.

To test this general hypothesis, a series of more specific hypotheses are written:

1. Patients who receive structured group teaching will score higher on the post-test than patients who receive the usual ward teaching.
2. Patients who receive structured group teaching will score higher than patients who receive structured individual teaching.

You might consider a series of teaching strategies to test the question, "Is structured group teaching more effective because of the teaching strategy or simply because the teaching is structured?" Hypotheses could be written to test specific teaching techniques such as the use of videotape versus lecture, videotape versus printed material, or other combinations of teaching methods.

To carry this study further, assume you found that structured teaching plus interpersonal interaction produced better learning. Now, you want to find out if knowledge about diabetes affects the patients' adherence to the treatment prescribed after returning home. Your hypothesis would read like this:

> Patients with greater knowledge of diabetes will have a significantly higher rate of adherence to the treatment regimen upon returning home than patients with lesser knowledge.

As you can see, with these predictive hypotheses you always provide at least one comparison group. Your specific hypothesis includes a prediction for what will happen to each set of comparison groups.

An entirely different study could begin with the following general hypothesis:

In hospitals where nurses have received assertiveness training, the nosocomial infection rate will be significantly lower than in hospitals where nurses have not received that training.

In this situation you assumed that assertiveness training produces assertive nurses, that assertive nurses will be more likely to demand that their patients' visitors follow rules of cleanliness, and that following rules of cleanliness leads to fewer nosocomial infections.

Once again, this example consists of a chain of assumptions or connections to explain the cause-and-effect relationship between nurses' assertiveness and hospital infections, not directly tested in this study. Support is either found for each of these assumptions in the research literature, or it will be necessary to test each assumption before embarking on the study as proposed. The first step would be to test the effectiveness of assertiveness training in producing assertive nurses. The next step would be to test the relationship between assertiveness and patient protectiveness. In this case, the hypothesis might read as follows:

Nurses who receive an assertiveness training program will have a significantly higher patient protectiveness rating than those who do not receive the training.

At this point, you may find you can support the rest of your assumptions from your own previous research findings or from the published research literature. In other words, you are able to demonstrate that patient protectiveness leads to following rules of cleanliness and that good aseptic technique reduces the incidence of nosocomial infections. Now you are ready to test directly the relationship between assertiveness and nosocomial infections in the first hypothesis:

In hospitals where nurses have received assertiveness training, the nosocomial infection rate will be significantly lower than in hospitals where nurses have not received that training.

Depending on the level of knowledge about a topic and the amount of research that has preceded your work, the specificity of your hypothesis will vary. In studies based on physiological measures, for example, the hypotheses are very specific. Nursing research on human behavior is generally less specific. The following hypotheses were written for a nursing study to test the effect of ice water on the blood pressure and pulse rate of healthy subjects:[4]

> Subjects consuming ice water will have significant increases in systolic and diastolic blood pressure and pulse rate compared with the same subjects consuming comparable volumes of room temperature tap water.

To test this general hypothesis, the following specific hypotheses were developed:

1. Subjects ingesting 240 cc ice water within five minutes will have a significant increase in systolic blood pressure compared with the same subjects consuming 240 cc room temperature water within five minutes.
2. Subjects ingesting 720 cc ice water within ten minutes will have a significant increase in systolic blood pressure compared with the same subjects consuming 720 cc room temperature water within ten minutes.

These hypotheses were repeated using diastolic blood pressure and pulse rate as the dependent variables. As you can see, three independent variables were tested: amount of water, temperature of water, and time taken to drink the water. There were three dependent variables, as well: systolic blood pressure, diastolic blood pressure, and pulse. The investigators were interested in grouping these independent variables in different ways to test their influence on the three dependent variables. This study could have been carried on until all possible combinations of the three independent variables had been exhausted.

EXAMINING THE COMPONENTS OF A HYPOTHESIS

Because Level III studies are designed to test theory, the way the hypothesis is written will greatly affect the study design. Writing the hypothesis correctly will save effort later.

The way hypotheses are written is similar to that of the examples we have considered in the preceding pages. For example:

> Nurses who receive assertiveness training will have significantly higher patient protectiveness ratings than those who do not receive the training.

---

4. Siegel, M.A., and Sparks, C., The effect of ice water ingestion on blood pressure and pulse rate in healthy young adults, *Heart and Lung*, 1980, *9*(2), 306–309.

The first clause of a hypothesis will identify both the sample and one position of the independent variable. In the previous hypothesis, this clause is "nurses who receive assertiveness training." "Nurses" is the sample, and "receiving assertiveness training" is one position of the independent variable.

The next clause specifies the direction the dependent variable is expected to take as a result of the independent variable. In the example, this clause is "will have significantly higher patient protectiveness ratings." The dependent variable is "patient protectiveness ratings," and the direction in which it is expected to change is "significantly higher." The last clause of the hypothesis provides the other position of the independent variable. In this case, "those who do not receive the training" specifies the group that will provide the comparison as another position of the independent variable.

A well-written hypothesis will contain all three clauses. The first describes the experimental group, the second specifies the expected result, and the third describes the comparison group. Here is another example:

Clause 1: "Subjects ingesting 720 cc ice water within ten minutes"

Clause 2: "will have a significant increase in systolic blood pressure"

Clause 3: "compared with the same subjects consuming 720 cc room temperature water within ten minutes"

Dividing your hypothesis into three components and checking that each component includes the necessary information will make writing the hypothesis easier.

THE SIGNIFICANCE OF THE STATEMENT OF PURPOSE

Once your statement of purpose has been written as a declarative statement, a question, or a predictive hypothesis, your decision about where your question belongs in the research literature, as well as the degree of sophistication of the study, is final. You are now committed to a particular plan of action.

STATING THE PURPOSE OF THE STUDY: A SUMMARY

1. The purpose of a study should include
    a. what you intend to do to collect the data,
    b. where you intend to collect the data,
    c. who you intend to collect the data on.

2. Purposes can be written as statements, questions, or hypotheses.

3. *Writing a Purpose as a Statement* (Level I questions):

   Example: The purpose of this study is to explore and describe the value orientations of Hutterian women in western Canada.

   Example: The purpose of this study is to explore and describe childbirth customs of the village Igbo of eastern Nigeria.

4. *Writing the Purpose as a Question* (Level II questions):

   Example: The purpose of this study is to answer the question: Is there a significant relationship between perception of postoperative pain and length of convalescence among abdominal surgery patients at Waverly Hospital in eastern Oregon?

   Example: The purpose of this study is to answer the question: Is there a significant relationship among health problems, health services sought, and types of abuse among battered women in Alberta?

5. *Writing the Purpose as a Hypothesis* (Level III questions):

   To write the purpose as a hypothesis, you need to include three clauses:

   a. The first clause gives the first position of the independent variable plus the sample.

   b. The second clause gives the dependent variable.

   c. The third clause gives the second (contrast) position of the independent variable.

   The research hypothesis (written as the purpose of the study) is always written positively. The null hypothesis (there will be no relationship between the independent and dependent variables) is used only for statistical data analysis purposes.

   Example: The purpose of this study is to test the following hypothesis: Nurses who receive assertiveness training will have significantly higher patient protectiveness ratings than nurses who do not receive assertiveness training.

   Example: The purpose of this study is to test the following hypothesis: Decubitus ulcers treated with topical regular insulin will have a significantly faster rate of healing than decubitus ulcers treated with any other method.

   Example: The purpose of this study is to test the following hypothesis: Persons with Type II diabetes who have a greater knowledge of their disease will have a significantly higher rate of adherence to the treatment regimen than persons with lesser knowledge.

RECOMMENDED READINGS

Armstrong, R. L., Hypothesis formulation. In S. D. Krampitz and N. Pavlovich (eds.), *Readings for nursing research,* St. Louis: Mosby, 1981, Chap. 4.

Munro, B. H., *Statistical methods for health care research* (3rd ed.), Philadelphia: Lippincott, 1997.

Polit, D. F. and Hungler, B. P., *Nursing research: Principles and methods* (6th ed.), Philadelphia: Lippincott, 1999.

Wandelt, M., *Guide for the beginning researcher,* New York: Appleton-Century-Crofts, 1970, 63–100.

CHAPTER 6

Defining Your Terms

In our discussion about writing a research question, the question was divided into its component parts, the stem question and the topic. The stem question directs the research process, while the topic is the actual focus of the study. The same stem and topic are then used to formulate the purpose of the study. The literature review has been done in relation to the topic—who has studied it, what was said about it, how the variables were measured, and whether or not the variables you are using have been put together in the same way before. The information you found on the topic has helped you determine the exact purpose of your study. Now you need to be more precise about the variables themselves.

Recall that we defined a variable as anything that varies, or any property that takes on different values. Before you can define your variables, you must decide exactly what you want to know. Suppose you are interested in anxiety. You know that anxiety can be short-term or long-term, acute or chronic, normal or abnormal, perceived by an observer or reported by an individual, manifest or latent, mild or severe. The aspect of anxiety in which you are interested and the ways in which it varies is what you are going to measure. The aspect of anxiety that you are going to measure and the method you will use constitute its *operational definition*. Operational definitions describe *what* you are going to measure and *how* you will measure it. They involve deleting all aspects of the variable except those in which you are interested, and then specifying how they will be measured.

As an example, your definition of anxiety might read, "vague feelings of alarm that persons report when faced with a stressful situation"; or it could read, "behavioral manifestations of persons subjected to stress, which can be identified by grimaces, muscle tensing, and palmar sweating." Still another definition might say, "a trait possessed by all persons to some degree, which is reflected in their responses to questions about their view of life in general."

Each definition measures a completely different concept of anxiety. The first measures people's reports of how they feel. The second measures an observer's perception of the individual's behavior. The third requires that the researcher infer how the individual feels from his or her responses to questions. None of these is a perfect measure; none is better than others.

Your operational definition must specify what *you* want to study and how *you* want to study it, and nothing more.

During the development of the problem, you dealt with the whole realm of literature and theory about anxiety. You decided which frame of reference you wanted to assume. Now, you must eliminate everything except that which fits your frame of reference and represents what you will be measuring. In other words, the operational definition isolates the central component of the variable under study and excludes all other components of that variable.

Theoretically, your operational definitions can be anything you want them to be, as long as they are consistent with your conceptual/theoretical framework (if you have one). They should have logical, empirical meaning and should define your concepts explicitly and precisely. In addition, they should relate directly to the theory on which they are based.

For example, Uphold and Susman[1] define marital adjustment as: "An ongoing process which involves adaptation between husband and wife to the point where there is 'satisfaction, consensus, cohesion, and affectional expression'"; and they measure marital adjustment with Spanier's Dyadic Adjustment Scale.[2] This operational definition clearly specifies the definition of the concept and puts it into the context of the theoretical framework of the study.

Operational definitions of terms, therefore, first define the term and then state how the term will be studied in this particular research project. Just as the definition is written in the context of the study, so is the operationalization of the definition. Usually, your operationalization refers to the method you will use to collect the data on that variable and can be either a single method

---

1. Uphold, C. R., and Susman, E. J., Self-reported climacteric symptoms as a function of the relationships between marital adjustment and childrearing stage, *Nursing Research,* 1981, *30*(2), 84–88.

2. Spanier, G. B., Measuring dyadic adjustment: New scales for assessing the quality of marriage and similar dyads, *Journal of Marriage and the Family,* February 1976, *38,* 15–28.

or multiple methods. Let's say you wanted to study patients' attitudes toward bed baths. You know that such attitudes are feelings, beliefs, or ideas about bed baths, but how do you intend to find out about those feelings? Generally you will ask patients about their attitudes. But you can ask directly or in a questionnaire—either one is appropriate. Your "operationalization" of attitudes is to state whether you plan to interview or hand out a questionnaire.

Similarly, if you are studying stress, you can operationalize your definition by using an interview, questionnaire, observations, or even physiological measures such as blood pressure, urinalysis, or pulse rate. But however you decide to study stress, state it briefly as the operational part of your operational definition of the term. And that's what is meant by an operational definition of terms: (1) what you intend to study, specifically, and (2) how you intend to study it.

The rest of this chapter will focus on how precisely you want to study or measure your terms and what these terms mean. If your study is at Level I, you are interested in doing an exploratory or descriptive study and you intend to describe your variable in great detail. At Level I you are not concerned with precision of measurement. But, as you proceed through Level II and Level III studies, the requirement for precision of measurement increases, so that at Level III your operationalization must be precise and clear.

Here is how it works.

After completing your literature review on your topic and learning all there is to know about your variable(s), you made your final decision as to the level of knowledge about the topic and the level of design you were determined to use. On the basis of all this decision making, you wrote the purpose of your study as a statement (Level I), as a question (Level II), or as a hypothesis (Level III). From your review of literature and your statement of the purpose of your study, you are now going to develop operational definitions of terms for your variables, concepts, or topics.

> Level I: The purpose of this study is to explore and describe the reasons parents give for taking their children to alternative health care centers in Los Angeles for treatment of leukemia.

In this purpose, the variable you need to define is "reasons." The rest of the purpose is either the sample or the dependent clause describing reasons. But your study is about people's reasons for their behavior. Therefore, you will need to define what you mean by reasons, in the context of the rest of the purpose. For the above study you may define reasons as "statements made by parents to explain their process of decision making in relation to their child's health care." To operationalize this definition, you simply need to add how you intend to elicit those statements. The operational definition then becomes: "statements made by parents to explain their process of decision making in relation to their child's health care as elicited by a semistructured interview." Another example might be:

> Level I: The purpose of this study is to explore and describe the types of medication errors made by medication nurses at X hospital.

Here you will define what you mean by "types of medication errors" and how you intend to measure them. You could say that types of medication errors are "descriptions of a situation in which a medication was given to a patient, later discovered to be an error." This definition could then be operationalized by adding "as written on incident reports over a six-month period filed in the office of the chief nurse."

At Levels II and III, the operational definitions become even more specific.

> Level II: The purpose of this study is to answer the question: "Is there a significant relationship among ethnicity, maternal diet, and full-term newborn birthweight at Community Hospital in Las Cruces, New Mexico?"

In this purpose, three variables need operational definitions. The following examples are simply one way of studying these variables. Ethnicity is defined as "self-identification of cultural background, ethnic identity, or national origin as checked off on the admission sheet of hospital X." Diet is defined as "the major food categories consumed each day as recorded in a food diary kept by pregnant women from the beginning diagnosis of pregnancy to termination." Newborn birthweight is defined as "the weight in grams or pounds/ounces of all full-term infants (actual weeks of gestation) whose mothers participate in the study as recorded immediately after birth on the neonates' charts at hospital X."

Another example might be the following:

> Level II: The purpose of this study is to answer the question: "Is there a significant relationship between obesity and heart disease among adults of all ethnic groups in greater Chicago?"

For the purpose of this study, heart disease could be defined as "a diagnosis of some form of heart ailment (as given in the cardiology diagnostic manual) listed on the final diagnosis page of all patients' charts for 1983 at hospital X." Obesity would be defined as "the weight of an individual listed on the chart at time of admission that is fifteen percent or more over the ideal weight, as defined by insurance standards."

At Level III, terms are much more specific because you know so much more about them. For example, because a great deal of research and theory has been done on vitamin C, we can write a hypothesis for an experimental study.

> Level III: The purpose of this study is to test the following hypothesis: Periodontal patients who receive 1,000 mg of vitamin C daily will have a significant reduction in dental plaque formation compared to patients who receive no vitamin C.

The independent variable here is "vitamin C," which can be defined as "a vitamin supplement synthetically produced by brand X and given daily to experimental groups of patients in amounts of 'none,' 1,000 mg., 2,000 mg., or 3,000 mg., for a period of 12 months." The dependent variable, "dental plaque formation," can be defined as "the formation of calcified dental plaque that is manually removed by a dental hygienist or dentist during routinely scheduled dental hygiene visits, graded, and recorded on patients' charts every three months for a period of 12 months."

Once you have written your purpose and have operationally defined your terms, you will have a clear idea of what your research study is about. The rest of your research plan is simply filling in the detail.

TYPES OF VARIABLES

When the research plan hypothesizes relationships between variables, it is necessary to clarify expected relationships by categorizing them as *independent* or *dependent*. The terms come from experimental research, where an independent or experimental variable is introduced into a controlled setting, and the result is measured. This result—the response to the independent variable—is the dependent variable. Changes in the dependent variable are considered to be caused by the introduction of the independent variable. When the hypothesis does not predict a causal relationship but simply an associative one, as you may see in the literature, the independent variable can still be identified as the one that came first in time and is thought to be affecting the response (dependent variable). For instance, in the finding, "turnover of staff nurses was significantly higher in units where the leadership style was authoritarian," a relationship was found between "turnover of staff" and "authoritarian leadership." No direct cause-and-effect relationship is specified, because too many other possible variables could be working with authoritarianism to bring about turnover. The hypothesis, however, implies that authoritarianism is affecting turnover. Therefore, authoritarianism is the independent variable and turnover is the dependent variable.

One easy way of differentiating between independent and dependent variables is to remember that independent means standing alone and dependent means relying on something.

Two other types of variables need to be considered in research at Levels II and III. *Intervening* variables are those thought to affect the relationship between the independent and dependent variables. In Level III studies their action must be highly controlled or accounted for. *Extraneous* variables are all those that are not of direct interest to the researcher but that could affect the variables measured. When hypotheses are tested, the major purpose of the research design is to control the extraneous variables so that the effect of the independent variable on the dependent variable can be estimated. In testing the effect of authoritarian leadership on nursing staff turnover, some extraneous variables would need to be controlled: nurses' age, educational background, marital status, and number of children. All of these variables could affect turnover.

DEFINING THE INDEPENDENT VARIABLE

In research, the independent variable is the cause or influencing variable by which the subgroups in the sample are distinguished. In other words, the researcher must be able to divide the sample into alternative groups based on this variable. For example, authoritarian/nonauthoritarian and smoking/non-smoking are both instances in which the independent variable is divided into two categories. Or you might wish to establish more than two categories: light, medium, and heavy smokers, based on the number of cigarettes smoked per day. In some studies, the independent variable may be divided into numerous precise classes, such as multiple dosage levels of a drug or exact monthly income. In defining the independent variable, the researcher decides on the categories for the sample. In doing this, there are three important objectives to keep in mind.

First, the various subdivisions or categories of the variable must be clearly distinguished from one another, and they must be mutually exclusive. There may not be a single case in which a subject would easily fit into more than one category at a time. The number of cigarettes per day constituting a medium smoker must be clearly distinguishable from that constituting a light smoker. The method of measurement for the categories must be clearly defined so that others reading the study can replicate the results. If the number of cigarettes is to be counted for a week and then divided by seven days, the procedure must be clearly stated and understood.

Second, the distinction between the categories should mean something in terms of the research problem. If age categories are developed to test the idea that children of different ages respond differently to health teaching, then the age categories must have some meaning in light of developmental theory. It is not enough just to set age categories by five-year increments; the categories selected must relate to the theory behind the study.

Third, the definition of the independent variable must remain constant during the data collection, as well as during the analysis of the data. If a nursing intervention is introduced to reduce pain in postoperative patients, and, part way through the study, it becomes apparent that the intervention is not working, it may not be increased or decreased, nor may it be changed to another intervention, in order to improve the results. A study that shows *no* difference between the intervention and nonintervention groups makes an important contribution to nursing theory.

A more subtle alteration in the definition of the independent variable can occur in this example. If several members of the nursing staff are required to carry out the intervention, perhaps even the entire staff of a particular unit, it may happen that some nurses do not follow the protocol of the study unless the researcher is actually present. When this happens, an alternative version of the independent variable is present, and its effect is being combined with that of the true variable. If the researcher is unaware of the problem, the relationship that emerges between the independent and dependent variables might be a spurious one.

The definition of the independent variable is critical to studies in which the purpose is stated as a question or a hypothesis. When a study is testing the independent variable as the cause or the dependent variable as the effect of the independent variable, then the description and definition of the independent variable are mandatory. On the other hand, in exploratory studies all variables are assumed to be independent. This is simply due to the lack of knowledge about the variables (see Table 6.1). Therefore, when a variable's status is unknown, the variable is treated *as if* it were independent.

TABLE 6-1	Definition of the Independent, Dependent, Intervening, and Extraneous[1] Variables	
Independent Variable	**Intervening Variable**	**Dependent Variable**
Stands alone	Comes between the independent and dependent variables	Is affected by the independent variables
Cause	May interfere	Effect
Comes first	Comes between	Comes later or last
	Can mask the effect of the independent variable	

1. *Extraneous variables* are variables you feel may influence or mask the dependent variable and is another name for an intervening variable. Unlike independent variables, extraneous variables are not of primary importance to the study, however they may be interesting or helpful in understanding the findings.

HOW VARIABLES ARE MEASURED

Variables are measured according to what you want to know about them as well as according to the amount of knowledge available from the literature. The four basic types of measurement are: *nominal, ordinal, interval,* and *ratio* scales. Each type of measurement dictates the way you collect your data and, subsequently, the way you analyze your data. So it's best to know, right at the beginning, exactly what these terms mean, how they are used, and what they do to the rest of your research plan. Although there are four levels of measurement, only the first three will be discussed in detail. Because there is little significant difference, for research, between interval and ratio scales, these levels of measurement will be discussed together.

The way you study your variable depends on what you want to know. Your choice of measurement scale depends on the answer you want from your data. If you want great precision, you will choose an interval (or ratio) scale. If you want to rank people or things in some order, you need an ordinal scale. If you simply want to contrast things and don't care much about either precision of measurement or ordering from small to large or bad to good, you will choose the nominal scale.

There are other reasons for choosing a particular scale or scales to measure your variables. One reason has to do with the variable itself. Sex is measured only in nominal scales as there are only two possible categories, male and female. Similarly, membership in a political party is measured only in nominal scales because Republican, Democrat, or Independent is a named category with no numerical significance. Other variables are numerical scales such as distance, temperature, and time. As numerical scales, distance can be given in precise measurement of miles or kilometers; time can be given in hours and minutes; temperature can be precisely calibrated in degrees. Each of these scales can be manipulated mathematically. Yet, at the same time, each of these three variables can be viewed nominally. Time can be viewed as morning or afternoon; temperature can be given as cold or hot. How and when you will use a nominal or a numerical scale depends on your particular study and what you want to know. That is why your literature review is so important; it should have told you the level of measurement of your variables in previous studies so you can decide how to measure your variables in this study.

Another factor in choosing how to measure your variables depends on how you collect your data. If you plan to use unstructured observations, your data will be either nominal or ordinal. If you use unstructured questionnaires, interviews, or projective tests, your data will still be at the nominal or ordinal level. If, however, you plan to use hospital records on blood gases, urinalysis, or EKGs, you will find that you have precise numerical scales to work with.

So your choice of measurement is dependent on your level of study, how you want to collect your data, and how your variables will occur naturally.

Finally, your choice will depend on the degree of precision you need to answer your original question.

Here's how it works.

Nominal Scale

When objects, events, or people are classified into two or more categories, and there is no difference in size or magnitude of the categories, then the variables are measured on a nominal scale. A nominal scale is a *qualitative* scale in that the qualities of a variable are examined rather than its quantities. The classic example of a nominal scale is the variable "sex." Everyone can be categorized as male or female. There is no magnitude to maleness compared with femaleness. They are *contrasting* categories, labeled with a descriptive title.

The only specified relationship between the categories in nominal scales is that they are different from one another: they contrast with one another. There is no suggestion of any magnitude or quality differences. Nominal scales can have as few as two categories or many categories, as in a taxonomy of diagnoses. The categories must be exhaustive so that all variations of your variables can be classified somewhere. When developing your categories, you must exhaust the possibilities as to where your sample will fall on that variable. If you planned to collect data on marital status and left out the category "single," you would lose part of your sample. What of the people who are "never married" as opposed to those who were formerly married but are now "divorced" and are, therefore, "single" again? When you decide to use a nominal scale, you should have some idea of the possible categories.

Finally, nominal scales demand a system of classification that is mutually exclusive. Each person must fit into one, and only one, category of a given variable. There must be no question where each person fits. A person cannot be part Republican and part Democrat. A person must be one or the other. If you are a Republican, you are not a Democrat or an Independent. If you are a nurse, then you probably are not an engineer or an accountant. If you are looking for the presence or absence of a particular trait, a person who has a little of that trait is classified along with the person who has a lot of it. Nominal scales do not allow for "a little bit" versus "a lot" as there is no magnitude to a nominal scale.

Ordinal Scale

Ordinal scales differ from nominal scales in that they rank a variable on a scale of increasing magnitude. Ordinal scales, like nominal scales, are generally named categories that, in addition, follow a particular ordering system. For example, to measure age on an ordinal scale, you would develop categories such as young, middle-aged, and old. The magnitude alters with the age of the individual, because the old person is older than the middle-aged person, who is older than the young person. You do not attempt to specify how much older the elderly person is than the young person. The number of years is not relevant here; what is relevant is the system of ranking. Just as with a nominal scale, the ordinal scale categories must be mutually exclusive. An individual cannot be rated as both young and middle-aged. The difference between the categories must be clearly established so that every person in the sample falls into only one category.

Many nursing studies use ordinal scales. In attitudinal research, people are asked to rank their opinions (on the basis of whether they agree or disagree with a statement) on a scale from "strongly disagree" to "strongly agree," with several points in between (the classic Likert scale). We can measure the success of nursing interventions by the level of comfort or discomfort expressed by the patient or by the degree of learning that has occurred. Any variable that can be ranked from "none" to "a great deal" can be measured on an ordinal scale.

Interval (and Ratio) Scale

In contrast to nominal and ordinal scales, the interval (and ratio) scale is a quantitative numerical scale. Its significant feature is that the numbered intervals between points are equidistant, whether those intervals are measured in miles, centimeters, pounds, or degrees. (There is little significant difference, for research, between interval and ratio scales. The only thing you need to remember is that ratio scales have an "absolute zero" and interval scales do not. Otherwise, the scales are treated identically in data analysis.) The intervals can be added or subtracted to provide each subject with a score on the variable being measured. The scores can then be analyzed statistically to determine whether subjects are significantly different from each other.

Interval scales are used when precise information about variables is needed. You must know enough about the variable to develop a precise form of measurement. Therefore, the use of interval scales for variables that are being explored for the first time must be ruled out.

Most nursing research utilizes nominal and ordinal scales, the most commonly used scales in behavioral and social research. Increasing use is also being made of interval and ratio level data, especially in nursing research involving biological and physical sciences. Later you will see how the measurement scale of your variables affect the possibilities for data analysis.

Let's look at an example.

If you wanted to do a study on runner's fatigue and you decided to test fatigue levels by the presence of blood in the urine, you could set up your study on the basis of a nominal scale: "the presence of blood" in the urine versus "no observable blood" in the urine. This scale would not measure the amount of blood in the urine or the degree of fatigue expressed in terms of severity of bleeding. What is desired in this case is a mutually exclusive statement on the presence or absence of blood, so a nominal scale is used.

If you want to measure the presence of blood on an ordinal scale, you could rank the amount of blood by the color of the urine: from "none" (clear yellow), to "a little" (pink), to "moderate" (light red), to "much" (bright red), to "a lot" (dark red). Now there is *magnitude* to the measurement of blood in the urine, although it is not known how much blood is classified as "moderate" versus "a little."

Using this same example, an interval scale also could be used. Here you would test samples of urine for the number of red blood cells present, a precise measurement of the amount of blood. Now you can describe subjects by their precise amount of hematuria. (With this example, you can trace the development of knowledge about the variable through the levels of measurement. If there were no precise way to measure blood in the urine other than gross observation, you would not be able to use a numerical scale.)

You may wonder what scaling has to do with operational definitions. Every variable in the written purpose must be defined according to a nominal, ordinal, interval, or ratio scale. The way you define your variable is the way you will measure it. The way you plan to measure it determines the methods of data collection you will use. This decision, in turn, requires certain forms of data analysis. Therefore, when you define your terms according to a particular scale, you determine the rest of your study.

At Level I exploratory levels of research, you have either one variable or one sample that you intend to explore and describe. Because you probably know little about either, you may not know whether an interval or ratio scale should be used. You must know something about your variable to determine if it can be studied quantitatively, but you must know much more to be able to choose the appropriate numerical scale. As a result, Level I studies generally use either a nominal or an ordinal scale. When exploring at the most elementary level, you will frequently start with a nominal scale. Does the variable exist? What is it? When does it exist? Where is it? Who has it? How often does it occur? Each of these questions can be answered by a word or a name of something; therefore, a nominal scale is appropriate.

In Level II studies where you are looking at the relationship between two or more variables, you need to decide which scale would be most appropriate for each variable (because you can study each variable on a different scale) so that you can plan your data analysis.

For example, if you were looking at the relationship between distance running and hematuria, you would be at Level II. Although you have a hunch that increased running causes bloody urine, you cannot prove it. First you must do a descriptive survey of runners to see if there is a relationship between running and hematuria. Using the same example:

The purpose of this study is to answer the question: "Is there a significant relationship between the number of miles run each week and the amount of hematuria among marathon runners?"

You will count the number of miles per week per runner from "zero" (the runner may not have run at all for a week) to the highest number achieved by one of the runners for one week. You will take urine specimens daily to perform blood counts. These data also will range from zero to the highest actual number for any one runner in one week. You will have two ratio scales as both variables have absolute zeros.

Had your purpose been to test the relationship between miles run per week and the presence or absence of blood in the urine as reported by the runner, you would have had a ratio scale for number of miles and a nominal scale for presence or absence of blood in the urine.

If you wanted to conduct a Level III study, you would first verify the relationship between running and hematuria. Your hypothesis would predict that hematuria occurs, for example, when an individual runs more than 50 miles each week or that the amount of hematuria for a runner will progressively increase in weekly increments from 100 miles per week as the base.

In this case you state that the amount of running causes hematuria and that a specific number of miles run is necessary for such a physiological condition to occur. You also state that the more one runs, the more blood will be found in the urine. You must have a physiological theory of distance running related to hematuria in order to hypothesize that increased running causes more blood in urine. To make this prediction you have to know that excessive running causes hematuria, that running is the independent variable, and that hematuria is the dependent variable.

Hypotheses predict relationships, thus you, the researcher, must know which variable is the cause and which is the effect. Every study has an independent variable: one you *assume* is independent as there are no others (Level I); one you *think* is independent, but you are looking for proof (Level II); and one you *know* is independent and can be manipulated (Level III). The level of knowledge about your topic indicates which variables are independent and which are dependent. If you are testing at Level III, your knowledge also tells you which variables are intervening or extraneous.

When defining your terms, keep in mind how you intend to measure your variables and whether the variable is dependent, independent, or extraneous. Remember, also, to define your terms according to the needs of your study. Here is an example:

Level I: The purpose of this study is to explore and describe the characteristics of runners at UCLA.

The critical term to define is "characteristics." Characteristics could be defined as "traits, qualities, or properties that distinguish an individual or a group, such as standard demographic data that are descriptive of certain classes of people—age, sex, marital status, education, and occupational status—as well as number of miles run per week, type of clothing worn, time of run, and so on." Most of these characteristics are nominal. Your definition of "runners" probably would include a minimum number of miles run per week and the speed of the run. In another example:

> Level II: The purpose of this study is to answer the question: "Is there a significant relationship between miles run per week and weight loss among distance runners in Denver?"

Here you could define weight loss as "none," "little," and "much" or, "under 5 lb.," "5 to 10 lb." or according to actual number of pounds lost. (Of these three definitions of weight loss, the last is a numerical scale while the first two examples are ordinal.)

For a Level III study predicting that successful dieting is accompanied by regular exercise, "successful dieting" might be defined as "weight loss of 10 lb. or more that was not regained one year following the end of the dieting program." In this case the scale would be a nominal scale of "yes" or "no"—if the individual was successful or not. "Regular exercise" must be defined according to what constitutes exercise and what is meant by regular exercise.

In a Level I study, the only term needing definition is the variable or concept under study. So when your purpose is "to explore and describe the value orientations of homeless men,"[3] the only variable to be defined either conceptually or operationally is value orientations. Although "homeless men" needs definition as well, this is better dealt with in the section on sample. If you have a Level I study, you will define only one variable or concept in the statement of purpose. The sample will not be defined under "Definition of Terms."

Many people planning a Level I study define their sample under Definition of Terms simply because this group of people has never been studied or because their study has been so variable. Homeless men are a good example of a population that has no real parameters. When a national census is taken, it is difficult to establish how many members of the population are homeless when the criteria for inclusion in the census requires a home address. In the same way, a study dealing with menopausal women would require a definition of the sample simply because there are no census materials on them. The authors had the same difficulty in their study of successful dieters (National Center for Nursing Research, Grant #1-RO1-NU01169–01) as every study used different parameters of what was "successful" and what was "unsuccessful."

Where do these definitions belong when you are planning your research? At the very beginning of your thinking and planning process, when you are writing out your question and your working definitions, you need to define

---

3. Downing, C. K., and Cobb, A. K., Value orientations of homeless men, *Western Journal of Nursing Research*, 1990, *12*(5), 619–628.

your target population (see Chapter 8). You need to consider the criteria for those who will be included in your study group and for those who will not. Try to use mutually exclusive characteristics to describe your study population. Then, when you write the proposal itself (see Chapter 13), you will describe these characteristics in the section on Target Population. The criteria for the selection of particular characteristics has already been discussed in your problem simply because you need to talk about the people you want to study before you actually study them. In the chapter on Definition of Terms, therefore, you will not find a section to describe your sample as part of the definition of terms.

TERMS THAT NEED DEFINITION

The purpose of your study states exactly what you intend to measure. Because of the specific nature of the purpose, every variable should be operationally defined. The economy of words in a statement of purpose necessitates operational definitions.

This chapter has focused on the operational definitions of the independent and dependent variables as the critical issues for the project. Remember, in a descriptive study, all variables are assumed to be independent; therefore, all variables need definition. In an experimental design, you as investigator are theoretically in complete control of the independent variable; therefore, you must know everything you can about it. Your study describes the effect of the independent variables on the dependent variable. You also need to define the possible intervening or extraneous variables to show your reader that you have considered them.

WRITING OPERATIONAL DEFINITIONS: A REVIEW

1. First, write out what the term (or variable) means in relation to the purpose of the study. This is the conceptual definition of the term.

    Example: The purpose of this study is to explore and describe <u>successful dieting programs</u>. (The terms to be defined are underlined.)

    <u>Dieting programs:</u> A fee-for-service regimen established to assist persons to lose weight.

    <u>Successful:</u> A dieting program that has a high percentage of clients who were able to achieve their goal weight and keep that weight off for one year or more.

2. Second, write out how you intend to study that definition or how you intend to measure the variable. This is the operational part of the operational definition of the term.

Example: The purpose of this study is to explore and describe <u>successful</u> <u>dieting programs</u>. (The terms to be defined are underlined.)

<u>Dieting programs:</u> A fee-for-service regimen, established to assist persons in losing weight, as listed in the Yellow Pages of the Pacific Telephone directory of the northwestern San Fernando Valley.

<u>Successful:</u> A dieting program that has a high percentage of clients who were able to achieve their goal weight and keep that weight off for one year or more as measured by the successful dieters questionnaire sent to all program participants in the previous year.

3. Combine both parts of the definition to form the operational definition of the term or variable.

    <u>Example: Successful Dieting Programs:</u> Fee-for-service regimen, established to assist persons in losing weight, that has a high percentage of clients who were able to achieve their goal weight and keep that weight off for one year or more as measured by the successful dieters questionnaire sent to all program participants from programs listed in the Yellow Pages of the Pacific Telephone directory of the northwestern San Fernando Valley.

4. Operationally define every major variable in your purpose whether the purpose is written as a statement, a question, or a hypothesis.

5. Your sample *should not be* operationally defined.

6. Additional examples of operational definitions:

PURPOSE OF THE STUDY

The purpose of this study is to explore and describe the value orientations of Hutterian women in western Canada.

DEFINITION OF TERMS

Value orientations: A 23-item ordinal scale instrument designed to elicit an individual's beliefs about the best way to solve four basic common human problems.

PURPOSE OF THE STUDY

The purpose of this study is to answer the question: Is there a significant relationship between level of stress and coping strategies in hospitalized patients?

DEFINITION OF TERMS

Level of stress: The number and intensity of events, perceived by the patient as causing strain or tension, that occurred during the past 12 months as measured by the Holmes and Rahe "Significant Life Events" scale.

Coping strategies: A person's customary pattern of adapting to or dealing with perceived stressful events as measured by a rating scale evaluating both the number of strategies and the frequency with which the individual uses them.

PURPOSE OF THE STUDY

The purpose of the study is to test the following hypothesis: Nurses who have had assertiveness training will have significantly higher patient protectiveness ratings than those who do not have assertiveness training.

DEFINITION OF TERMS

Assertiveness training: A program designed to increase an individual's ability to select assertive behaviors when faced with a conflict situation. The experimental group will receive a four-day program in assertiveness training.

Patient protectiveness rating: A nine-item ordinal scale to measure a nurse's feelings of responsibility for preventing harm from occurring to the patient.

RECOMMENDED READINGS

Abdellah, F. G., and Levine, E., *Better patient care through nursing research*, New York: Macmillan, 1965, Chap. 7.

Diers, D., *Research in nursing practice*, Philadelphia: Lippincott, 1979, Chap. 9.

Johnson, B. A., Johnson, J. E., and Dumas, R. G., Research in nursing practice: The problem of uncontrolled situational variables, *Nursing Research*, July/August 1970, *19*, 337–342.

Kerlinger, F. N., *Foundations of behavioral research* (3rd ed.), New York: Holt, Rinehart and Winston, 1986.

Munro, B. H., *Statistical methods for health care research* (3rd ed.), Philadelphia: Lippincott, 1997.

Polit, D., and Hungler, B., *Essentials of nursing research: Methods and applications*, Philadelphia: Lippincott, 1985, 80–87.

Polit, D., and Hungler, B., *Nursing research: Principles and methods* (6th ed.), Philadelphia: Lippincott, 1999.

Summers, S., Level of measurement: Key to appropriate data analysis, *Journal of Post Anesthesia Nursing,* 1991, *6*(2), 143–147.

Waltz, C. F., Strickland, O. L., and Lenz, E. R., *Measurement in nursing research*, Philadelphia: F. A. Davis Company, 1991.

Wandelt, M., *Guide for the beginning researcher*, New York: Appleton-Century-Crofts, 1970, 101–126.

CHAPTER 7

The Research Design: Blueprint for Action

The preceding chapters have taken you through the process of deciding *what* you want to study. The remaining chapters will help you decide *how* to study it. You are ready to take the work you have already done—your stem question, your topic, your operational definitions, and your statement of purpose—and lay them out into a working plan, a blueprint for action.

As with any blueprint, you start with an overall picture of the design and then go on to show close-up pictures of each section. In that way, you won't get bogged down in details before you have visualized the end result. If you tried to design a kitchen by starting with a detailed plan for the spice cupboard and then tried to fit the rest of the kitchen around it, you would be in trouble. Similarly, the research plan will suffer if you start by minutely describing the sample before you know what the overall plan is to be. The result would be a research design planned to fit the sample instead of a sample selected to meet the needs of the design.

The purpose of a research design is to provide a plan for answering the research question. The major concern within the blueprint, or plan, is to specify the control mechanisms you will use in your study so that the answer to the question will be clear and valid. The concept of control in research is an extremely important one, and the extent to which you can achieve control will depend on the level of your study. *Control* refers to the control of the variables under study and variables that may possibly affect the study. Control is attained by (1) allowing for *no* variation; (2) *specifying* the variation to be allowed; or (3) *distributing* the variation equally. Laboratory settings, for example, provide for control by allowing no variation. Homogeneity of the sample allows for no variations on some characteristics, while matched samples ensure that some characteristics are identical. Randomization distributes variation equally.

In experimental studies, control is a major requirement; the only thing that is allowed to vary in the pure experiment is the dependent variable. The experimenter manipulates the independent variable and observes the effect on the dependent variable, with nothing else varying. Extraneous variables are controlled *only* if the groups are formed by random assignment and are kept intact. Any other form of group assignment or any drop out from the group diminishes control over extraneous variables. Variables are said to be distributed normally among groups or throughout the sample by either random assignment to groups, in experimental designs, or by the use of probability samples in comparative and correlational designs.

Another type of control is to build extraneous variables into the design. This is accomplished in one of two ways: by writing the variable into the study as part of the purpose as an alternate independent variable or as an intervening variable; or by collecting data on the variable and then analyzing it at the end of the study during the data analysis. When variables are built into the design, the problem and definition of terms need to reflect that fact; there needs to be literature review on all variables; there needs to be discussion on how the data will be collected and analyzed. When variables are collected as demographic data, they are later treated as intervening variables between and among all other variables during data analysis. These techniques are used to specify the variance that is allowable.

Allowing for no variance is accomplished with homogeneous samples in which everyone is alike on one or more dimensions. When everyone in the sample is the same gender, or has the same disease, or is of the same racial or ethnic group, we have a homogeneous sample *on that variable* because that particular variable is not allowed to vary or is specified as having no variance.

Variables on which data are collected, analyzed, and simply described at the end of the study are not considered "intervening"; they are called "extraneous" variables.

DESIGNING YOUR STUDY FROM THE QUESTION

All research designs fall into one of two categories: descriptive or experimental. The choice of which to use is made during the development of the problem. Descriptive designs result in a description of the data, whether in words, pictures, charts, or tables, and whether the data analysis shows statistical or merely descriptive relationships. Experimental designs result in inferences drawn from the data that explain the relationships between the variables. If the topic is appropriate for Level I or II, the design will be descriptive; if your study is at Level III, an experimental design is best.

"What" questions invariably lead to descriptive designs; "why" questions are always experimental. Thus, the choice of design is made when the question is finalized; now it needs to be given a name and to be developed into a detailed plan of action.

The design is a set of instructions to the researcher to gather and analyze data in certain ways that will control who and what are to be studied. Unwanted or extraneous variables can thus be controlled, the variance of specific variables is enhanced, and the possibility of error in measurement is minimized. In other words, the design makes it possible for you to isolate the variables you are interested in from all other variables and to measure them accurately so that your data are reliable and valid.

The design chosen must be the best way to answer the question; it must fit the level of the question. Variables about which nothing is known need to be questioned at a basic level, and the answer is a description of those variables.

The design always builds on previous findings, except in replication studies. If you feel the results of previous research require further support, your study may replicate the previous research, following the design *exactly* as it was in the original study.

CHARACTERISTICS OF RESEARCH DESIGNS

When you read research studies that specify the design being used, you can make judgments about the adequacy of the design to answer the question, and you can evaluate the study in relation to its "goodness-of-fit" with the requirements of the design. When a research report does not specify the design being used, then you have to guess what the researcher intended to do and then evaluate the study in relation to your best guess. Obviously, it is easier to evaluate a study when the writer tells you in advance the name of the design rather than your having to decide on the type of design being used. To help you select a design that meets the requirements of your stated purpose, and evaluate studies more easily, the following areas need to be considered.

The Setting for the Study

Will your study be conducted in a laboratory setting or "field" setting? When you are planning a study, the setting in which it will be conducted is a first order of decision making. If your study will be conducted in a laboratory, you will have far greater control than if your study is conducted in a natural setting. If you are doing research in a laboratory, but do not build in the controls usual to this setting, then you are wasting your setting and could have done the study anywhere.

Laboratory studies are designed to be more highly controlled in relation to both the environment in which the study is conducted and the control of extraneous and intervening variables. You are familiar with physiological laboratory experiments, chemistry and physics experiments, as well as psychological and microbiological experiments. All are laboratory experiments designed to control the possibility of extraneous variables influencing the effect of the independent variable on the dependent variable. In the laboratory setting, it is possible to control environmental variables, such as temperature, humidity, light, and sound, as well as physiological variables such as nutrition and hydration of the subjects during the experiment.

All other studies, not conducted in laboratories, are called *field studies,* which simply means they occur somewhere other than in a controlled laboratory setting. "Field studies" occur in natural settings and use a variety of methods such as field experiments, participant observations in villages or hospital wards, interviews in the home or office, questionnaires sent to research subjects, and, in fact, anything at all that does not occur in a controlled laboratory setting.

Timing of Data Collection

What type of study do you plan to conduct in relation to time? Do you plan to look into the past, study present behaviors, predict future events? There are several design labels that focus on the timing of your data collection. Those looking at events that are underway or expected to occur in the future are called *prospective* or *longitudinal studies.* Those focusing on events that have occurred in the past are called *retrospective, ex post facto,* or *historical studies.* Those in which data collection is strictly in the present time are called *cross-sectional studies.* You may find these labels useful in designing your study, since they may help you to clarify how the timing of your data collection fits into your design. They are also terms that you will see in the literature, and an understanding of how they are meant to be used will help you in critiquing research reports.

Of the three labels for studies that focus on events in the past, the first is the *retrospective* study. This term is used by epidemiologists to describe a cause-effect study in which the effect is known (such as lung cancer) and the cause is sought. Social scientists use the label *ex post facto* to describe this same type of study. In other words, a phenomenon that occurs in the present is thought to have a cause that can be found (retrospectively) in the past. Many early studies of diseases (such as alcoholism, obesity, lung cancer, and diabetes) were retrospective (or *ex post facto*) studies.

Historical studies, on the other hand, are often descriptive studies that ask people to recall events, other people, and memories from the past, or refer to written historical documents and artifacts to reconstruct past events.

Studies that look to the future are called *prospective* or *longitudinal* studies. These terms generally mean the same thing, but epidemiologists are apt to use "prospective," whereas social scientists use "longitudinal," to describe studies that are designed to follow the subjects for a period of time, obtaining repeated measurements, and establishing changes in the variables over time. In this type of study, the sample is chosen on the basis of the presence of a presumed causative (independent) variable. The sample is followed to find out if the dependent variable occurs and/or changes over time. Prospective or longitudinal studies can be very expensive. They can require a considerable investment of time because the researcher must wait for the presumed effect to occur and therefore must be prepared to follow the subjects for long periods, sometimes many years. The strength of these designs is that they have more control over extraneous variables than do retrospective studies.

Cross-sectional studies collect data one time only and are meant to obtain a "cross-section" of the population at a given moment in time. The result is a measurement of what exists today, with no attempt to document changes over time either in the past or the future.

The decision you make as to whether you will do a retrospective or a prospective study is based on whether you are looking for causes in the past (retrospective) or present-day causes for future effects (prospective); or looking for descriptions of events and things that occurred in the past (retrospective) or following people into the future to describe events as they occur (prospective); or using one measurement time to describe what exists today (cross-sectional).

Sample Selection

When you choose a sample to be studied you need to be aware of whether or not it will be a random sample and the degree to which it is accessible to you.

In sample selection, randomness refers to the principle of randomization, which states:

> Since, in random procedures, every member of a population has an equal chance of being selected, members with certain distinguishing characteristics—male or female, high or low intelligence, Republican or Democrat, dogmatic or not dogmatic, and so on and on—will, if selected, probably be counterbalanced in the long run by the selection of other members of the population with the "opposite" quantity or quality of the characteristic.[1]

---

1. Kerlinger, Fred N., *Foundations of behavioral research* (3rd ed.), New York: Holt, Rinehart and Winston, 1986.

When you are selecting a random sample from a population, the idea is to have distinguishing characteristics randomly distributed in the sample so that the sample is representative of the population. In other words, the distribution in the sample approximates that in the population. In experimental research, when subjects are randomly assigned to groups, the principle is used to ensure that these distinguishing characteristics will be equivalently distributed among all the study groups so that the groups themselves can be considered equivalent at the beginning of the study, before the experimental treatment has been started. The purpose of randomization is to distribute extraneous or intervening variables throughout the sample in such a way that no particular group is favored more than another.

Randomness is generally associated with generalizability. The degree to which the sample represents the population affects the degree to which the study can be generalized to the same population. These ideas will be discussed in further detail later.

Accessibility of the sample refers to whether you can reasonably expect to find enough individuals, animals, events, or units of the population—whether they are available to you. If you were interested in studying populations with Toxic Shock Syndrome, or AIDS, or Bilharzia, you would need to have an accessible target population that would be large enough for your study. Because these are difficult-to-find populations, your ability to do the study may be inhibited.

Type of Data to Be Collected

In general, all data can be categorized according to whether it is collected as qualitative (qualities) or quantitative (numerical). All studies are categorized according to the type of data collected and will emphasize one over the other. Qualitative data have names or labels rather than numbers. Any attribute or variable having a number is called quantitative. Within quantitative data, there will be differences in the scale used to measure the variables (nominal, ordinal, or interval/ratio).

ISSUES OF CONTROL

Before discussing the individual research designs for each level of research, there are two concepts basic to the idea of control that you need to consider. These are internal and external validity.

Internal validity is defined as the extent to which the results of the study can actually be attributed to the action of the independent variable and not something else. In this case, validity refers to the truth of the findings as determined by the purity of the design. Internal validity is determined by the way the experimental and control groups are formed in an experimental design. If the investigator is able to say with perfect certainty that *all groups were equal at the beginning of the study, and no other variables were allowed to interfere with the independent variable,* then any change in the dependent variable can be attributed to the effect of the independent variable. The study then has internal validity. The degree to which that perfect certainty is compromised indicates the degree to which the study does not have internal validity. How much control can you plan to have over your experimental variables? Is this to be a relatively uncontrolled field experiment or a highly controlled laboratory experiment? With all of the methods you plan to use, be sure that nothing can interfere with the action of your independent variable to attain internal validity.

External validity refers to the degree to which the findings of the study are generalizable to the target population. The key issue here is the degree to which the sample represents the population. Random sampling is intended to produce a representative sample, providing the sample size is large enough to incorporate all the relevant extraneous variables. If the sample is not representative, then the results do not generalize and you can only describe what you have found in your sample. If you did generalize on the basis of a nonprobability sample, people would accuse you of making a "quantum leap" from the data to the conclusions. The reason for using random sampling is to promote the external validity of your results. Here the focus is on the degree to which your sample represents the target population accurately, so that the results you obtain can be applied to the entire target population. Chapter 8 will discuss in detail the strategies for attaining external validity through obtaining random or representative samples.

DESCRIPTIVE DESIGNS

No matter what method is chosen to collect the data, all descriptive designs have one thing in common: they must provide descriptions of the variables in order to answer the question. The type of description that results from the design depends on how much information the researcher has about the topic prior to data collection. Look at the design in the same way that you looked at the question. Level I questions, with little or no prior knowledge of the topic, lead to exploratory descriptive designs. Level II questions, where the variables are known but their action cannot be predicted, lead to descriptive survey designs.

Exploratory Descriptive Designs

At this level, the design is one of two basic models: exploratory or descriptive. *Exploratory studies* provide an in-depth exploration of a single process, variable, or concept, such as bereavement or role conflict. *Descriptive studies* examine one or more characteristics of a specific population, such as the value orientations of aboriginals in Canada or the indicators of health among new immigrants from Southeast Asia. Level I studies always involve one variable and one population.

When the purpose of a study is exploration, a flexible research design that provides an opportunity to examine all aspects of the problem is needed. As knowledge of the variables increases, the researcher may have to change direction. Ideas occur as data are collected and examined. The key to a good exploratory design is *flexibility.*

We emphasize throughout the book that the research process is dependent on what is known about the topic. The word "exploratory" indicates that not much is known, which means that a survey of the literature failed to reveal any significant research in the area. Thus, you cannot build on the work of others; you *must* explore the topic for yourself.

Even though we talk about the exploratory study as an entity in itself, it should be remembered that it is an initial step in the development of new knowledge. Because of the flexibility of this type of design, very few, if any, variables are under the researcher's control. They are said to be under the control of the situation—in other words, observed as they happen or as the researcher comes upon them. As a result, no inferences can be drawn from the data. The data may lead to suggestions of hypotheses for further study or to an idea for a conceptual framework to explain the action of the variables, but the exploratory question must be followed by higher-level questions if new knowledge is to be gained.

In nursing research, there are many topics for which the level of knowledge is such that exploratory studies are required. For instance, a research question might be, "What is the reaction of patients to being transferred from room to room during hospitalization?" This is a Level I question. If the literature review reveals no information on this topic, the purpose of your study will be to explore and describe patients' reactions to being moved from room to room during a hospital stay. In this type of study, you may *not* ask, "What is the 'effect' of moving patients from room to room?" To ask questions about effect, you must know the cause and have sufficient information to predict the effect; or you may know the effect, in which case you must be able to predict the cause. Either option requires a lot of information. You do not have this type of information in our present example. You have no idea whether moving patients has any effect on anything at all. And if there is an effect, you have no idea of its extent. Perhaps it will be temporary annoyance, a mild disorientation, a severe setback in convalescence, an increase in sensory disturbances, or a loss of social relationships—the list of possibilities could fill volumes. To find out what the patients' reaction actually is, you will have to explore all these possibilities. That means asking open-ended questions and being prepared to shift gears, depending on the patients' initial response. You will need to observe patients being moved and describe what you see; you will need to interview patients and families and ask what their reactions are; you will want to question nurses, ward clerks, physicians, and others who are in contact with the patient to see what their experiences have been. Your methods and questions will change depending on what you find out as you go along. Thus, it is imperative that the design be flexible.

The results of this study will provide detailed descriptions of all the observations made by the researcher, arranged in some kind of order. Conclusions drawn from the data include some educated guesses or hypotheses for further study. A relationship between the observations made and a concept such as territorialism might be proposed. Or, perhaps, a relationship with systems theory might be seen. Further research would be required to test these proposals. This is the purpose of exploratory research.

The basic exploratory design requires the personal involvement of the researcher with a small number of people (usually less than 25); uses purposive or theoretical sampling; occurs in a small, circumscribed geographical setting; and uses either field notes or audiotaped transcriptions of interviews. The strongest exploratory design is based on repeated interviews, observations, or both of the same people or phenomena. In this design, more than any other, the data control the investigator, and not the reverse. Underlying this design are the following assumptions: the topic has never been studied before; the sample has personal experience in or knowledge about the topic; and the sample is able to talk about the topic.

The exploratory design is also known as qualitative research when the samples are deliberative or convenient; questions and observations are qualitative; and the analysis of data is via verbal description and, perhaps, preliminary or tentative theorizing about the findings. Examples of exploratory/qualitative designs include ethnomethodology, grounded theory, and phenomenology. Exploratory designs, by their nature, are not replicable.

Exploratory designs, as opposed to descriptive designs, include a beginning exploration of an idea or concept; an attempt at discovery rather than description; an attempt to find meaning in the data; and an immersion in the area studied.

Descriptive studies differ from exploratory studies in several ways. They are studies of known variables in unknown populations, whereas the exploratory study collects in-depth data on a single abstract concept or process variable. In the descriptive study, there may be literature on the variables but the variables have not been studied in a particular population. For example, in Brink's 1984 study of the value orientations of the Annang of Nigeria, the tool used to measure value orientations had been used previously in a comparative study of five cultures in the United States,[2] but nothing was known about this variable for the Annang. For this study, a tool was available to measure a

_____

2. Kluckhohn, F. R., and Strodtbeck, F. L., *1961 Variations in value orientations*, New York: Row, Peterson and Company.

known variable in an unknown population. Some flexibility is built into a descriptive study because there is little information on the population, and available tools may prove inadequate to measure the variables; but descriptive studies do not have the degree of flexibility found in exploratory studies.

Another descriptive design is the census or population study. This descriptive design is used in the collection of census data every ten years by the United States Department of the Census. In this type of descriptive study, the total population is surveyed using structured data collection methods. In this instance, the purpose is to compile a complete description of the population to record changing trends in population characteristics for ten-year periods. Each census, however, is an individual descriptive study. The purpose is not to look for relationships among variables, but rather to provide a descriptive data base for the population. These studies do not have a theoretical or conceptual base. A recent study by Williams reported characteristics of college freshmen choosing nursing as a major.[3] The results were compared to similar studies done of college freshmen over time to look at changing patterns of characteristics. Census studies will always be fairly structured in design compared to exploratory studies. They usually have large samples (or total population) and the type of data to be collected will always be predetermined. The usual form of data collection is structured questionnaires, although there may be some open-ended questions to account for areas in which the researcher may be unsure of the potential responses.

The results of a descriptive study will provide detailed information on the variable(s) under study. No relationships among variables are predicted in these studies, although comparisons over time or among whole populations are frequently made during a secondary analysis and associations between demographic characteristics and the study variables are often sought.

The purpose of the purely descriptive design is to describe a single variable or a single population. The basic assumptions of this design are that (1) *one* variable exists in the population; (2) the variable may have been studied in other populations (in other words, there is a literature base for the study) but has not been studied in *this* population; (3) the variable is a *new* variable (such as toxic shock syndrome) or a *new* population (such as recent discoveries in the highlands of New Guinea or the Philippines) requiring complete description; (4) although a theoretical or conceptual framework may form the basis for the study, the intent is not to theorize or conceptualize; (5) in the absence of a theoretical or conceptual framework, a thorough rationale for the study is required based on the known research or literature on the variable; (6) if the population parameters are known, a probability sample is the basic sampling frame; (7) if the population parameters are not known, population characteristics from other studies on the same (or similar) variable can be used; and (8)

---

3. Williams, R., Characteristics of college freshmen who aspire to a nursing career, *Western Journal of Nursing Research*, 1988, 10(1), 15–23.

the purpose of the study is to describe the variable as it exists in the specific population. Data are controlled through the sample selection methods and the conditions under which variables are observed and measured.

Several types of descriptive designs usually are associated with a specific discipline, such as ethnography (anthropology), census studies (government), demography (sociology), and ethology (the observation of animal behavior). Each design has its own rules, although all must meet the criteria for a descriptive design.

Methods of data collection in descriptive designs include observation (both participant and nonparticipant observation); questioning in the form of either interviews or questionnaires; physiological measures; and available data such as artifacts and written records. The level of measurement can be either quantitative or both quantitative and qualitative. Data analysis involves, therefore, verbal description of the findings, content analysis to organize the findings into a framework, and descriptive statistics, as in measures of central tendency.

Sampling includes the total available population, as in census studies, probability sampling techniques, and convenience sampling through (1) formal interviewing of key informants, (2) informal interviewing with available subjects; and participant observation. Remember that sample size and data collection methods have a negative relationship. In other words, the smaller the sample size, the larger the number of unstructured questions that can be used. The larger the sample size, the smaller the number of unstructured questions that can be used in data collection.

In single method (i.e., questionnaires) descriptive studies (such as census studies and demographies), questionnaires/interviews usually have face and content validity. In ethnographic studies, validity of data in an unknown culture is established through triangulation of data collection methods such as interviews with observation and available data. In single method descriptive studies (i.e., interviews), face and content validity of the data is established through repeated interviews. In historical research, the document review is the literature review. The study involves making connections among pieces of data according to chronology. Each piece of data must be validated (contextually, comparatively, and by the source).

Descriptive designs differ from correlational designs by studying only one variable or one population; making no attempt to find statistical relationships; having either or both qualitative and quantitative data; using data collection instruments whose validity may not be well developed; and by not requiring a conceptual framework at the beginning of a study.

These designs are most useful when the variable has not been described for the population or when population parameters have not been established. It is, however, unethical to use these designs when the instrumentation is neither valid nor reliable or when there is no possibility of producing usable results. It is impossible to use a descriptive design when the variable does not exist in the population or when the population refuses to be studied.

Both exploratory designs and descriptive designs meet the criteria of a Level I study based on little prior knowledge of the variable or the population under study. Neither design is looking for cause-and-effect relationships, but instead are studies of single variables or single populations.

Descriptive Survey Designs

The primary designs at Level II are the correlational and comparative surveys. The major differences between them stem from the level of knowledge of the topic. *Correlational designs* have a conceptual base and are looking for cause-and-effect relationships in the results but cannot specify the direction of the relationship at the beginning of the study. In contrast, *comparative designs* can specify cause and effect at the beginning of a study and are based on a theoretical framework. Both the comparative and correlational designs are based on an accurate description of the variables as they occur naturally. The major difference between the comparative and the experimental design, and the reason the comparative design is placed at Level II, and not Level III, is that the independent variable is *not manipulated*.

Questions at Level II ask, "What is the relationship between or among variables?" You know what the variables are, and you know how to measure them, so you are beyond the scope of an exploratory study. The variables you are interested in have been studied before, either independently, as in an exploratory study, or with other variables, so that there is sufficient information to ask a question about the relationship between then. You are able to relate the variables in your study to a concept or conceptual framework so that the study does build on previous work. The major consideration is *accuracy* in the measurement of the variables.

Designs for studies at Level II require a descriptive survey. The design dictates how the variables are to be measured in testing their relationship. In this design, the variables are partly controlled by the situation, as they are in exploratory designs, but they are also partly controlled by the investigator, usually by the method of choosing a sample for the study. For example, in a study of the relationship between educational level of nurses and ability to make sound judgments about patient care, the investigator controls the first variable by selecting a sample of nurses with all types of educational backgrounds. The judgments of these nurses are then analyzed. The nurses' judgments will be examined in relationship to their educational level. The purpose of the study will be accomplished by seeing if the occurrence of sound judgment is related to educational background.

Surveys cover all types of studies in which a group of people are compared on two or more variables. Some descriptive surveys look at a specific population, such as nurses, to see whether their attitude toward some issue, such as abortion or women's rights is related to their age or educational background. Others take two or more groups, such as blacks, whites, and Hispanics, and see if they differ on some variable, such as life expectancy or the incidence of a particular health problem. Still others take a small patient population, such as renal dialysis patients, and study their coping mechanisms in relation to their acceptance or rejection of a transplanted kidney. All of these are descriptive surveys. Just as with exploratory designs, the answer is in descriptive form, but the description is of the relationship between the variables rather than of the variables themselves.

Many research questions ask about variables that cannot be subjected to experimental manipulation, either because the variables cannot be manipulated or because to look at them outside their natural setting would be meaningless. For example, in looking at factors leading to mental illness, it would be unethical to isolate a single factor, such as poverty, and manipulate it to see if it results in mental illness. An experimental design would require that subjects be assigned to groups and required to live at different levels of poverty. After the specified length of time had passed, the groups would be examined to see if mental illness had developed. The absurdity of such an approach is obvious.

Rather than using experimentation to discover the causes of mental illness, you start with the effect and select a sample of mentally ill patients. Then you look for variables that might be related to mental illness. You might find a significant relationship between poverty and mental illness. You might also establish that poverty precedes mental illness in time. However, you might discover that well-to-do persons are less likely to be diagnosed as mentally ill even when they have the same symptoms as persons at the bottom of the poverty scale. The type of health care available to persons of different economic levels is different, as are educational opportunities and many other factors. Thus poverty cannot be isolated as the single cause of mental illness. Other variables cannot be controlled or ruled out as possible causative factors either. This is the chance you take when trying to establish causality: alternative explanations are always possible in descriptive surveys. Subjects differ on many factors, only a few of which can be controlled.

Although absolute proof of causality cannot be established in a descriptive survey, it is possible to accumulate extensive evidence to support causality. Much of the research on cigarette smoking and lung cancer was done using descriptive surveys. No experimental research has been or will be done with human subjects to see if lung cancer can be caused by introducing cigarette smoking. But, by showing that cigarette smoking is the one variable preponderant in persons with lung cancer, support grows for the theory that the disease can be caused by smoking.

Many variables of interest to nursing researchers cannot be experimentally manipulated. Attitudes, beliefs, or behaviors are concepts that are often thought of as causal in health, illness, response to treatment, and other effects. The descriptive survey can be of great value in the study of these variables.

Correlational designs are studies of the relationship of two or more variables. An outcome variable may be known but the causative variable is unknown or thought to be a combination of several variables. Two variables may be known to coexist but research has not shown any relationship between them or established the direction of their relationship. In other words, you may not know if the variables are positively or negatively correlated. These are field studies that may be cross-sectional, prospective, or retrospective. The concept of control in these studies will focus on reliability testing of data collection instruments and sample selection procedures. The central issue in correlational designs is to establish generalizability to the target population or external validity.

The purpose of correlational designs is to establish definitively the strength and direction of the relationship between two or more variables based on the findings from previous research. These designs are different from comparative designs because they do not require a theoretical framework or explanation; they only look for relationships among variables. They may not be able to establish (from the literature) which variable is independent and which is dependent at the beginning of the study. They require large probability samples. They are similar to comparative designs in that there is no control over the independent variable; in other words, there is no manipulation, and they require reliable and valid measurement of variables based on previous research literature on the study variables.[4]

All correlational designs demand a conceptual framework or an explanation of why the researcher thinks these variables are related to one another and how. The basic assumptions of the design are that the variables exist in the population; the sample represents the population (probability sampling); the variables can be measured accurately, on a numerical scale; and there is no manipulation of variables.

Variations of the classic design include systematic or convenience samples, (which must provide detailed information on the population); time series; and designs that are either retrospective or prospective. Data collection methods must be quantitative, with reliable and valid measurements. Each subject is measured more than once (multiple measurements on each subject). Because of the type of data collected and the size of the samples, data analysis usually involves multivariate statistical techniques, such as correlational analysis, regression analysis, and factor analysis.

Researchers generally use correlational designs when they are not sure if the variables are related to each other; when they think the variables are related to each other, but are not sure how they are related; or when they think variables are related to each other, but do not know how strong that relationship really is. It is unethical to use correlational designs when the instrumentation is neither valid nor reliable and when there is no possibility of producing usable results. It is impossible to use correlational designs when there has been no previous research on the variables; when variables cannot be measured numerically; and when the sample is too small.

When critiquing correlational designs, focus on the sampling strategies used as well as the measurement of variables.

---

4. Data analysis is a correlational statistic.

Comparative designs are usually field studies in which the independent variable already exists and the sample is selected on the basis of the independent variable. For example, the sample is divided into groups at the beginning of the study based on the age of the subjects. The comparative design is distinguished from the quasi-experimental design by not having researcher manipulation of the independent variable.

The comparative design, like the correlational design, is a descriptive design because it does not control or manipulate the independent variable. Therefore, a comparative design cannot prove or disprove theory. It does, however, provide information about naturally occurring phenomena in a way that is impossible for experimental designs. To use this design, it must be possible to find naturally occurring groups that differ on the independent variable.

Just like the experimental design, the comparative design must have the following characteristics: (1) at least two known and previously studied variables: an independent variable that is believed to be causative, and a dependent variable that is believed to be the effect; (2) the dependent variable is the only variable that is measured; (3) the design is theory based; and (4) the design uses a predictive hypothesis rather than a simple statement of relationship.

Unlike the experimental design, (1) the independent variable is observed as it occurs naturally in the population; (2) the independent variable cannot be manipulated in reality or ethically; (3) the design cannot test theory directly; (4) the design is based on a research question, such as "What are the differences between groups when the groups represent different positions of the independent variable?" and (5) the design attempts to represent the population through probability sampling.

The classic comparative design is similar to the experimental design with two groups: a treatment group and a control group. After the change or intervention has occurred naturally, the dependent variable is measured with either a ratio or interval level measurement tool, which has been previously tested and found to be both valid and reliable. An example of a two-group comparative design would be the classic study of smokers versus nonsmokers (the independent variable) on their length of life (the dependent variable), based on the predictive hypothesis that nonsmokers would live longer than smokers. The study would have been designed on the basis of findings from a correlational survey answering the question, "What is the relationship between smoking and general health?"

Variations in the design: The comparative design has more than one form. The study can be retrospective if the sample is selected on the basis of the dependent variable. The sample could have consisted of individuals with a variety of cancers (the effect or dependent variable). Their past histories would have been examined for their smoking history (the assumed cause or independent variable). Another variation could be a time series comparative design in which an effect had been noted in a hospital chart (e.g., staphylococcus infection) as occurring on a specific date in the patient's stay. Multiple observations are made before and after the onset of the infection. A third variation could be the study of existing multiple treatment groups, such as nursing management systems in the same or different hospitals compared to one or more patient outcomes.

In the comparative design, control over the data is accomplished through the sample selection methods, the conditions under which variables are observed and measured, and by the statistical techniques used to analyze the data.

There are several sampling issues in comparative designs. The most desirable sample is the stratified random sample, a probability sample based on a known population. The second option, based on unknown population parameters, is the quota or nonprobability stratified sample drawn on the independent variable. Samples may be either proportionate to the total population or groups of equal size. The third and most common sampling type is the convenience sample: runners versus nonrunners, normal weight versus obese subjects. If the samples are not representative of the population (i.e., probability sampling), then the groups must be equivalent on all relevant variables except the independent variable.

When collecting data for a comparative design, all methods of data collection are acceptable. At this level of design, the reliability and validity of the measurement instruments are critical because the validity of the results will depend on accurate discrimination between groups. The best measurements are on ratio or interval scales. A nominal or ordinal scale can be used if it is a numerical scale. It is always best to use known data collection instruments that have been previously tested.

Data analysis procedures involve looking at the differences between two groups. If we assume probability sampling and interval/ratio levels of measurement, then the t-test is the appropriate test, because it compares the mean scores on both groups and examines the probability that this magnitude of difference could have happened by chance. If we used multiple groups, and the independent variable was categorical, then the ANOVA is appropriate. This tells us if multiple group means are statistically different from one another. If we have only one independent variable, then we can use the "One-way ANOVA." If our independent variable is quantitative, such as level of income, and the dependent variable is also quantitative, use a regression analysis.

EXPERIMENTAL DESIGNS

All experimental designs have one central characteristic: They are based on manipulating the independent variable and measuring the effect on the dependent variable.

Control is achieved in experimental designs by eliminating all sources of variation except that which the researcher introduces. In a study designed to measure the outcome of an intervention, for example, everything that happens to the subjects during the study must be equivalent for both the experimental and control subjects except the fact that the experimental subjects receive the intervention and the controls do not. This ensures that differences between these groups, following the intervention, can be attributed to the effect of the intervention.

Even with perfect control of the independent variable, however, the assumptions of cause and effect cannot be met unless the experimental and control groups are equivalent to one another before the intervention is imposed. Extraneous differences between the groups could affect the outcome of the experiment, which would then falsely be attributed to the success or failure of the intervention. These extraneous variables are considered to be *controlled* when the sample is randomly assigned to the experimental and control groups, and the groups remain intact for the duration of the experiment. Other forms of assignment to groups and large dropout rates diminish the confidence of the investigator in the results of the experiment.

Another type of control is achieved by building extraneous variables into the study as independent variables, and therefore being able to measure their effect on the dependent variable(s). This method is generally used in Level II studies where random assignment to groups is not possible. Each additional variable added to the study will increase the cost of the research; therefore, adding variables must be done with care.

The classic experimental design consists of the experimental group and the control group. In the experimental group, the independent variable is manipulated. In the control group, the dependent variable is measured when no alteration has been made on the independent variable. The dependent variable is measured in the experimental group the same way, and at the same time, as in the control group. The prediction is that the dependent variable in the experimental group will change in a specific way and that the dependent variable in the control group will not change.

	Independent Variable	*Dependent Variable*
Experimental Group	Changed	Measured
Control Group	Unchanged	Measured

When data are analyzed, only the measurements on the dependent variable for the two groups are contrasted.

For example:

Independent Variable	*Dependent Variable*
Preoperative teaching	Postoperative pain, medication consumption
No teaching	Postoperative pain, medication consumption

A number of variations are possible. First, there are designs in which there is one control group and two or more experimental groups, and the independent variable is manipulated in several different ways. For example:

Independent Variable	*Dependent Variable*
Usual preoperative teaching	Postoperative pain, medication consumption
Structured preoperative teaching	
Lecture/Discussion	Postoperative pain, medication consumption
Videotape/Discussion	Postoperative pain, medication consumption

The hypothesis would predict which of the three teaching methods would be most "successful" (that is, the group with the lowest pain medication consumption post-operatively). The point is to contrast the three groups.

Another, more sophisticated design would pretest all three groups on the content to be taught. After the teaching (manipulating the independent variable), the subjects would again be tested on the same content (the dependent variable). The scores for each subject before and after the teaching would be compared. The differences among groups would then be placed side by side to see which teaching method was most effective. Following the surgery, pain medication consumption would be compared among all groups (the second dependent variable). Each subject would be examined in relation to knowledge and consumption of pain medication. With the addition of pain medication consumption as a dependent variable, knowledge of the subject would become an intervening variable between preoperative teaching and medication consumption. The design would look like this:

	Experiment			*Medication*
Pretest	*Teaching*	*Post-test*	*Surgery*	*Consumption*
O_1	Group 1	O_2	Control	O_3
O_4	Group 2	O_5	Exp 1	O_6
O_7	Group 3	O_8	Exp 2	O_9

We simply have added several other variables to the classic experimental design and measured them as well, as in the first design. In addition, we have added groups to the design and tested/compared them as well.

Each group is tested or observed (O) three times: pretest, after the teaching program, and after the intervening variable of surgery. Group 1 is the control group and does not receive any form of experimental teaching. Following the teaching, each group is tested on their knowledge base (second set of Os). The third set of Os follows the surgery and tests the amount of medication consumed. Subjects therefore can be compared to themselves, to others in their group, and to other groups.

The most critical characteristic of experimental designs is investigator manipulation of the independent variable; it is always manipulated, altered, or changed in some way in the experimental group. In true experiments there is always a control group and random assignment of subjects to groups. The theoretical base for the study predicts the direction of the change in the dependent variable as a result of the change in the independent variable. The distinguishing feature between true experiments and quasi-experiments is that the quasi-experiment does not have random assignment to groups and/or does not have a control group.

Features of the True or Classic Experiment

1. Subjects are randomly assigned to groups (R)
2. The experimenter manipulates the experimental variable (X)
3. There are at least two groups: experimental (X) and control (C)

The control group is used to measure the dependent variable when the independent variable has not been applied. The experiment is based on the assumption that there will be a difference in measurement of the dependent variable depending on the manipulation of the independent variable.

The following are some examples of experimental designs where R = random assignment to groups; X = experimental group; C = control group; O = measurement or observation before or after the experimental manipulation.

After Only Design

R X O_1
R C O_2

In the After Only Design, there are two groups, random assignment to both groups, experimental manipulation of one group, no manipulation of the other group, and both groups tested.

Before-After Design

R O_1 X O_2
R O_3 C O_4

In the Before-After Design, both groups are tested at the same time on the dependent variable both before and after the experimental manipulation in the experimental group.

Solomon Four Group Design

R O_1 X O_2
R O_3 C O_4
R . X O_5
R . C O_6

In the Solomon Four Group Design, the After-Only and the Before-After designs are combined into one design. The rationale for this combination is that subjects have been known to do better on a measurement the second time they are tested no matter what has happened between testing periods. There is some learning that occurs simply with familiarity with the measuring instrument or the experience itself. For this reason, this design compares the scores of groups who have not had a pretest (After-Only) with the scores of the two groups who have been pretested. In this way the two experimental groups are contrasted and the two control groups are contrasted to verify the difference in the post-test as a result of the pretest. Then the After Only groups are contrasted and the Before and After Groups are contrasted on the dependent variable. Finally the two experimental groups together are contrasted with the two control groups' scores.

Although this may sound like a pointless exercise, it really isn't. Remember that the true experimental design is expected to be the most highly controlled laboratory study possible. As a result, a number of statistical analyses are required in all types of combinations to test the hypothesis.

Quasi-experimental designs are based solely on experimenter manipulation of the independent variable and lack at least one characteristic of the true experiment.

Features of the Quasi-experiment
1. Experimental manipulation of the independent variable
2. No random assignment to groups, and/or
3. No control group(s)

The quasi-experimental design looks much like the experimental designs above; simply remove the "R" for random assignment to groups and the same type of experiments are possible. Instead of random assignment, you may substitute matched groups or you may have convenient groups. A quasi-experimental design without a control group might look like this:

$$O_1 \ O_2 \ O_3 \ O_4 \ X \ O_5 \ O_6 \ O_7 \ O_8$$

In this example, the experimental group serves as its own control in a time series design with one or more measurements before the experiment and one or more measurements after.

Sometimes a true experimental design is simply not possible to carry out. Many nursing studies are forced into quasi-experimental designs by the nature of the study or the natural clinical setting. A study of a new nursing intervention on an in-patient unit might use a quasi-experimental time series design like the one above to test the old intervention over time before instituting a new one and then testing the new one over time. Or if two nursing units were fairly similar in their type of patient population, two wards might be used for comparison, both using different nursing interventions. Both wards would serve as a comparison group for the other in Before-After designs without random assignment to groups.

The limitations of the experimental design are that some variables are simply not amenable to manipulation (such as age, sex, and ethnicity). Other variables (such as smoking to cause cancer, use of a placebo in place of a contraceptive device, nontreatment of a disease for which a cure is known) are not experimentally ethical. Sometimes experiments are impractical, sometimes they seem artificial or contrived, and sometimes the Hawthorne effect (discussed later in this chapter) causes people to change their behavior.

A major purpose of the experimental design is to eliminate alternative explanations or hypotheses to account for the findings. It is the controlled setting, the contrast groups, and the control over the experimental variable that allow for acceptance or rejection of the hypothesis being tested. Although the experiment may have turned out correctly, there is still the outside chance that something other than the experimental variable caused the effect in the dependent variable. As a result, we always hold that we *tentatively* accept the findings in the light of current evidence, always subject to change with new knowledge.

CONTROLLING UNWANTED INFLUENCES

To obtain a reliable answer to the research question, the design must indicate how it will control or eliminate possible unwanted influences. The amount of control that the researcher has over the variables being studied varies, from very little in exploratory studies to a great deal in experimental design, but the limitations on control must be addressed in any research proposal.

These unwanted influences stem from one or more of the following: extraneous variables, bias, the Hawthorne effect, and the passage of time. These four will be discussed in turn, along with some suggestions for controlling their effects. You will need to identify those that seem relevant to your question and show how you will control their effects.

Extraneous Variables

As explained in Chapter 6, extraneous variables are variables that can interfere with the action of the ones you are studying. They could as easily have been chosen as independent variables had you been interested in them because of their known effect on your variables. Because they are not part of your study, their influence must be controlled.

In the research literature, you will see extraneous variables also referred to as intervening, environmental, organismic, confounding, or demographic variables. Each term, however, defines a slightly different class of extraneous variables. Intervening or confounding variables, found in Level III experimental designs, directly affect the action of the independent variable on the dependent variable. They must be controlled in the design even though they are not of prime interest to the researcher as they will affect the results of the experiment. Environmental variables are those that occur in the study setting. They include economic, physical, and psychosocial variables. Organismic variables refer to person characteristics such as physiological, psychological, or demographic. Demographic variables are descriptive characteristics such as age, sex, marital status, and education.

Your literature review should help you determine which extraneous variables might be present in your study. As an example, look at the question, "What are the relationships among style of leadership, educational opportunities on the job, and the job satisfaction of staff nurses?" Many factors are known to influence job satisfaction. Why not choose age, marital status of the nurse, the amount of independence on the job, or the level of education of the nurse as independent variables? Any of these could qualify, but, because you are not interested in them, they are not directly a part of your study. They are extraneous to your study and you want to be sure they do not interfere with the relationship between style of leadership and job satisfaction and between educational opportunities and job satisfaction.

Extraneous variables usually are not a problem in Level I studies. Because you are studying only one variable in depth, these variables are assumed to be independent. They could all be extraneous variables as well. That is why an exploratory descriptive study explores *in depth:* all variables must be accounted for and taken into consideration in order to be described adequately.

At Level II, when you do not know which variables are independent and which are dependent, you must assume that there may be variables that have not been accounted for that may be related to the dependent variable. Some variables have been shown to be related to one of your variables in other studies. These are *known* extraneous variables and must be considered when designing your study, so that their effect on your variables can be controlled. At Level II, it is sometimes difficult to establish which one is the independent variable, even after confirming that there is a significant relationship between two variables. Unless you can demonstrate that one variable precedes the other in time, it may be impossible to determine which is the independent variable. Therefore, it is important to control extraneous variables when you can identify what they are, so that you can isolate the relationship between the ones you are interested in studying.

At Level III, where you are predicting the relationship, you must be very careful to control all possible extraneous variables that might intervene in your test. These variables can be identified from the literature on your topic.

Methods of controlling extraneous variables include randomization, homogenous sampling techniques, matching, and building the variables into the design.

RANDOMIZATION. Theoretically, randomization is the only method of controlling all possible extraneous variables. The random assignment of subjects to the various treatment and control groups means that the groups can be considered equivalent in all ways at the beginning of the experiment. It does not mean that they actually *are* equal for all variables. However, the probability of their being equal is greater than the probability of their not being equal, if the random assignment was carried out properly. The exception lies with small groups where random assignment could result in unequal distribution of crucial variables. If this possibility exits in your study, perhaps one of the other methods of control would be more appropriate. In most instances, however, randomization is the best method of controlling extraneous variables.

The principle of randomization applies to both Level II and Level III studies. In Level II studies, a random sampling technique results in a normal distribution of extraneous variables in the sample, which approximates the distribution of those variables in the population. Probability theory demonstrates that this will happen in 95 random samples out of 100 from the same population. The purpose of randomization at Level II is to ensure a representative sample so that your result can be generalized from the sample to the population.

At Level III, randomization comes into play when you randomly assign subjects to experimental and control groups, thus ensuring that the groups are as equivalent as possible prior to the manipulation of the independent variable. Random assignment ensures that the researcher was not biased in putting certain people into the experimental groups. Instead, each subject had an equal chance of being in any of the groups at the beginning of the assignment process.

Here is one method of random assignment. This method is called "systematic assignment to groups with a random start," and is used when the sample is expected to arrive sequentially, such as patients do in an emergency room on any given day. When the first patient who meets the criteria for the sample arrives, that person is randomly assigned to one of the groups. This assignment can be done by flipping a coin, or by drawing a number out of a hat. If the study has four groups, and the first patient is assigned to group 2, the next patient goes to group 3, the next to group 4, the next to group 1, and so on. With this method, you make no choice as to which group a patient will be in, and the groups will be of approximately equal size at any given time during the study. This is important if you expect it to take a long time to fill the groups to the desired size.

If all the subjects are available at the beginning of the study, you can place tickets in a box with group numbers representing the way you want the subjects distributed (that is, thirty subjects per group divided into four groups), and then have each subject draw a number. If you use this method, and subjects arrive sequentially over a long period, you might end up with one group filling sooner than the others, which could introduce some bias into your study.

Whichever method is used, every precaution must be taken to remove subjectivity from the assignment of subjects to groups. Clinical studies, for example, have been seriously affected by having professional staff reassign subjects away from the protocol. Abbey[5] reported having to cancel a clinical experiment because the nursing staff, believing that the experimental variable was highly successful, began assigning patients whom they felt would benefit from it rather than following the protocol for random assignment. Such decisions should not be made by clinical staff, so the research design must be carefully monitored to make sure the system is carried out.

HOMOGENEOUS SAMPLE. One simple and effective way of controlling an extraneous variable is not to allow it to vary. Choose a sample that is homogeneous for that variable. For instance, if you are concerned about the effect that the patients' cultural backgrounds might have on your study of pain, choose a sample from only one cultural group, such as all Chinese-Americans or all Mexican-Americans. In this way, you have eliminated the possible effect that the subjects' cultural backgrounds might have on their responses to pain, as they all represent the same culture. This method has one serious drawback, however: the ability to generalize the findings is limited. As you might expect, if you study only Mexican-Americans, then your results apply only to Mexican-Americans and not to African-Americans, Asians, or Native Americans. If the sample is limited to one age group, the results apply only to that age group, as the relationship you find between your variables might be different for other age groups. You will not know; you can only guess.

For instance, in the example on job satisfaction, the sample could be limited to nurses with generic bachelor's degrees or to nurses over 50 years of age. On the other hand, the study could be of nurses on night shift or nurses who are in critical care units. The sample is being made homogeneous for certain variables and not others. Saunders's[6] study explored and described bereavement of widows, contrasting the modes of death of the husbands to see if there was any difference in the bereavement process. The sample was made as homogeneous as possible by choosing husbands (at the time of their death) who were Caucasian, Protestant, and within a ten-year age range (30–39) to

---

5. Abbey, J., A study of control of shivering during hypothermia. Paper presented at the second annual Octoberquest Nursing Research Conference, Los Angeles, October 1980.

6. Saunders, J., A process of bereavement resolution: Uncoupled identity, *Western Journal of Nursing Research,* Fall 1981, 3(4).

control for the possible intervening variables of ethnicity, religion, and age. The results of studies such as these can then be generalized only to the population from which the sample was selected.

MATCHING. When randomization is not possible, or when the experimental groups are too small and contain some crucial variables, subjects can be matched for those variables. The experimenter chooses subjects who match each other for the specified variables, such as sex, age, and diagnosis. One of these matched subjects is assigned to the control group and the other to the experimental group, thus ensuring the equality of the groups at the outset.

In a study on postoperative convalescence in Anglos and Mexican-Americans, Williams attempted to match her sample on class, number of generations in the United States, type of surgery, age, and level of education. In this study, Williams[7] was seeking the relationship between ethnicity and convalescence, holding all of these possible intervening variables constant.

The process of matching is time-consuming and introduces considerable subjectivity into sample selection. Therefore, it should be avoided whenever possible.

If you use matching, limit the number of groups to be matched and keep the number of variables for which the subjects are matched low. Matching with more than five variables becomes extremely cumbersome, and it is almost impossible to find enough matched partners for your sample. Matching may be used in all research designs (besides Level III) when you are looking at certain outcomes and want to have as much control as possible.

BUILDING EXTRANEOUS VARIABLES INTO THE DESIGN. When extraneous variables cannot be adequately controlled by randomization, they can be built into the design as independent variables. They would have to be added to the purpose of your study and tested for significance along with your other variables. In this way, their effect can be measured and separated from the effect of the variables you wanted to study initially. Particularly in experimental designs, but also in descriptive surveys, the effect of these variables can be removed statistically from the total action of the variables. This method adds to the cost of the study because of the additional data collection and analysis required. Therefore, it should be used with caution.

In exploratory descriptive studies where the nature of the variables is not known, extraneous variables are said to be built into the design. The purpose

---

7. Williams, M., A comparative study of postsurgical convalescence among women of two ethnic groups: Anglo and Mexican-American. In M. V. Batey (ed.), *Communicating nursing research*, Boulder, Co.: Western Interstate Commission for Higher Education, 1972, 59–73.

in these studies is to identify the relevant variables and assess their relationship in the data analysis. Therefore, it is essential that you treat all variables as independent during the data collection so that no data that later might point to relationships between variables will be overlooked. The separation of extraneous variables from independent and dependent variables is part of the analysis of data in exploratory research.

Bias

Bias results from collecting the data in such a way that one answer to the research question is given undue favor over another. Bias can be introduced into a study at any point, from the initial writing of the research question to the conclusions of the research report, and must be constantly guarded against when you are developing your research project. All researchers are biased in relation to their own studies as a natural outcome of their intense interest in their research topics. We all know how we would like our studies to come out and what we think we will find when we collect and analyze the data. We are therefore obligated to avoid influencing the outcome in any way, even unconsciously. The results must be an objective reporting of the real situation. Because most researchers are scrupulously honest in the accuracy with which they handle their data, we will only deal with the two areas where bias can easily be introduced (even by the most honest researcher) if care is not taken. These are during the sample selection and data collection phases of the project. (The other area of concern is the interpretation of data, which we do not deal with in this book, but you need to be aware of when you are critiquing research reports.)

Because you know what you would like your results to be, you want to avoid unconsciously swaying the study in that direction. During sample selection, if you are not able to use random sampling techniques, it is only too easy to acquire a biased sample if you are not careful. Always take precautions to maintain objectivity whenever you can, and use methods to predetermine who will be in your sample; do not wait until you are face-to-face with potential subjects to decide. For example, if your plan is to interview hospitalized patients on a particular unit, choose the room numbers you will visit from an available list, and then ask all patients in those rooms to be interviewed. If an interviewer arrives on a nursing unit to select patients without these kinds of guidelines, he or she may end up choosing patients who look as if they would enjoy being interviewed—a biased sample! Another biased sample could result from asking a staff member to recommend some patients for interview, as you would not know the staff member's criteria for the recommendation. Any time random selection is not possible, make your choice of subjects as objective as possible by reducing the number of choices available to you by setting predetermined guidelines.

Bias during the data collection phase of research means that the researcher is either influencing the responses of the subjects in some way, or is selectively recording data according to conscious or unconscious predispositions.

In the first case, the subjects' responses are influenced in any one direction by the way in which data collection is approached. This is easiest to do in an interview, where subjects can be given the impression that one response will be received more favorably than another or that one response represents the "best" choice. Careful training and monitoring of interviewers is required to prevent undue influence from affecting interview responses.

The second case refers to selective recording of data by the researcher. This can occur in observational studies and in reviewing audiotapes, audiovisual tapes, and written documents even when structured tools are used to record the data. Selectively focusing on some parts of the data and overlooking significant opposing views can be easily done by persons eager to prove a point. Everyone must guard against this happening by building in checks and balances—such as having an impartial colleague periodically work along with the researcher. Other checks and balances are discussed in Chapter 10, in the sections on reliability and validity in participant observation. You cannot completely eliminate bias from an exploratory study because of the essential flexibility of the design. You can, however, plan for as much objectivity as possible and keep in mind the limitations of this design when drawing conclusions from your data.

In other levels of designs—descriptive survey designs and experimental designs—the complete elimination of bias from the data collection becomes more critical. The influence of the investigator's bias in an exploratory study, though difficult to eliminate, can at least be described along with the data. If, however, inferences are to be drawn from the data, there is no room for bias. Therefore, every precaution must be taken to prevent influencing the data collection process.

The Hawthorne Effect

The Hawthorne effect refers to the effect that the knowledge of being the subjects of a research study has on the subjects' responses. In experimental studies, care needs to be taken that the resultant changes in the dependent variable can be attributed to the independent variable and not to the special attention given to the subjects in the experimental group. When testing the effect of nursing interventions, it may be wise to equalize the amount of nursing time spent with patients in both the experimental and control groups, to rule out the possibility that the patient is responding to the interaction with the nurse rather than to the intervention. The control group can be thought of as a "placebo" group in which nursing interaction is provided without the experimental variable.

In the early stages of nursing research, many studies capitalized on the Hawthorne effect without realizing that they had done so. These early clinical studies used a two-group experimental design in which the control group received the usual nursing care and the experimental group received the full force of a deliberate nursing intervention. In every case, the experimental group was significantly different from the control group. Because of the Hawthorne effect, these studies did not prove anything except that deliberate nursing actions do make a difference. They did *not* prove which interventions were better than others.

To minimize the Hawthorne effect in experimental designs, or at least to account for them, try to use more than one experimental group and preferably those who are competitive with the point you are trying to make. For example, in a patient teaching study, have several experimental groups who receive different teaching methods; or, have a group that receives individualized attention from a nurse for the same length of time as the experimental group receiving the experimental variable. Otherwise, you will prove, once again, that patients appreciate being noticed, even as research subjects.

Time

This category is used to cover those factors resulting from the fact that life goes on during the research process. Events that occur just before or during the study period can affect the responses of subjects, yet have nothing to do with the study—for example, an earthquake, a race riot, or a movie on television. These events can produce changes in attitudes, feelings, and behavior; if the researcher is unaware of their effect, they can lead to erroneous conclusions. Interviewing patients about sensory disturbances during the aftermath of an earthquake would produce some interesting data. But the data would be related to the earthquake rather than to being a patient. If you are questioning people about controversial issues in order to assess their attitudes, it would be wise to check the television schedule for the week of your data collection to avoid coinciding with a special program on your topic.

Developmental or maturation processes also can influence the variables you are planning to measure, particularly if your subjects are very young or very old. This is of special concern when it is necessary to have a long interval between data collection times. The use of control groups may be necessary to rule out the possibility of developmental changes. A special counseling program for disadvantaged students, for example, is expected to ease the students' adjustment to nursing school. A control group would give substance to the fact that the special counseling program did ease adjustment and that the students' adjustment was not due simply to the social experience that the school provides.

LEVEL OF STUDY AND DEGREE OF CONTROL

In Level I studies, where as much flexibility as possible is encouraged, the concept of control of the variables in the design has little relevance. What is needed at Level I is the concept of control of external influences on the research process itself. Here you are concerned with the biases of the researcher and how to control or minimize them. You are expected to keep a journal of events that occur when you are doing exploratory research, so that you can account for possible alterations in the study that may be related to these events. The Hawthorne effect occurs in Level I studies when the subjects react to being studied. It is controlled over time, when the presence of the investigator becomes so familiar that the subjects become unaware they are being observed.

At Level II, you are more concerned with controlling extraneous variables in the design and conduct of the study. When you are looking for significant relationships between two or more variables, you must be sure you have accounted for all other variables that might influence the interaction of the variable you are studying. These are accounted for by random sample selection and by collecting data on key extraneous variables so that their effect can be measured. At Level II, you are not as concerned with the bias of the investigator since the objectivity of the structured data collection methods tends to minimize investigator bias.

In experimental studies at Level III, you must be careful to control extraneous variables that occur as a result of time, the Hawthorne effect, or sampling. To accomplish this control, you attempt to keep the experimental conditions identical for the various groups in your design. You begin by randomly assigning the sample to the groups so that they will be equivalent at the beginning of the experiment. In addition, you may select a relatively homogeneous population to begin with so that some extraneous variables do not have to be considered. Next, make sure that the treatment of the groups throughout the collection of the data continues to be the same in every respect except for the application of the independent variable. Data on the dependent variable are collected in the same way from all groups. An excessive drop-out rate from one of your groups may be an indication that the experimental conditions are not being maintained for all groups and that some subjects are dissatisfied with their role in the study.

In summary, the research design provides the blueprint for the research plan specifically in terms of the control mechanisms that will be used to provide a clear and accurate answer to your research question. The level at which you can study a given research topic is based on the level of knowledge already in existence about that topic. This will also affect the degree of control you can achieve over the variables in your study. To gain sufficient depth of information, the flexibility that is required for a Level I exploratory study will limit the degree of control over the study conditions. In order to achieve maximum control, every detail of a study must be planned in advance. Therefore, at Level I, control is limited to the choice of the initial sample and most commonly results in a homogeneous sample.

At Level II, the major concern is to maximize the external validity of the results; therefore the critical control mechanism is the random selection of subjects from the population. When this is not possible in a Level II study, it is always considered a serious limitation in the design. Also at this level, you will be concerned with maintaining consistent conditions throughout the study so that bias in data collection will be minimized.

Experimental designs require maximum possible control over extraneous and intervening variables so that internal validity can be maximized. You want to be able to say with some assurance that the results are an accurate reflection of the action of the independent variable. Thus random assignment to groups is essential, as is maintaining consistent study conditions for all groups. When planning a Level III study, your goal is to be able to foresee every detail of the design so that unwanted influences can be avoided.

Regardless of the level of study you are planning, the design phase will require significant time and effort on your part to think through the elements that will be required to provide the answer to your question. This time is well-spent, however, in terms of the time and effort it saves later when you are carrying out the steps in your plan.

RECOMMENDED READINGS

Bailey, P. H., Finding your way around qualitative methods in nursing research. *Journal of Advanced Nursing*, 1997, *25*, 18–22.

Barhyte, D. Y., Redman, B. K., and Neill, K. M., Population or sample: Design decision, *Nursing Research*, 1990, *39*(5), 309–310.

Barrett, E. A., Unique nursing research methods: the diversity chant of pioneers. *Nursing Science Quarterly*, 1998, *11*(3), 94–96.

Beck, S. L., The crossover design in clinical nursing research. *Nursing Research*, 1989, *38*(5), 291–293.

Behi, R., and Nolan, M., Causality and control: Threats to internal validity. *British Journal of Nursing*, 1996, *5*(6), 374–377.

Brink, P. J., Exploratory designs. In P. J. Brink and M. J. Wood (eds.), *Advanced design in nursing research* (2nd ed.), Thousand Oaks, Ca.: Sage, 1998, 141–160.

Brink, P. J., and Wood, M. J., (eds.), *Advanced design in nursing research* (2nd ed.), Thousand Oaks, Ca.: Sage, 1998.

Brink, P. J., and Wood, M. J., Correlational designs. In P. J. Brink and M. J. Wood (eds.), *Advanced design in nursing research* (2nd ed.), Thousand Oaks, Ca.: Sage, 1998, 160–167.

Brink, P. J., and Wood, M. J., Descriptive designs. In P. J. Brink and M. J. Wood (eds.), *Advanced design in nursing research* (2nd ed.), Thousand Oaks, Ca.: Sage, 1998, 287–307.

Brown, S. R., and Melamed, L. E. *Experimental design and analysis,* Newbury Park, Ca.: Sage, 1990.

Buckwalter, K. C., and Maas, M. L., Classical experimental designs. In P. J. Brink and M. J. Wood (eds.), *Advanced design in nursing research* (2nd ed.), Thousand Oaks, Ca.: Sage, 1998, 21–62.

Campbell, D. T., and Stanley, J. C., *Experimental and quasi-experimental design for research,* Chicago: Rand McNally, 1963.

Cohen, M. Z., Kahn, D. L., and Steeves, R. H., *Hermeneutic phenomenological research: A practical guide for nurse researchers.* Thousand Oaks, Ca.: Sage, 2000.

Conlon, M., and Anderson, G. C., Three methods of random assignment: Comparison of balance achieved on potentially confounding variables, *Nursing Research,* 1990, *39*(6), 376–379.

Cook, T. D., and Campbell, D. T., *Quasi-experimentation: Design and analysis issues for field settings,* Chicago: Rand McNally, 1979.

Corben, V., Misusing phenomenology in nursing research: Identifying the issues. *Nurse Researcher,* 1999, *6*(3), 52–66.

Crosby, F. E., Ventura, M. R., and Feldman, M. J., Examination of a survey methodology: Dillman's total design method, *Nursing Research,* 1989, *38*(1), 56–58.

Egan, E. C., Snyder, M., and Burns, K. R., Intervention studies in nursing: Is the effect due to the independent variable? *Nursing Outlook,* 1992, *40*(4), 187–190.

Field, P. A., and Morse, J., *Nursing Research: The application of qualitative approaches,* Rockville, Md.: Aspen Systems, 1986.

Glass, L., Historical research. In P. J. Brink and M. J. Wood (eds.), *Advanced design in nursing research* (2nd ed.), Thousand Oaks, Ca.: Sage, 1998, 183–200.

Goodwin, L. D., and Goodwin, W. L., Qualitative vs. quantitative research or qualitative and quantitative research?, *Nursing Research,* 1984, *33*(6), 378–380.

Guiffre, M., Designing research: Expost facto designs. *Journal of PeriAnesthesia Nursing,* 1997, *12*(3), 191–195.

Hagemaster, N., Life history: A qualitative method of research. *Journal of Advanced Nursing,* 1992, *17,* 1122–1128.

Jacobsen, B. S., and Meninger, J. C., The designs and methods of published nursing research: 1956–1983, *Nursing Research,* 1985, *34*(5), 306–312.

Knaak, P., Phenomenological research, *Western Journal of Nursing Research,* 1984, *6*(1), 107–114.

Maas, M. L., and Buckwalter, K. C., Quasi-experimental designs. In P. J. Brink and M. J. Wood (eds.), *Advanced design in nursing research* (2nd ed.), Thousand Oaks, Ca.: Sage, 1998, 63–104.

Meininger, J. C., Epidemiologic designs. In P. J. Brink and M. J. Wood, (eds.), *Advanced design in nursing research* (2nd ed.), Thousand Oaks, Ca.: Sage, 1998, 210–234.

Morse, J. M., and Bottorff, J. L., The use of ethology in clinical nursing research, *Advances in Nursing Science,* 1990, *12*(3), 53–64.

Oberst, M. T., Bias in clinical samples, *Research in Nursing and Health,* 1991, *14*(2), iii, iv.

Pallikkathayil, L., and Morgan, S. A., Phenomenology as a method for conducting clinical research, *Applied Nursing Research,* 1991, *4*(4), 195–200.

Patton, M. Q., *Qualitative evaluation and research methods* (2nd ed.), Newbury Park, Ca.: Sage, 1990.

Roper, J. M., and Shapira, J., *Ethnography in nursing research,* Thousand Oaks, Ca.: Sage, 2000.

Rossi, P. H., and Freeman, H. E., *Evaluation: A systematic approach,* Thousand Oaks, Ca.: Sage, 1979.

Sarnecky, M. T., Historiography: A legitimate research methodology for nursing, *Advances in Nursing Science,* 1990 *12*(4), 1–10.

Sharp, K., The case for case studies in nursing research: The problem of generalization, *Journal of Advanced Nursing,* 1998, *27,* 785–789.

Sheldon, L., Grounded theory: Issues for research in nursing, *Nursing Standard,* 1998, *12*(52), 47–50.

Strauss, A., and Corbin, J. M., *Basics of qualitative research: Grounded theory procedures and techniques,* Newbury Park, Ca.: Sage, 1990.

Waltz, C., and Bausell, R. B., *Nursing research: Design, statistics and computer analysis,* Philadelphia: F. A. Davis, 1981, Chaps. 8–11.

Wood, M., Evaluative designs. In P. J. Brink and M.J. Wood (eds.), *Advanced design in nursing research* (2nd ed.), Thousand Oaks, Ca.: Sage, 1998, 124–138.

Wood, M. J., and Brink, P. J., Comparative designs. In P. J. Brink and M. J. Wood (eds.), *Advanced design in nursing research* (2nd ed.), Thousand Oaks, Ca.: Sage, 1998, 143–159.

Wooldridge, P. J., Leonard, R. C., and Skipper, Jr., J. K., *Methods of clinical experimentation to improve patient care,* St. Louis: Mosby, 1978.

Zeller, R., Good, M., Anderson, G. C., and Zeller, D. L., Strengthening experimental design by balancing potentially confounding variables across treatment groups, *Nursing Research,* 1997, *48*(6), 345–348.

Selecting the Sample

When you stop to think about the population for your study, you will realize that by now you have already given considerable thought to this topic in the process of developing your question into a research problem and in planning the design for your study. All along you have had a picture in the back of your mind of the group of subjects that would provide the data for your study. Usually, in nursing research, the subjects are people, but they can also be events, animals, places, or objects. For simplicity's sake, in this discussion, we will proceed as though the subjects were always people.

The *total population* (or universe) can be defined as everyone in the world who meets the criteria for the people you are interested in studying. To decide who makes up this group, you need to look back at the purpose of your study. Perhaps you have said you would be studying pregnant teenagers, or preterm infants, bereaved widows, people with diabetes, hospitalized in-patients, or the general public. Now is the time to describe these people as fully as possible in relation to: who they are, where you will find them, and when they will be found. Your total population could be all members of a village or tribe, all citizens of a town or city, all members of the United Nations, all individuals with breast cancer, all members of a single racial or ethnic group in the United States, or all students in baccalaureate nursing programs. Some of these represent very large groups of people, others are quite small. As you begin to describe your total population more fully, you will begin to eliminate some people as possible subjects. Perhaps you will be studying pregnant teenagers, but are only interested in girls between the ages of ten and fourteen who are in their first trimester. Now you have narrowed your focus considerably and have eliminated most of the pregnant teenagers in the world from eligibility for your study. Or perhaps you now realize, because of the conceptual framework you have used for your study, that you really want to concentrate on girls who reside in juvenile halls. This has further delineated your population. Now your total population looks like this: "Pregnant girls, ages ten to fourteen, in the first trimester of pregnancy, who are incarcerated in juvenile halls in the city of Los Angeles." This is the group from which you would like to sample and to whom you would like to generalize your results, so you have answered the "who, where, and when" part of the definition of your population. You can now call this your target population.

The *target population* is always the "theoretically available" group to whom you expect to generalize your results. Sometimes this group is identical to the total population with which you started. For example, if your total population had been the current active members of the West Coast Cocker Spaniel Club, your task would now be simple. To answer the questions of "where" and "when," you would obtain a mailing list of the current members from the club secretary and could draw your sample from that list at any time during the current fiscal year. Your total and target populations are identical. The same would be true if your task were to conduct the United States Census in 1990. Your total population would be everyone residing in this country at the time of the census in 1990, and your target population is this same group. This was not true for the population of pregnant teenagers that we previously described. It took several steps to get from the universe of pregnant teenagers to the target population that represents the group you really wanted to study. Even now, however, the target population of juvenile-hall pregnant teenagers in one city is too complex for you to handle, and so you begin to limit, or target, your study to an even more accessible group. The total population of pregnant teenagers becomes more specifically targeted to one specific juvenile hall in your city to which you have access. Remember, the target population is the group that is theoretically available to you and to which you plan to generalize your results. The more you limit, or target, this population, the smaller the group to whom you can generalize in your final analysis. One specific juvenile hall in your city is not representative of your original total population, and so you must change your idea of the total population to include inmates of just one juvenile hall. Some of the considerations you will make in targeting your population stem from your own resources. Can you get to the population once you have defined it? Are the subjects in your geographic location or do you have funds and transportation to get to them? Can you get permission to study the subjects you have targeted? Your study population is dependent on your resources, including the amount of time and money you have available to do research. If you want to study current college presidents, the total population in the world is very likely too much to handle so you may limit your target population to U.S. college presidents and sample from that group. You may decide on Eastern college presidents or presidents of colleges in your own state. Each subsequent geographical narrowing targets the population further and with each narrowing you limit further the group to whom you will generalize your results. At the same time, you are making your sample selection more and more reasonable. Think of targeting as narrowing or limiting the total population into something reasonable.

One further consideration needs to be made when you are finalizing the definition of your target population, and that is to *make sure the population will be accessible to you when you get ready to select your sample and collect your data.* This is the single most serious problem facing any researcher. Nothing is more discouraging than finding that the subjects you need are either not accessible or not available when you need them. Sometimes it is a problem of getting permission to access the subjects. Several students have recently tried to access a population of AIDS patients for research and have found that these patients are very protected by the organizations responsible for their care; although as nursing graduate students they could get permission to give nursing care through the home health agency, they were not allowed to collect data for research. For your own population, you must give serious consideration to whether once you get to them, you will have permission to study them. Will they talk to you? If the target population is not accessible to you, you cannot proceed.

The question of availability must also be considered. Are you sure there will be enough subjects available from which to draw your sample? How many pregnant girls are there at juvenile halls between the ages of ten and fourteen at any given time? Perhaps even the entire population will not provide you with enough data to do your study. One of the authors traveled to London to look up some archives in the British Colonial Office only to find that the files had been destroyed by treaty. The targeted files were not available. These are questions that can be investigated before "casting your target population in cement." It is much better to discover these kinds of problems during the process of defining your population rather than after the study is under way.

Once you have completely defined your target population, you can choose your sample from that group. The population is the group of people you are interested in studying; the sample merely represents them. Be as detailed as you can about who qualifies to be in your population, and your sample selection will be easier.

If you plan to replicate another study, remember that the population in your study must closely approximate the population used in the original study. The setting in which you find the subjects will be different, but all other aspects of the original population should be identical. For instance, if the original study used nurses from two-, three-, and four-year programs; any age, sex, race, or ethnic background; working at UCLA Hospital within three years after graduating from nursing school—your replication study must use a population as close to this one as possible. Perhaps you are doing the study in Seattle and want to use nurses working at the University of Washington Hospital. This change is acceptable provided that you keep the other characteristics of the population the same.

When you replicate a study that has been (or is being) done by another researcher, you cannot possibly use the exact target population the other researcher used (or is using) because you are not in the same place at the same time. In a sense, the difference in time and location validates the findings. In multiple concurrent replication studies[1] and clinical trials, the replication of a research project occurs simultaneously in multiple settings. Several investigators conduct the same study, using the same design, at different locations. Each of them can generalize only to his or her own target population; however, the total population can be expanded through comparison of the concurrent replication studies.

Where your subjects will be found is a major element in your population description. If you are interested only in ICU nurses at Battleground Hospital, say so. If you are interested in nursing staff or patients at a particular nursing home or day-care center, specify where the population will be found. Populations must be defined according to location as well as to the time when the study will be done.[2]

TYPES OF SAMPLES

Once you have set up the criteria for inclusion in your sample by describing the population in detail, you must determine next whether yours will be a *probability* or *nonprobability* sample (see Table 8.1). In probability sampling, each element in the population has a known probability of being included in the sample. In nonprobability sampling, this probability is unknown. Some individuals may have no chance of being included, whereas others are sure of being subjects in the study, but these chances are not known to the researcher.

With probability sampling, the sample is much more certain to be representative of the population, making it possible to estimate the degree to which the findings differ from those that would have been obtained if the whole population had been studied. In addition, it is possible to calculate the necessary sample size for the margin of error you are willing to accept.

---

1. Brink, P. J., and Wood, M. J., Multiple concurrent replication, *Western Journal of Nursing Research,* 1979, *1*(2), 117–118.

2. The research proposal must identify the specific population to be studied, even though you may not be specific later in a published article, in order to protect the anonymity of the subjects.

TABLE 8-1	*Sample Selection*

Probability Sampling	*Nonprobability Sampling*
ASSUMPTIONS	
A complete listing of all members of the target population is available.	No list of all members of the target population is available, or availability is expected to be sequential.
Researcher knows the probability of each subject being in the sample.	There is no way to estimate that all members of the population have some chance of being in the sample.
Systematic Sampling with Random Start	*Nonprobability Systematic Sampling*
Obtain listing of the population.	No list of population.
Begin sampling with a random start.	Begin with first available subject.
Select every *nth* subject from the list until predetermined number has been reached.	Select every *nth* subject until enough subjects have been obtained.
Simple Random Sampling	*Convenience Sampling*
A specified percentage or number from the population is determined in advance.	A minimum number of subjects (or time frame) is determined in advance.
All members of the population are assigned a number (such as a Social Security number).	Every person who meets the criteria is asked to participate.
From a table of random numbers, select from the population until sample size is reached.	Researcher goes to setting and selects sample from persons meeting the sample criteria.
Each member of the population has an known chance of being selected.	The actual population is unknown; other terms for convenience sample are available sample, accidental sample, deliberate sample, chance sample.
Stratified Random Sampling	*Quota Sampling*
Divide population into strata based on the sample criteria.	Make up a list of the criteria needed to divide the sample into groups (such as age, sex, education).
Draw a predetermined number from each group, using simple random sampling technique.	Decide on the number from each group you want in the sample, then go to the setting and select a convenience sample until you have filled your quota in each group.

(continued)

TABLE 8-1	*Sample Selection* (Continued)

Cluster (Multistage) Sampling	*Network Sampling*
List the relevant geographic locations of the populations (states, counties, cities).	Locate an individual or group meeting the sample criteria who agrees to be in the study (or a person known by persons who meet the sample criteria).
Draw a simple random sample from that list until your predetermined number is reached.	Obtain from the first and each subsequent member of the sample the names of (or a method of contacting) other individuals meeting the sample criteria.
List the sample obtained according to the next relevant criterion (such as schools, health care facilities).	Continue the above until the predetermined number has been reached or until all contacts are exhausted.
Draw a simple random sample from the new list until the predetermined number is reached.	
Repeat the above until all relevant criteria have been exhausted. At the last stage, list all members of the population and draw a simple random sample to the predetermined number.	

Nonprobability sampling, on the other hand, may or may not accurately represent the population. It is usually more convenient and economical and allows the study of populations when they are not amenable to probability sampling or when it is not possible to locate the entire population.

Probability Samples

The probability sample reduces the possibility of bias in sampling and ensures a more representative sample, as the probability of each person in the population being selected for the sample is known. There must be an available listing of all members of the population from which the sample can be drawn. This available list of the population is the single most important criterion in determining whether probability sampling is possible for a given study. If it is, then one of the three types of random sampling can be used. If there is no list, a nonprobability sample is required. Sample size is discussed later in this chapter.

SIMPLE RANDOM SAMPLES. The basic probability sampling design is the simple random sample, which gives every element in the population an equal chance of being selected. First draw up a numbered list of the population. Then refer to a table of random numbers. Beginning at some arbitrary point on the page, move up or down the column of random numbers one by one, counting off enough to complete your sample size. Now look for numbers from your population list that correspond to the random numbers, and they become your sample. Tables of random numbers can be found in many statistics books and provide a good method of taking simple random samples. There are also computer programs that will generate random samples for you.

Examples of population lists that can be used by nurses for simple random samples are members of a state or national nursing organization; all students enrolled at a university; all nurses with a current nursing license; all members of the county heart association; all babies born in the county or state during a given day, month, or year; all nursing schools accredited by the National League for Nursing; all hospitals over 200 beds licensed in a given city or state; all records of patients admitted (or discharged) with a given diagnosis within the last year at a given hospital; all incident reports related to medicine errors within a hospital or series of hospitals. There are many more possibilities; the key element is that a listing of all members of the population be available.

The following are some examples of how to draw simple random samples. Remember that in a simple random sample each element in the available population should have an equal chance of being selected.

1. Example 1. From an available population of all in-patients at Walter Reed Army Hospital on December 1, 1988, and using the last four digits of the patient registration number, begin at the top of the fifth column of a table of random numbers and proceed down the page until fifty numbers have been selected. Select ten more numbers to serve as replacements. Alternatively, using the last four digits of the patient number, use the computer program to generate a random sample of patients.

2. Example 2. From an available population of all students in a research class at Azusa Pacific University, all students in the class agreeing to participate in the research project will pull a slip of paper out of a box. Thirty percent of the slips of paper will state, "You are a member of the sample!" Five percent of the slips will state "You are an alternate." The rest of the slips will be blank. There are just enough slips for the number of students in the class. As each student selects a slip, the content of the slip is recorded. During the selection process the probability of each student being in the sample or an alternate can be calculated. Again, the alternate list is used for replacement purposes and is used from first to last.

3. Example 3. From a target population of all currently registered graduate nursing students at the University of Alberta, and using a table of
random numbers, select ten percent of the listed registration numbers
on November 11, 2000. An alternate list will be established by selecting
a further five percent at the same time as replacements for those in the
first list who decide not to participate in the study. Alternates will be
approached in the order in which they were selected from the table of
random numbers.

If a simple random sample is both possible and appropriate to your study,
there is no better method of selecting subjects. Objectivity can be obtained and
much bias eliminated, thus strengthening the results of the study.

STRATIFIED RANDOM SAMPLES. This method is based on the same principle
as the simple random sample, except that before the sample is drawn, the population is divided into two or more strata or groups. A simple random sample
is then taken from each group. For instance, if having equal numbers of men
and women is vital to your study, you can divide the population into two
groups according to gender and then draw an equal number of subjects from
each. Remember that the variable chosen as a criterion for stratifying a sample
must be important to the purpose of the study.

In a study of the relationship between educational preparation and nurses'
behavior, a stratified random sample would be very appropriate. If a simple
random sample of nurses is taken, the proportions of subjects from each type
of educational background will not be equal; in fact, some might be missing
altogether. Therefore, it makes sense first to divide the population into strata
according to educational preparation and then draw random samples from
each group. The probability of being selected can be calculated for each element in the population, even though it may not be equal among groups.

Like simple random samples, this method requires a complete listing of
the population. It also requires information on the criterion for stratification.
So if you plan to stratify by educational preparation, your list of the population
must include information about educational preparation. The ease with which
you can obtain the necessary information about the sample may help you
decide whether to use stratified random sampling. Stratified sampling simply
allows you to control the size of the sample from each stratum but does not
increase the validity of your answer.

The whole point of stratifying a sample is to make sure that certain characteristics of a population are in the study. If you were interested in a study of
diabetic behavior and you wanted to be sure that you had specific groups
included, such as type of diabetes or age of onset (childhood or adult), you
would want to stratify your sample on that basis. This way, you are sure spe-

cific characteristics will be present in the sample. Sometimes studies are strati-fied by gender to be sure of equal representation.

Sometimes the question is asked: Should I use equal numbers in my strata or should I use percentages of my population? The answer is up to you. Do you want to have a particular number of subjects in your final sample or is total sample size irrelevant for your study (outside of the computation of error and levels of confidence)? In other words it makes no significant difference whether you use ten percent or a total of ten in each stratum as far as the sam-pling technique is concerned. It makes a difference in relation to your compu-tation of the size of the final sample you wish to have. Frequently, too, the dif-ference will be determined by the number of strata and their complexity.

If you were studying the nutritional status of school-aged children (K–6), you might want to be sure you included both boys and girls as well as the major ethnic or racial groups represented in your school. First you stratify your school by grade:

$$K \quad 1 \quad 2 \quad 3 \quad 4 \quad 5 \quad 6$$

Then you stratify by sex:

K	1	2	3	4	5	6
M F	M F	M F	M F	M F	M F	M F

If you wanted to include ethnic or racial groups, you would have to decide which ones you wanted to be sure to include. If your school had a substantial proportion of children who were black (B), Spanish (S), and white (W), you might want to be sure each major group was represented also and so your stratification plan would look like this:

K		1		2		3	
M	F	M	F	M	F	M	F
B S W	B S W	B S W	B S W	B S W	B S W	B S W	B S W

This is the way you plan out your stratification procedures prior to doing any form of data collection. As you can see, the more you stratify, the more complex your sample becomes. The only reason for stratification in a study of this nature is to ensure representation of the major elements in the popula-tion. Otherwise, if you had simply drawn a simple random sample of all chil-dren in the school, your final sample may not have had any kindergartners, or may have had an overrepresentation of Spanish children, or may not have had enough boys. You could have stratified simply on the grade, or simply on sex, or simply on ethnic group, but if you wanted to ensure representation of ethnic group and sex at each grade, this is the way you would have to plan it out.

CLUSTER SAMPLES. In large-scale surveys, when the population represents broad geographic areas or large numbers of people, simple random samples and stratified samples can be very expensive. A nationwide sample of nurses might necessitate sending interviewers to scattered localities across the country, and the expense could become prohibitive. A cluster sample would reduce the expense while allowing the results to be generalized. The *cluster sample* method is also called *multistage* sampling, because the process of sampling moves through stages until the final sample has been selected.

Starting with the overall population for the study, such as all nursing students in the state, you would proceed as follows.

Prepare a list of counties and draw a random sample. Prepare a list of nursing schools in those selected counties and take a random sample of the schools. Then prepare a list of students from these schools and make a random selection of a sample of students. This three-stage process yields a representative sample of nursing students in this state, yet the location of the students is limited first to the counties selected and then to the schools selected from those counties. The savings in time, travel, and expense can be enormous by using cluster sampling.

As with simple and stratified random sampling, cluster sampling requires that lists of elements in the population be available. In cluster sampling, however, complete lists of the final subjects are not necessary until you reach the final stage; then, you need only obtain complete listings of the elements needed for that stage.

Nonprobability Samples

The use of nonprobability samples is often a necessity in nursing research as in other disciplines. Some populations do not have lists available. For instance, if your population is defined as women in menopause, you will not find a list of names from any single source. Nor will you find complete listings of populations of heroin addicts, alcoholics, or persons with upper-respiratory infections. These populations have no central registry, no gathering place, and unless you redefine your population to include only those receiving some type of treatment, you will have no way to locate a list of the population. This is not to say that you cannot obtain samples of these populations but, rather, that the sample cannot be a probability sample and will have to be obtained by some more deliberate method. Keep in mind that the sample must fit the purpose of the study. Therefore, your goal must be to find the sample that best represents your population rather than one that uses the most sophisticated sampling

articularly useful with patients when
t available.

ce sample (sometimes called an "avail-
ple that happens to be available at the
a convenience sample of patients, you
atients who happened to come into the
se the first 50 people who came into the
irday night. There is no way of estimating
ple, but it is possible to plan for objectivity,
selected by the researcher.
es are convenience samples because of the
gh treatment centers. You will probably not
in for treatment, and you may have to wait
tients to arrive before the sample selection is
rget population is defined as new diabetics
an outpatient clinic, it may take considerable
iew diabetic patients to present themselves for
outpatient department. However, you can esti-
it will take to obtain your sample, as you know
iany patients usually arrive at the clinic each

nience samples are: all male Caucasian patients
Care Unit for myocardial infarction during the
iers whose premature infants are born during the
tween the ages of two and four who are admitted
rhaphy during the study period.

NETWORK SAMI ‿   nonprobability sampling technique that is seldom
discussed in the literature is network sampling.[3] This is a method that is useful
in studies where it is difficult or impossible to locate the population. You may
know that the population exists but have no idea where to look for a sample.
Network sampling takes advantage of the fact that all human beings have
social networks; everyone has friends that have certain characteristics in common. For this technique, you need only locate one individual who has the
desired characteristics and then ask that person to help you get in touch with
friends who would also meet your sample criteria. Network sampling is
extremely useful in finding socially devalued urban populations such as
addicts, alcoholics, child abusers, and criminals, because these people do not
readily reveal themselves to strangers or outsiders. It is also useful for finding
groups such as successful dieters, widows, women experiencing menopause,

---

3. Saunders, J. M., *Personal communication,* 1981.

and so on. These groups are hard to locate by the usual methods, but by finding a link in the social network, one subject will lead the researcher to others. Sometimes, it is the only way to locate a difficult-to-find population.

QUOTA SAMPLES. Like the convenience sample, the quota sample uses available subjects, but it takes additional steps to ensure inclusion of representatives from certain elements in the population. It can ensure that these elements are present in the same proportion in the sample as they appear in the population. This method is used when a convenience sample does not provide the desired balance of elements. For example, the postpartum unit in your hospital may have a patient population that is predominantly Hispanic, therefore, whites and blacks do not appear in sufficient numbers in this convenience sample. To counteract this problem, ethnic percentages are specified so that the proportion of each group in the sample represents the ethnic breakdown of total population.

Like stratified random sampling, quota sampling allows you to control the numbers of sample subjects with desired characteristics. When you have several independent variables (for example, age, education, diagnosis, ethnic background), you will have to ensure that you have enough subjects in each category of independent variable so that you have enough data to analyze the relationships among your variables. For example, if you plan to categorize education according to levels in order to analyze the differences among them, you must have a sufficient number of subjects in each category for your analysis to be valid. In this instance, a quota sample would be appropriate, and it might be a good idea to have equal numbers of subjects in each group instead of groups proportionate to the population distribution of educational level, to simplify the data analysis. Whether you decide to use a proportionate quota sample or an equal number depends on your research question. Whichever sampling technique best answers your question is the one to use.

SYSTEMATIC SAMPLES. You will find reference to systematic samples in published research reports and other research texts. Systematic sampling is the selection of every *nth* member of the available population, after beginning with a random start. If you used a telephone book or a list of students, you might select every fifth or every tenth person on the list. If you wanted to interview people on the street you could decide to approach every third person. If you were interviewing in-patients you could select every other room or every room with an even number and interview every patient in the window bed. These are all predetermined methods of selecting a systematic sample that are obviously not probability samples but are not as subjective as convenience samples. The purpose here is to try to avoid the simple human biases that creep in to nonprobability sampling techniques: interviewing people who make eye contact or smile at you; interviewing your friends; interviewing people who look good; and so on. The decision about who will be in the sample is predetermined rather than left up to the researcher at the time of selection. Systematic sampling is a type of nonprobability sampling technique that is intended to control investigator bias in sample selection but does not meet the criteria for probability sampling since it does not control for environmental bias and does not ensure random distribution of extraneous variables. In addition, a systematic sample can introduce bias into the sample, if there is some bias to the order in which the population is listed. In using the telephone book, for example, the sample can omit entire ethnic groups and overrepresent others because of the alphabetical listing of the names. Choosing every other patient room in a hospital unit sounds objective, but there may be some bias of which you are unaware in the way patients are assigned to rooms. Therefore, you cannot know the distribution of the extraneous variables in your study, which is the important point in probability sampling.

SAMPLE SIZE

The best advice for the novice researcher is to use as large a sample as possible. Large samples maximize the possibility that the means, percentages, and other statistics are true estimates of the population. They give the effects of randomness a chance to work. The chance of error goes down in direct proportion to the increased size of the sample. However, practical considerations are important too—for example, how many people are available from your resources?

With random samples, it is possible to set the size of the sample according to how accurately you want to estimate the actual population parameters, or how much sampling error you are willing to accept. The basic formula for computing the sampling error for a sample estimate of a population parameter is as follows:

$$\text{sampling error} = \frac{\text{variability of the measurement values among the sampling units}}{\sqrt{\text{size of sample}}}$$

It is possible to devise a number of sampling plans that will ensure that your estimates will not differ from the corresponding actual population figures by, say, more than five percent (sampling error) on more than ten percent of the possible samples that you might draw from the population (level of confidence). You can also devise plans that will produce correct results within two percent, ninety-nine percent of the time. In practice, of course, we do not repeat the same study on an infinite number of samples drawn from the same population, but it is possible to predict the probability that the sample will produce data within five percent of those resulting from a study of the whole population.

If you attempt to predict the necessary sample size for your study using the formula, you will see that the larger the percentage of possible error you are willing to accept, the smaller your sample can be. Therefore, the more accuracy you are trying to achieve, the larger the sample should be. However, this formula is applicable only to probability samples. When you do use it, you must know the variance of the measurement you plan to use with your population. This means that the measurement must be at least at an interval scale, so that the variance can be calculated. The measurement must also have been used before with the same or a similar population so that the variance is known. You will find that if the variance is small, the sample size need not be as large as when the variance is large. When none of the measurements varies too far from the mean for the population, it takes only a small sample to obtain measurements that accurately reflect the population. But if there is a lot of variation in measurements, a larger group will be needed to incorporate the entire range of scores in the sample.

Another way to estimate the size of the sample you will need is to do a *power analysis.* A power analysis is a method of estimating that the sample is large enough to assume that your statistical analysis is meaningful and large enough to detect errors. A power analysis is itself a statistical analysis based on several factors: the amount of error you are willing to tolerate, the level of significance of the test (usually described as the *p* level), the size of the sample, the type of statistical test, and the effect size. A power analysis accounts for all these factors. If you know any three factors, the fourth can be calculated. There are books of tables and computer programs that estimate power based on these factors. (An excellent article on power analysis by Polit and Sherman is listed at the end of the chapter in the recommended readings.)

If you know that you can obtain a probability sample and you know the variance of the measurement you plan to use, you can decide on your margin of error and select the optimal sample size to use. But, as mentioned before, there are practical factors that sometimes limit your ability to decide on sample size. If you have access to a group of women undergoing assertion training and they meet your criteria for inclusion in your sample, you will probably use the group for your study, no matter how large or small it may be. The practical factor influencing your decision is availability. If there is one such group available, take it. If there are many such groups available, you can plan for the best sample size.

When you have some choice in planning sample size but cannot use probability sampling, then the size of sample will depend on the number and type of variables that you plan to measure—your goal once again being to ensure sufficient data for your analysis. If you plan to look at the relationships between variables, a handy rule of thumb is to plan for at least five observations for each category of each variable. If you plot your variables in a chart or table, you can see how many subjects you will need in order to have enough data. For instance, Table 8.2 shows the relationship among sex, age, and postoperative anxiety level. With these variables divided into three categories each, you would need at least 90 subjects. Each variable is then measured once for each subject.

If you plan to measure the same variable many times for the same subject over a period of time, then each measurement can be counted in the same way as you counted subjects in the last example. Look at the table again. If

TABLE 8-2	*Relationship among Age, Sex, and Postoperative Anxiety Level*					
	Males			Females		
Anxiety Level	Age			Age		
	20–30	31–40	41–50	20–30	31–40	41–50
Low	5	5	5	5	5	5
Medium	5	5	5	5	5	5
High	5	5	5	5	5	5

anxiety level is to be measured five times for each subject, you will need only one subject for each of the five observations; therefore, the minimum sample size becomes 18. In exploratory studies, you will frequently make multiple, in-depth observations of the same subjects, which means that a small sample size will produce a large quantity of data.

LEVEL OF STUDY AND SAMPLE SELECTION

The type of sample you plan to select depends on the level of study you have chosen to do. Level I exploratory descriptive studies require nonprobability samples for several reasons. First, there is usually an insufficient amount of information about the problem and the population to allow you to plan a probability sample. Second, because of the exploratory nature of the study and the flexibility of the data collection methods, it is rarely possible to generalize beyond the immediate sample. As is true with all sampling techniques, your major interest is to represent the population to the best of your ability. The reason for a representative sample at Level I, however, is to enhance your interpretation of the results and to give you a base on which to build further studies rather than to generalize to a broader population. Therefore, convenience, network, quota, and systematic samples are perfectly adequate techniques.

At the early stages of exploratory research, you begin with convenience sampling or network sampling in order to find subjects for the study. If you are studying patients on a ward or nurses in a hospital, you may use convenience sampling. But, if you are interested in people out in the community who are not easy to locate, you may have to advertise in newspapers for volunteers and ask people to refer their families and friends to you, using any network system to which you have access. Probability sampling is not possible in these studies.

At the exploratory level, the sample size is usually quite small because you are interested in doing an in-depth study. Sometimes, you find that the entire population is very small and end up studying everyone. If, for example, you were interested in toxic shock syndrome and wanted to explore the characteristics of the women who died from it, you would not wait for a large sample; rather, you would begin to study all the victims there were. Five women may be a small sample, but at the time of your study, they might constitute the entire known population.

Another facet of sample selection in exploratory descriptive studies is the amount of time you have to spend collecting your sample. If your resources are limited, you must plan your study within a reasonable length of time. Your plan may call for a statement such as, "as many as possible from January to June who meet criteria, with a minimum of five." In this way, you have established a minimum sample size but will do your best to get a larger sample if you can. In a study of out-of-body experiences following cardiac or respiratory arrest, Joy[4] found that only the pulmonary arrest patients recall these experiences twenty-four hours later. Although she interviewed twenty-four postarrest patients over a six-month period (all that survived), her sample reporting out-of-body experiences was only three. At this point, the resources of the researcher determine whether to proceed with the study or whether to stop and analyze the experiences of three patients.

In using the multiple concurrent replication concept for exploratory studies, the sample size can be expanded considerably by having several investigators work at different locations, collecting data on different groups of people at the same time. In this way, also, the bias of the individual investigator can be described and accounted for because each one will be slightly different from the others.

Finally, the exploratory descriptive design is the most suitable for the case study approach using one subject or one small group (a total population) that the investigator studies in depth. This is the basis for biographical accounts and early studies of nursing interventions. Level I descriptive designs that look at the characteristics of a single population typically use either a total population or a simple random sample.

At Level II, the best approach to sample selection is the probability sample. Survey designs are based on the concept of generalizing to populations from samples. They also utilize nonprobability techniques when a probability sample cannot be obtained. At this level, any deviation from the probability sample must be explained as a limitation of the design, because any such deviation diminishes the confidence you can have in the relationships you find. Remember that at Level II you are looking for significant relationships between variables and that these relationships are meaningful only if you can apply them to populations (external validity). Level II studies utilize all three forms of probability sampling techniques, depending on the question asked.

Comparative designs are always found at Level II. The purpose of the comparative design is to compare groups to see if they are significantly different on some characteristic or trait. Usually the groups utilize a stratified random

---

4. Joy, F., *Patients' arrest experiences,* unpublished Master's thesis, University of California, Los Angeles, 1979.

sample technique and are formed at the beginning of the study during sample selection. There are times, however, when the groups are not identifiable until the data have been collected using a simple random sample. In this case, during data analysis the groups will be separated on the variable and then compared. So a Level II comparative survey can use either a stratified sample or a simple random sample with subsequent data analysis to form comparative groups.

Level III is similar to Level I in that nonprobability convenience sampling is the most usual. In experimental designs, the investigator must have full control of the variables. As far as the sample is concerned, this control is maintained through assignment to groups. (See Chapter 7.) The first concern in an experimental design is that the various experimental and control groups be equivalent at the beginning of the study so that the effect of the independent variable can be measured. To ensure the equivalence of the groups, the members of the sample are randomly assigned to the various groups, thus producing groups that have equal distribution of the key variables (internal validity). This works well provided that the sample is large enough. If it is not, the researcher must ensure the distribution of key variables by some other method. Matching and selecting from a homogeneous population are two such methods. The use of random assignment at Level III provides control of sample variables essential to the experimental design. These samples are not, however, probability samples. In experimental designs, samples are obtained by asking people who meet the criteria to consent to be subjects—convenience samples. In clinical studies, the criteria for being in the sample usually involve being a patient with a particular problem at a given time. It is difficult, if not impossible, to obtain a random sample of patients who are in need of treatment at the time of the study. Frequently, the subjects are obtained sequentially, as they arrive for treatment. The population is unknown; therefore, probability sampling is impossible.

The main purpose of random sampling is to allow the results from the sample to be generalized to the population (external validity). Although it might seem advantageous to be able to do this at Level III, in reality it is usually impossible. Because of the researcher's concentration on control of variables, the sample is usually not representative of the population. The major emphasis is on identifying the effect of the independent variable on the dependent variable and on controlling all possible variables that might intervene in that relationship. As a result, the sample is selected to hold many variables constant; therefore, many elements of the population are not included.

RECOMMENDED READINGS

Beck, C. T., Achieving statistical power through research design sensitivity, *Journal of Advanced Nursing*, 1994, *20*, 912–916.

Charman, L., Sampling: Who and how many?, *Nursing Standard*, August 1990, 4(45), 38–39.

Chein, I., An introduction to sampling. In C. Selltiz, L. S. Wrightsman, and S. Cook (eds.), *Research methods in social relations* (3rd ed.), New York: Holt, Rinehart and Winston, 1976, Appendix A.

Cochran, W. G., *Sampling techniques* (2nd ed.), New York: Wiley, 1963.

Coyne, I. T., Sampling in qualitative research. Purposeful and theoretical sampling; merging or clear boundaries? *Journal of Advanced Nursing*, 1997, *26*, 623–630.

Crosby, F., Ventura, M. R., Finnick, M., Lohr, G., and Feldman, M. J., Enhancing subject recruitment for nursing research, *Clinical Nurse Specialist*, 1991, *5*(1), 25–30.

Ford, J. S., and Reutter, L. I., Ethical dilemmas associated with small samples, *Journal of Advanced Nursing*, 1990, *15*(2), 187–191.

Hauck, W. W., Gilliss, C. L., Donner, A., and Gortner, S., Randomization by cluster, *Nursing Research*, 1991, *40*(6), 356–358.

Ingram, R., Power analysis and sample size estimation, *NTResearch*, 1998, *3*(2), 132–141.

Kachoyeanos, M. K., The significance of power in research design (Part I), *MCN*, 1998, *23*(2), 105.

Kachoyeanos, M. K., The significance of power in research design (Part II), *MCN*, 1998, *23*(3), 155.

Lentz, M. J., Time series—Issues in sampling, *Western Journal of Nursing Research*, 1990, *12*(1), 123–127.

Morse, J. M., Strategies for sampling. In J. M. Morse (ed.), *Qualitative nursing research: A contemporary dialogue* (rev. ed.), Newbury Park, Ca.: Sage, 1991, pp. 127–145.

Lipsey, M. W., *Design sensitivity: Statistical power for experimental research*. Newbury Park, Ca.: Sage, 1990.

Polit, D. F., and Hungler, B. P., *Nursing research: Principles and methods* (4th ed.), Philadelphia: Lippincott, 1991.

Polit, D. F., and Sherman, R. E., Statistical power in nursing research, *Nursing Research*, 1990, *39*(6), 365–369.

Roper, J. M., and Shapira, J. *Ethnography in Nursing Research*, Thousand Oaks, Ca.: Sage, 2000.

Ruth, M. V., and White, C. M., Data collection: Sample. In S. D. Krampitz and N. Pavlovich (eds.), *Readings for nursing research*, St. Louis: Mosby, 1981, Chap. 12.

Sharp, K., The case for case studies in nursing research: The problem of generalization, *Journal of Advanced Nursing*, 1998, *27*, 785–789.

Sheldon, L., Grounded theory: Issues for research in nursing, *Nursing Standard*, 1998, *12*(52), 47–50.

Waltz, C., and Bausell, R. B., *Nursing research: Design, statistics and computer analysis*, Philadelphia: F. A. Davis, 1981, Chap. 3.

Williamson, Y. M. (ed.), *Research methodology and its application to nursing*, New York: Wiley, 1981, Chap. 9.

Yarandi, H. N., Planning sample sizes: Comparison of factor level means, *Nursing Research*, 1991, *40*(1), 57–58.

Zeller, R., Good, M., Anderson, G. C., and Zeller, D. L., Strengthening experimental design by balancing potentially confounding variables across treatment groups, *Nursing Research*, 1997, *48*(6), 345–348.

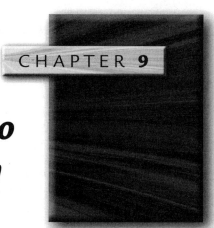

CHAPTER 9

Selecting a Method to Answer the Question

Observation

Questionnaires and Interviews

Available Data

Physiological Measures

Recommended Readings

The actual method you choose to collect your data depends on several factors. First, it depends on the level of your question, or how much is known about your variables. In a Level I study, you want to amass as much information as possible, and you are not sure what results to expect. In this case, the best methods are those such as unstructured observation, open-ended interviews and questionnaires, participant observation, and the use of written, available data. The advantage of these methods is flexibility because you may have to change the questions you ask or the situations you observe as you find out more about the variables.

In a Level II study, in which you are looking for relationships among variables, you must have accurate techniques for measuring your variables. Your data must be quantifiable, as you are looking for statistical relationships among the variables. Here, structured observation, questionnaires, and interviews can be used. Written, available data and projective tests may be considered. Questions and observations must be comparable from one subject to the next; even open-ended questions must be the same for each subject. The criterion here is accuracy rather than flexibility.

In Level III studies, you control the situation and the variables. Therefore, the method must be structured. Any method that produces structured, quantifiable data can be used. Conditions and measurements must be identical for all subjects, as inferential statistics will be used to test the hypotheses.

Another consideration in selecting a method is which instruments are available and have already been tested and evaluated in measuring your variables. During your search of the literature, some instruments may have come to light that other investigators have developed to measure the variables you are studying. If this is so, by all means use one of these instruments. Using an already tested instrument provides another link between your study and a growing body of knowledge about your variables. You will be adding to this body of knowledge with your data. But be sure that the instrument fits your definition of the variable. Does it measure exactly what you want to know? Only you can decide. Remember that it is possible to adapt an instrument to fit your question, provided you obtain permission from the person who developed it.

Developing your own instrument is not too difficult if you want to measure relatively concrete things like demographic characteristics, level of knowledge of a particular topic, or other factual reporting. If, however, you are attempting to measure an abstract concept such as hope or grief, measurement becomes more complex. In this case, the development of measuring instruments is a science of its own, which is why beginning researchers should not attempt to develop their own instruments to measure complex concepts.

Instrument or tool development is a specialty area of research requiring advanced skill and experience. Where does it fit in the research paradigm? Exploratory studies can provide the basis for tool development by providing an in-depth description of the concept. For example, the concept of hope could be described as it is perceived by patients in a variety of settings and with various diagnoses and prognoses. From this exploratory work, the investigator might develop a theoretical perspective of the concept of hope. From this theoretical perspective, a tool might be developed to measure levels of hope. Using this approach, instrument development belongs following Level I studies and must be done prior to Level II or Level III studies in which the level of hope is to be measured. Before the instrument is used, it must be tested extensively to establish its reliability and validity (see Chapter 10); this process becomes a study of its own.

If the literature review does not reveal any tools to measure a complex concept, the beginner should consider whether a Level I study would be more appropriate. If the study really belongs at Level II or III, there should be literature representing previous research on the concept, and a tool will be found that can be used or adapted for use in your study. This chapter focuses on some general guidelines for devising your own instrument or in evaluating one for your study.

OBSERVATION

Observation is a method of collecting descriptive behavioral data and is extremely useful in nursing studies because one can observe behavior as it occurs. Observation stops being a normal part of everyday life and becomes a research method if it is systematically planned and recorded and if both observations and recordings are checked for their validity and reliability. These factors make the difference between simply observing the world around you and collecting research data through observation.

Observation may be the only way to gather some data. If the information you need cannot be obtained by asking questions, through available records, or by directly measuring some quality of the subject, you may have to observe the behavior of the subject and record what you see. Studying the behavior of infants, psychiatric patients, and dying patients; examining the verbal or nonverbal interaction between individuals or within groups; looking to see if people behave as they say they will—these are all well suited to observation.

In nursing studies, observation can provide a rich source of data that describe patient responses. Observation can be used alone or with other methods, and it will assist you in interpreting the results obtained through other methods.

For example, you can use observation in conjunction with interviews to validate self-report information. Many obesity studies are based on self-report (interviews about the individual's personal dieting/weight history) in conjunction with observation (observing the person's appearance and behavior during the interview), plus physiological measures (weighing the individual on a scale). Observations are frequently used when questionnaires or interviews cannot be done because the subject is not able to respond to questions. Observation has produced excellent studies of infants (refer to the incredible work of Gesell and Spock), as well as studies of people who do not speak English, and brain-damaged individuals who have lost the ability to speak.

The act of observation itself is usually interactive. Unless you are behind a two-way mirror or viewing a videotape, you are a part of what you are observing. In addition, the act of observing is selective. It is impossible to observe everything that is happening at one time. Finally, the act of recording observations is also selective—you can *never record everything* you observe. Look at the following diagram adapted from Hunter and Foley.[1]

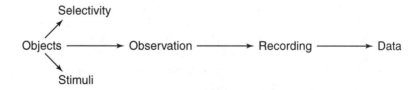

---

1. See Hunter, D. E., and Foley, M. B., *Doing anthropology: A student centered approach to cultural anthropology,* New York, Harper & Row, 1976, for a more detailed discussion on how to observe, the rationale and theory of observation, and how to take field notes on, as well as how to interpret, observations.

Objects in the environment impinge on your consciousness as stimuli, some of which you select out to observe and others which you do not. Some nurses, for example, have a tendency to observe interpersonal interactions and to neglect the physical environment in which they occur. Some nurses will observe nuances of facial expression but ignore room temperature, the passage of time, light sources, or weather. Another nurse might walk into a room, observe the equipment in great detail, and fail to notice the patient in the bed. So out of innumerable objects to observe, certain things are selected for observation. In addition, you will find that not all observations can possibly be recorded. Certain observations are selected out to be recorded, and these then become the "data base." The way in which we select observations and record them is not random. Selectivity is highly patterned both by our culture and by our individual preferences.

All behavior can be observed from two points of view: (1) the insider's or actor's point of view or (2) the outsider's or observer's point of view. *Both points of view are true.* No two human observers observe the same thing or observe in exactly the same way. Observation is an expression of individuality, personality, preconceptions, and values. As an exercise, observe a social situation with two other people and then compare notes. You may be surprised at the results. (See Hunter and Foley.)

Human behaviors can be looked at as individual acts, unrelated to the setting, or they can be examined in the context in which they are occurring. For example, let us say you were observing the way in which people walk up and down a flight of stairs at your school. The basic elements of the behavior are in the stepping procedures, either up or down. If you see a person alone, going up or down stairs, it is easy to examine the basic elements of how it is done. When you begin to observe the individual in relation to others, however, you begin to see patterns to the behavior that give you the idea that there are rules governing the behavior. You may notice that most people walk up on the right and walk down on the left side of the stairwell. You may also notice that if anyone walks up and down the stairs in a different pattern there are bodily collisions. You may begin to assume that there are rules governing on which side of the stairs one walks. You may also find that at certain times of the day, everyone is going up, and the stairs are treated as a "one-way street." Someone attempting to go the other way will be trampled in the traffic. The people in the setting may not be aware of the "rules." A stranger may not know the rules and always walk the wrong way until he or she becomes familiar with how things are done.

Recording observations provides a description of the behavior and the setting. The act of description (or recording) is in itself an analytical process that breaks down the observation into its most indivisible or basic parts and demonstrates how the parts fit together. Always record the behavior first, in the same way that you record behavioral data in the nursing process, and avoid labeling the behavior until you are ready for the analysis phase of your study. Labels represent a synthesis of your thinking or a conclusion that you have drawn from your observation. For example:

The boy was too weak to hit the ball very far.

The woman was too lazy to clean her house.

Both "weak" and "lazy" are labels or concepts that stand for generalizations and value judgments. They are not descriptions of what was seen, heard, touched, tasted, or felt. After many subsequent observations, you will not remember when you go back and read your notes what those words meant. Was the woman disheveled? Did the boy look thin and pale? Did he move slowly and without vigor?

The value of observation in research is that it provides the context in which social interactions occur. When you are observing a behavior, describe the setting from both the actor's and the observer's perception of the environment. Look for such things as the geographical setting, the time of day, the activity within the setting, the people present, and the relationships among them. Break up your observation into equal time periods. Try to discover the frequency with which situations are encountered in a typical setting. Develop an observational record chart with one observation per actor in every setting.

Notice the way the following recording of a Little League ballgame is described. One activity or unit of behavior is listed per line. The focus is on the boy exclusively.

Boy hit ball.

Boy threw bat down.

Boy ran to a bag.

Another form of recording is the paragraph summary in which overall impressions of a basketball game are listed. You might select one person or several persons to observe in the activity and summarize their activity in a paragraph. You might select a family observing a basketball game, or a player on the team, or even the concessionaire. This data will be quite different from the very focused recording of the baseball game. Using the paragraph summary, you will notice how much more detail you are able to rely on later when it comes to data analysis.

Observe yourself as an observer. Try some of these observational exercises. Investigate the material objects in the setting such as all the objects in the area where you brush your teeth. Observe other people's responses to you when you behave out of context (try walking up the down escalator).

The observational technique you use depends on the purpose of the study. If detail is not your interest, you need not have detailed observations and notes. But as in levels of measurement, detailed notes can be grouped into general statements, but general notes can never result in detailed analysis. Determining the appropriate observational technique ultimately depends on the research question being asked. Clinical studies that combine observation with another method of data collection make the most of the opportunity to study patient responses and will provide a depth of data not possible with only one method.

When you plan to use observation as a method of data collection, you need to make two decisions before you proceed. First, how involved do you intend to become with the subjects as participants? Second, how structured do you intend your observations to be?

Degree of Investigator Involvement

In participant observation studies, the observer is involved in the setting with the subjects. Examples include observations collected by nurses in the course of their patient-care activities and studies where an investigator becomes part of the setting in order to collect data for research. In these studies, it is easy for bias to be introduced into the data collection process. Participant observers have unique opportunities to influence the behavior of their subjects; in fact, it is difficult to avoid doing so. If nurses are observing patient responses while they are giving patient care, it is easy to influence the patient's response through subtle changes in approach to the patient. Participant observers frequently influence the subjects' behavior by communicating their expectations to the subject. These influences are difficult, if not impossible, to control since objectivity is influenced by interaction with subjects. There will always be some bias in participant observation studies even though the investigator may make every effort to remain objective and not influence the behavior of the subjects. Through detailed recording, however, the influence of the researcher will be described as part of the data.

When the observer is not a participant in the setting but is merely viewing the situation, there is less likelihood of observations being directed. Frequently, there is some Hawthorne effect in the initial stages because the subjects are aware of being observed. This effect diminishes over time as subjects become accustomed to being observed. Nonparticipant observation studies can range from use of a one-way mirror for observing behavior to face-to-face observation of the subject. In any event, the observer must try to maintain the naturalness of the situation and be as unobtrusive as possible. The likelihood of subjects exhibiting normal behavior is directly related to the inconspicuousness of the researcher as observer. The goal in observational methods is always to maintain the normal environment of the subjects. This enables you to collect the type of data required by the study.

The advantage of nonparticipant observation is that the observed person will be less influenced by the researcher than one who is actively involved with the researcher. Participant observation, on the other hand, has the advantage of providing a more "normal" environment for the subject, because the observer either is a normal part of the environment or becomes so in the course of the study. In participant observation studies, the researcher begins the study as a stranger to the setting, so all subjects must "teach" the researcher how to behave "properly." By the time the researcher becomes familiar with the people and the setting, the subjects simply forget the researcher is there.

In many observational studies, the subject is frequently a stranger to the setting (for example, rooms with one-way mirrors) and alters behavior to meet the new and unfamiliar environment. If the researcher follows the subject about, a different dimension is added to the subject's life—namely, the researcher.

Determining the appropriate observational role (see Pearsall and Byerly, listed in the Recommended Readings) ultimately depends on the research question being asked.

Degree of Structure

Observational methods vary greatly in the amount of structure provided for the observer. They range from very unstructured observations, which attempt to provide as complete and nonselective a description as possible, to very structured methods, which provide a complete list of expected behaviors and require only that the observer check which ones occurred.

An unstructured observation method might be used to describe the behavior of nurses immediately following the death of a patient. It would involve a complete description of everything the nurse says and does at this time. Remember that complete recording of an event is virtually impossible. Even with videotaping, exact replication will not be obtained because of biases introduced by camera angle and lighting. Selectivity is bound to occur. This fact should be recognized if you use unstructured observation. Even so, a rich depth of material can be gathered from unstructured observation—a depth that will never result from the use of structured methods. As long as the researcher accounts for possible bias in both data analysis and interpretation, this valuable method can be used to great advantage in nursing research. Of particular value is the combination of unstructured observation with structured methods, which gives the data more depth.

Structured observation can take one of several forms, but perhaps the most common is the checklist. A checklist allows the researcher to record whether or not a given behavior occurs. The desired behaviors must be explicitly defined so that there is no question in the mind of the observer as to whether or not they occur. For instance, "unhappy" is not a sufficient description. As it stands, the observer would have to interpret observations in light of a personal definition. A good checklist would specify more operational definitions, such as "visibly crying," "refuses treatment," "turns back to nurse." These are all easily identifiable action definitions.

Structured observation requires a knowledge of the *expected* range of behaviors in a given situation. When developing a checklist, for instance, the researcher must list all the expected behaviors related to the variable being measured, so that the observer will be able to correctly identify all relevant behaviors in the subjects.

You can develop checklists for nursing studies when you know approximately what behaviors to expect. Sometimes a pilot study can be done with a few subjects to give you an idea of the kinds of behaviors you can expect. A checklist will simplify data collection. A checklist makes it difficult to record unexpected behaviors that are not included in the original list because the observer tends to watch for the expected behaviors on the checklist and can easily miss the unexpected.

An example of a checklist used in a nursing study is the following instrument to measure nurses' monitor-watching activity in a cardiac care unit (CCU):

1. Looks at monitor only (at nurses' station).
2. Looks at monitor, goes to bedside, does not talk to patient.
3. Looks at monitor, goes to bedside, talks to patient.
4. Goes to bedside, talks to patient without checking desk monitor.[2]

This instrument was developed to measure the number of instances in a given time period that CCU nurses behaved in one of the four ways listed above. In this study, the researcher was interested only in those four activities and, therefore, had no category for unexpected behaviors.

Structured observation, when appropriate, is an excellent method of collecting data. Many more subjects can be observed, in less time, than with unstructured observation, and the data analysis is much simpler. Taking results from a checklist merely involves counting how many times a particular behavior occurred. The results of unstructured observation, on the other hand, consist of quantities of descriptive data, as the observer was trying to record everything that happened. These data must be sorted out to see if there are any patterns to the observed behavior—a very time-consuming process.

---

2. Adapted from Stuart, I., *A study of the incidence of monitor watching and nurse-patient communication in a coronary care unit*, UCLA, unpublished Master's Thesis, 1975.

Timing of Observations

Since it is usually impossible to observe behaviors for extended periods because of fatigue and boredom, you must plan how and when you will make the observations. The two main methods are *time sampling* and *event sampling.*

In *time sampling,* it is customary to divide the day into units that are appropriate for your observation. For instance, in the previous example of the CCU nurse activities, fifteen-minute periods make sense, as they would allow ample time for a nurse to exhibit any or all of the expected behaviors. One minute would not be sufficient time for one of the behaviors to occur. Several fifteen-minute periods during an eight-hour shift would provide a good sample of an individual nurse's behavior. The periods can be either randomly selected or predetermined according to the daily routine of the CCU.

Event sampling is used when you need to observe an entire event in order to give the subject the opportunity to perform all the expected behaviors. If your purpose is to record breaks in sterile technique during dressing changes by student nurses, the sensible approach would be to observe entire dressing change procedures. Time sampling would make no sense for this study. Describing nurse/patient interaction during admission to the hospital is another instance when event sampling might be used.

In all of these examples, observation is the best, if not the only, way to gather the required data. If you want to know about breaks in sterile technique by student nurses, your alternative research method is to ask the student or the patient. But neither of these approaches is likely to produce the data you need. Observation is the best method.

Type of Observation and Level of Study

The level of the study will affect the observational technique you choose to measure your variables. Unstructured observation is a method for use in Level I studies where flexible exploration is needed. This type of observation is not appropriate for Level II and III studies where precision in measurement of the variables is required. We have emphasized the concept that each level of research builds on the preceding level. To carry this idea through to choosing data collection methods, we look at the ability to provide structure in measurement as dependent on knowledge about the topic and/or variables. It is not possible to develop a structured tool to observe behavior unless you can base the tool on previous descriptions of behavior under the same circumstances. Therefore, developing a tool for a Level II study requires the results of a Level I study on the same topic.

In the same light, the tool used in a Level III study must be precise enough to differentiate between experimental and control groups. The tool, therefore, must be highly structured and based on considerable knowledge of the variable. Remember, *the degree of structure increases with the level of the study* and the extent of research and theory available to explain the action of the variables.

QUESTIONNAIRES AND INTERVIEWS

When your objective is to find out what people believe or think, the easiest and most effective method is to ask questions directly of the person. The purpose of asking questions is to find out what is going on in the minds of subjects: their perceptions, attitudes, beliefs, feelings, motives, plans, past events, and recall. In research, questionnaires and interviews are the methods designed to collect primary self-reported data.

Asking questions can provide measurement of many concepts and variables important to nursing research. Nurses ask questions frequently as part of assessment and evaluation of patient care. Although nurses are more accustomed to the interview technique, they quickly see the value of questionnaires also and adapt easily to the idea that the patient's self-report is one of the most valuable data collection methods. The important thing to remember when choosing this method is that it must be the most appropriate one to measure the variables *as you have defined them.*

Whether you use the interview or questionnaire method (see Table 9.1), it must be because your operational definition calls for the subject's self-report. If

TABLE 9-1	*Criteria for Selecting the Interview or Questionnaire*
Advantages of the Interview	**Advantages of the Questionnaire**
1. The subject need not be able to read or write.	1. This approach is less expensive in terms of time and money.
2. The interviewer can observe the responses of the subject.	2. Subjects feel a greater sense of anonymity.
3. Questions may be clarified if they are misunderstood.	3. The format is standard for all subjects and is not dependent on mood of interviewer.
4. In-depth data may be obtained on any subject and are not dependent on predetermined questions.	4. Large samples, covering large geographic areas, compensate for the expected loss of subjects.
5. There is a higher response and retention rate.	5. A greater amount of data over a broad range of topics may be collected.

it does not, or if there is reason to believe that the person cannot give a valid response (for example, if you are trying to measure an unconscious process), then these methods are not appropriate.

The major difference between questionnaires and interviews is the presence of an interviewer. In questionnaires, responses are limited to answers to predetermined questions. In interviews, because the interviewer is present with the subject, there is an opportunity to collect nonverbal data as well and to clarify the meaning of questions if the subjects do not understand.

Advantages and Disadvantages of Interviews and Questionnaires

The written questionnaire has some advantages. For one thing, it is likely to be less expensive, particularly in time spent collecting the data. Questionnaires can be given to large numbers of people simultaneously; they can also be sent by mail. Therefore, it is possible to cover wide geographic areas and to question large numbers of people relatively inexpensively.

Another advantage of questionnaires is that subjects are more likely to feel that they can remain anonymous and thus may be more likely to express controversial opinions. This is more difficult in an interview, where the opinion must be given directly to the interviewer. Also, the written question is standard from one subject to the next and is not susceptible to changes in emphasis, as can be the case in oral questioning. There is always the possibility, however, that the written question will be interpreted differently by different readers, which is one reason for carefully pretesting questionnaires.

Interviews have many advantages, the most significant of which is questioning people who cannot write their responses (for example, patients with eye patches or in traction). This category also includes illiterate subjects or subjects who do not write as fluently as they speak. Oral responses from these individuals will contain much more information than would their written responses.

Another advantage of the interview method is that it usually results in a higher response rate than does the questionnaire. Many people who would ignore a questionnaire are willing to talk with an interviewer who is obviously interested in what they have to say. Hospitalized patients are a good example. Few patients refuse to be interviewed, but questionnaires left at the bedside or given to patients to take home have a much lower response rate.

When conducting an interview, you can be sensitive to misunderstandings by your subjects and provide further clarification if a subject misinterprets a question. In a questionnaire, on the other hand, you will not know whether the subject really misunderstood the question unless the response is quite bizarre. Even then, there is always some doubt as to what to do with such a response.

Another advantage of the interview technique is that you can plan to ask questions at several levels to get the most information from the subject. As an example, the sensory deprivation questionnaires developed by Jackson and O'Neil[3] start by asking the patient some ambiguous questions such as, "How have you felt for the last three days?" These are followed by more structured questions such as, "Did you experience anything out of the ordinary the last three days?" If no reports of sensory disturbances are elicited by these two sets of questions, the interviewer goes on to the very structured questions: "Sometimes people who are in the hospital with conditions like yours do have thoughts, feelings, and experiences which they wonder about. For example, they see things and wonder if they are real. If anything like this happened to you the last three days, would you describe it for me?" This approach is unique to the interview. The combination of structured and unstructured questions can provide depth and richness to the data and, at the same time, elicit data that are comparable from one subject to the next.

Types of Questions

When looking for a questionnaire or interview schedule to use in your study or when developing your own tool, you will have to consider the various kinds of questions that you can ask to obtain a range of data, and then decide which method is best suited to your variables. The content of the questions must be considered first, then the amount of structure in the format.

Question content or the purpose of the question falls into two basic categories: those aimed at *facts* and those aimed at *perceptions* or *feelings*. *Factual questions* ask subjects for information about themselves or about events or people about which they know something. Questions asking for demographic data (for example, age, marital status, income, and education) fall into this category. So do questions asking the individual to recall an event or sequence of events ("Tell me about the events leading to your coming to the hospital").

Nonfactual questions deal with the subjects' perception of what happened or their feelings about people, events, or things. They may also deal with the subjects' reasons for their behavior ("Why did you call the doctor at that particular time?"). In these kinds of questions, you are not interested in whether the subject's report is *accurate* but rather in the subject's *perception*, which may or may not accurately reflect the facts.

---

3. Jackson, C. W., and O'Neil, M., Experiences associated with sensory deprivation reported for patients having eye surgery, *Ross Roundtable on Maternal and Child Nursing*, Columbus: Ross Laboratories, 1966, 54–69.

The format of interviews and questionnaires, just as that of observational methods, can range from very structured to very unstructured, depending on how much is known about the range of possible responses.

Degree of Structure in Questionnaires and Interviews

Structured questionnaires and interviews are those in which the questions are presented in exactly the same way, with the same wording, and in the same order to all subjects. The questions are standardized to ensure that the subjects' answers can be compared. The questions can be asked by an interviewer or can be given to the subject as a "paper-pencil test"; in either case, the questions are asked in the same order for all subjects so that the order of the questions cannot affect the subjects' responses.

The most structured questions are *fixed alternative* questions in which the subject is asked to choose one of the given alternatives. Some examples of fixed alternative questions are as follows:

A. Check the response that best describes how you feel about the statement: "Alcoholism is basically a character disorder."
Strongly agree __ Agree __ Neutral __ Disagree __ Strongly disagree __
B. Which of the following is your choice of specialty area? Choose only one:
___ 1. Medical or Medical Intensive Care
___ 2. Surgical or Surgical Intensive Care
___ 3. Obstetrics: Labor and Delivery, Postpartum or Newborn Nursery, and area specialties
___ 4. Pediatrics and area specialties
___ 5. Psychiatric and area specialties
C. Which three of the following life events have been most difficult for you? Please rank your three choices in order from the most difficult (1) to the least difficult (3).
___ 1. Childhood
___ 2. Marriage
___ 3. Retirement
___ 4. Illness of self or spouse
___ 5. Death of spouse or other close relative
___ 6. Children leaving home
___ 7. Parenthood

Questions such as these are the same whether used in a questionnaire or in an interview. They are more commonly used in questionnaires but may be used in interviews, particularly if the subject is unable or unwilling to fill out a questionnaire.

In exploratory research, it may not be appropriate to structure the interview questions in advance, other than to decide on the opening statement or question. A flexible interview, properly used, can bring out much useful material because it allows the interviewer to pursue whatever seems important to the subjects and thus elicit the subjects' values, beliefs, and attitudes. Their responses will be completely spontaneous, self-revealing, and personal.

The flexibility of the interview is both an advantage and a disadvantage to the researcher. The results will not be comparable from one subject to the next because the interview format is never the same. However, the interview is invaluable in exploring the whole range of attitudes, thoughts, and feelings that exist for the topic.

Sometimes the interview has a focus, as in psychiatric evaluations, in which the interviewers have a list of topics to cover but can select their own method of eliciting the information. Also left up to the interviewer is whether to pursue an area of particular interest.

Another unstructured interview uses the nondirective technique. Here the initiative is almost completely in the hands of the subject. The interviewer's function is to encourage the subject to talk but with a minimum of guidance. The main function of the interviewer is to show interest in the subject and anything the subject cares to talk about, thus serving as a catalyst for the expression of the subject's feelings. This type of interview requires considerable skill on the part of the interviewer.

In a questionnaire, it is difficult to be unstructured. Some degree of structure is always required because you must set your questions in advance and cannot change them according to the subjects' responses. Questions that do not have fixed alternatives, however, are much less structured than those that do, because they require subjects to respond in their own words. The extent of the response that the subject must provide to answer the question will vary from a word to a sentence, a paragraph, or even an essay. The least structured questionnaires are those designed to elicit extensive response from the subject. For example:

Describe an event in your life that has had a significant impact on your present state of mind.

This questionnaire item is quite unstructured because it defines few parameters for the subject. The event described can be anything—a health problem, a social or cultural event, a positive or negative event. The choice is up to the subject.

Open-ended questions are less structured than the fixed-alternative kind and give subjects more leeway to provide their own answers. The question is designed to allow the subject a free response rather than a response limited to or guided by given alternatives. Some examples of open-ended questions are as follows:

1. How do you feel about abortions?
2. What do you think women should do to ensure equal rights?
3. What do you like most about nursing school?

Setting Up Your Data Collection Instrument

In this age of computer literacy, you will find it helpful to design your questionnaire format so that your data can be easily entered into the computer. When you are planning your format, remember that the computer reads only numbers, and that it is set up to read across columns of numbers, either singly or by two or more numbers grouped together. Each variable that you want the computer to read can be set up on your questionnaire in numerical form. For example, rather than setting up your questionnaire to look like this:

What is your current age _____ ?

You might set up the same questions to look like this:

What is your current age?   __ __

What you are doing is providing the correct number of spaces for marking a person's actual age. (If you are doing a study of children under ten you will need only one space. If you are doing a study of the very old, three spaces will be needed.) The placement of the lines at the far right of the page facilitates entry into the computer as your eye will simply run down the right side of the page rather than searching all over for the input. Normally, the first few digits will be used for the subjects' identification number, after which you begin to enter the data from your questionnaire. Remember, also, that the computer cannot handle blank spaces, so if you have allowed two digits to record age, and one of your subjects is only six years old, the age must be recorded as "06" in order not to leave any blank columns. The same procedure would be done if you were asking for a person's weight. Rather than ask:

What is your current weight _____ ?

Format the question instead:

What is your current weight, in pounds?   __ __ __

As you can see, these are obviously numerical answers. What would you do if you had nominal or ordinal answers? Setting up the questionnaire for these answers is more complex but similar. For example:

Please circle your current marital status:

Never married   Married   Divorced   Separated   Widowed

If you were setting this up for a quick computer scan your answer sheet would look more like this:

Please indicate your current marital status:

Never married	1. ___
Married	2. ___
Divorced	3. ___
Separated	4. ___
Widowed	5. ___

Once you have set up your questions and answers for easy input into the computer, go through the questionnaire and number each space consecutively just as the computer does, leaving room at the beginning of your numbering system for the number you have given to each individual in the sample—two spaces if you plan scores lower than 100, three if higher. You may want to leave other spaces as well. Remember always that your number system is zero to nine for any given space. If your number goes over nine you will need two spaces. If over 99, three, and so on. So plan ahead for data collection.

The most usual standardized or structured data you will plan to collect is the demographic data. Table 9.2 is an example of how to collect demographic data and how to set up the data collection sheet on each member of the sample.

INTERVIEWS. Although interviews and questionnaires can use the same questions, interviews are most effective when they are based on open-ended rather than yes/no or numerical answers. A major error that occurs with new researchers is to design an ordinal scale instrument and use it as the basis for an interview. Few people listening to an interviewer can remember the details necessary to answer the question. Likert scales were designed for questionnaires and are best limited to that method of data collection.

Projective Tests

There are times when the variables you are trying to measure are neither observable nor obtainable from the subject because they represent feelings or attitudes that the individual is unable or unwilling to report. Projective techniques are indirect methods of measuring these variables. They typically involve some type of imaginative activity on the part of the subject in response to an ambiguous stimulus. The use of these techniques requires intensive specialized training. Some nurses have this training, and others will have access to people who do; therefore, this discussion is appropriate.

TABLE 9-2	*Demographic Data Sheet*

Subject ID Number

$\overline{}_{1}\ \overline{}_{2}\ \overline{}_{3}$

Age (in years)

$\overline{}_{4}\ \overline{}_{5}$

Gender

  1. Male   2. Female

$\overline{}_{6}$

Ethnic/Racial Identity

  1. Native American   2. Latin   3. Caucasian

  4. Black   5. Asian/Pacific   6. Other _____

$\overline{}_{7}$

Marital Status

  1. Never Married   2. Married   3. Separated

  4. Divorced   5. Widowed

  6. Other (Please describe.)

$\overline{}_{8}$

Total Annual Income/Household

$\overline{}_{9}\ \overline{}_{10}\ \overline{}_{11}\ \overline{}_{12}\ \overline{}_{13}\ \overline{}_{14}$

Religion

  1. Catholic

  2. Protestant

  3. Jewish

  4. None

  5. Other _____

$\overline{}_{15}$

Education

(Circle *highest* degree.)

  1. High School diploma

  2. Certificate program (Please describe.)

  3. Associate of Arts/Science

  4. Baccalaureate (BA/BS/BEd, etc.)

  5. Master's (MA/MS/MEd/MPH, etc.)

  6. Academic doctorate (PhD, DSc, DNS, etc.)

  7. Professional doctorate (MD, ND, DDS, etc.)

  8. Other (Please describe.)

$\overline{}_{16}$

The stimuli used in a projective test must be capable of arousing many different reactions: for instance, an inkblot can appear to be many different things; a picture can elicit many different stories; toys can be used to portray many people and events. The subject's perception of the stimulus, the feelings it arouses, and the way the subject organizes his or her responses provide the data for analysis by an expert. The responses are not taken at face value but, instead, are interpreted according to predetermined conceptualizations.

The *Rorschach Inkblot Test* consists of ten cards, each of which depicts an inkblot. The subject is shown each card and asked, "What might this be?" The *Thematic Apperception Test (TAT)* provides a series of pictures about which the subject is asked to tell stories. Both of these frequently used techniques are designed to elicit a rich sample of responses from which a wide variety of inferences can be drawn. Other commonly used projective tests are word association, sentence completion, and figure drawing.

All projective tests rely on the fact that people often find it easier to be expressive when they are not talking specifically about themselves and their own feelings. Talking through the medium of the projective test allows the subjects to maintain a distance from their own thoughts and feelings, which enables them to talk impersonally about themselves. In addition, feelings of which the subject may not be consciously aware appear in the responses to the ambiguous stimulus.

If your operational definition calls for a projective measure, you will want to consider one of these approaches. Keep in mind, however, that most projective measures require the assistance of an expert to analyze the subjects' responses. If this help is not available, you may have to abandon this method of data collection even though it might be the most suitable.

Level of Question and Degree of Structure

With questionnaires, interviews, and observational methods, the level of the study is related to the degree of structure in the measurement tool. Unstructured interviews are appropriate for Level I studies but not for Levels II and III. Starting at Level II, questions must be standardized with fixed alternatives so that the responses of subjects can be compared. In addition, the responses at Level III must be sensitive enough to distinguish small differences between experimental and control groups; this task involves structured questions and answers. Therefore, *only* fixed-alternative questions may be used at Level III. You will find, when writing questions, that developing fixed-alternative answers requires a great deal of knowledge, because you need to provide an alternative to fit every response. You can do it only if you *know* the whole range of possible responses. That means previous research has provided you with the necessary range of responses. If this knowledge is unavailable, the topic is not appropriate for a Level III study.

Designing the Questionnaire or Interview Guide

If you have decided to use a questionnaire or an interview guide, here are some suggestions on how to go about it.

1. List your questions in the same order to provide consistency and also to prevent the interviewers from forgetting something or from changing the order from one subject to the next. When determining the best sequence for the content of your questions, use the following guidelines:

    a. Order your questions from impersonal to personal topics;

    b. Order from less sensitive to more sensitive (in this way the rapport with the investigator is established and trust developed prior to asking personal or sensitive questions);

    c. In a list of options, alphabetize the order to minimize bias;

    d. Earlier questions may influence later questions, so begin from general questions first, and move to more specific questions later;

    e. Begin questioning with questions that arouse interest;

    f. Group questions by topic.

2. In exploratory studies, be as unstructured as possible while getting at what you want to know—the more you know, the more structured you can become. Examples of unstructured open-ended interview questions are:

    Think back to the most difficult experience you ever had. Tell me about it.

    In your opinion, why do people commit suicide?

    If you had it to do over again, what profession would you choose:

    Nursing?

    Medicine?

    Another Health Science?

    Liberal Arts?

    Other?

    Why?

3. Base your questions on the literature as much as possible—if there is not enough literature, then ask logical questions—those derived from findings or unasked questions.

4. Start with topics you want covered. A handy rule is to follow the outline used in writing your problem. Give your initial questionnaire to others to critique prior to using it in your study (such as people who

write questionnaires, or people who know a lot about your topic). From their comments rewrite your questionnaire.

5. Pretest your questions on people similar to the sample you plan to study. Discuss the interview questions or questionnaire with the subject after the session is completed.

6. Remember, interviews take a long time.

AVAILABLE DATA

The health field offers a multitude of available data. Using this data is economical and has other advantages as well. Most official records have been collected over time, thus making it possible to follow trends. Time and money are saved by the availability of a large sample of records in one location.

The kind of available data that comes to mind for nursing research is the medical record. Hospitals keep medical records on hand for at least five years and have records dating back much further that are retrievable for research purposes. Also available through hospital records departments are admission rates by age, sex, diagnosis, and other variables such as data on length of stay, types of surgery performed, and so on. Much information about work patterns of nurses can be found in personnel records and in the records of staffing patterns kept by nursing departments.

Data from entire communities can be found in census records and in records from public health departments. These can be used to look for trends within a community or to compare one community with another.

Less frequently, data from newspapers, magazines, professional journals, textbooks, and the like are used for research purposes. In historical studies, personal documents such as autobiographies, letters, and diaries can provide a wealth of data. Mass communication can also provide useful information. For instance, consider the possibility of analyzing the image of the nurse as presented on television or in movies.

Unwritten sources of available data include television, motion pictures, tape recordings, photographs, and, in rare cases, a historian studying a culture without written records. The use of historical artifacts, buildings, architecture, clothing, and the like are examples of unwritten available data and are possible sources of data for nursing studies.

The major drawback in using available data, no matter how they were collected, is that they were not compiled primarily for your study and, therefore, may not quite fit your definition of terms. For instance, if you were collecting data on the number of times patients are transferred from room to room during their hospital stay, you might go to the hospital daily census as a source only to discover that this document lists only transfers from one nursing unit to another and not those made from room to room within the same unit. Hopefully, this is something you would find out before you began to collect data, but sometimes there is no way of knowing how the data were collected and how the recorders defined the categories of data. You can, therefore, obtain misleading results from available data.

For instance, suppose you wanted to compare the nurse/patient ratio among several hospitals in your area. Each hospital has data available that can be translated into a nurse/patient ratio. However, you might find that one hospital that appears to have fewer patients per nurse actually includes head nurses and unit secretaries in its staffing figures, whereas other hospitals do not. If you are not aware of how the data are reported, you may be misled by your findings.

When using nurses' notes as a source of data, you must take into account the fact that the nurses doing the recording had no common operational definitions for the terms used. Even simple terms like "slept well" have different meanings for different nurses. An operational definition established for research purposes has to specify exactly what is meant by "slept well" and how it is to be differentiated from "slept poorly" or other categories. Thus, "slept well" might become "when checked every half hour during the hours of midnight to 6 A.M., the patient was asleep." When operational definitions are not available, the individual data collectors use their own definitions. As long as this fact is taken into account, much valuable information can be found in nurses' notes and other such records.

The amount of structure used to collect available data can usually be determined from the method of data recording. If predetermined categories were used, such as checklists or fixed-alternative responses, the data will be more structured than if the recorder used a personal diary or journal to record the data. Looking at a medical record, you will find many examples of unstructured data. Progress notes and daily nurses' notes are usually written in the individual's own words. A physical examination, on the other hand, may be recorded on a checklist, with few statements by the individual. Vital signs, medication dosages, and surgical checklists are other examples of structured available data.

Many Level I and Level II studies can utilize available data; unstructured data will be appropriate only at Level I. Available data can never be used in experimental designs exclusively, because they have, by definition, already been collected and therefore cannot be manipulated to measure the effect of an experimental independent variable. In Level III studies, however, available data may be used to provide background information about the sample but not to provide measurements of the independent and dependent variables.

PHYSIOLOGICAL MEASURES

As a method of data collection, nurses have the opportunity to utilize a wealth of physiological measures. These provide objective data relating to patients' responses to nursing care and should not be overlooked as sources of valuable data. Physiological methods can be used alone or with other methods. They can be used as the data collection method for your study, or the results of physiological measures can be obtained from available records, such as patients' charts.

Physiological measures available to nurses range from simple (such as blood pressure, pulse, and temperature) to the more complex (measurement of sodium and potassium ratios in twelve-hour urine collections). Nurses can use measurements such as tidal volume and blood gasses to measure the response to treatment of respiratory patients. In a study of the physiological effects of shift rotation on ICU nurses, Tooraen used the measurement of seventeen hydroxycorticosteroids as an index of overall adrenal cortical secretory activity; rather than measuring it directly, however, she measured increases in sodium and potassium in the urine.[4]

With the complex monitoring equipment available in critical care units, nurses have the opportunity to study many variables that formerly could not be accurately measured. Instant and continuous measures of physiological response can be obtained for patients in critical care units. In addition, such equipment can be obtained through schools of nursing and medical centers for research with healthy subjects.

RECOMMENDED READINGS

Abbey, J. (Guest ed.), Symposium on bioinstrumentation for nurses, *Nursing Clinics of North America*, 1978, *13*, 561–640.

Allen, M. N., and Jensen, L., Hermeneutical inquiry: Meaning and scope, *Western Journal of Nursing Research*, 1990, *12*(2), 241–253.

Barriball, I. K. L., Christian, S. L., While, A. E., and Bergen, A., The telephone survey method: a discussion paper, *Journal of Advanced Nursing*, 1996, *24*, 115–121.

Beck, C. T., Opening student's eyes: The process of selecting a research instrument, *Nurse Educator*, 1999, *21*(3), 21–23.

Brink, P., Value orientations as an assessment tool in cultural diversity, *Nursing Research*, 1984, *33*(4), 198–203.

Byerly, E. L., The nurse researcher as participant-observer in a nursing setting. In P. J. Brink (ed.), *Transcultural nursing: A book of readings*, Englewood Cliffs, N.J.: Prentice-Hall, 1976, 143–162.

Cassiani, S. H. B., Zanetti, M. L., and Pela, N. T. R., The telephone survey: A methodological strategy for obtaining information, *Journal of Advanced Nursing*, 1992, *17*(5), 576–581.

Couper, M. R., The Delphi technique: Characteristics and sequence model, *Advances in Nursing Science*, 1984, *7*:72–77.

Crane, J. G., and Angrosino, M. V., *Field projects in anthropology: A student handbook* (2nd ed.), Prospect Heights, Ill.: Waveland Press, 1992.

Dagenais, F. and Meleis, A. I., Professionalism, work ethic, and empathy in nursing, *Western Journal of Nursing Research*, 1982, *4*:407–422.

---

4. Tooraen, Sister L. A., Physiological effects of shift rotation on ICU nurses, *Nursing Research*, 21, 5 (Sept.–Oct. 1972), 398–405.

Denny, E., Feminist research methods in nursing, *Senior Nurse*, 1991, *11*(6), 38–40.

Dobbert, M. L., *Ethnographic research: Theory and application for modern schools and societies,* New York: Praeger, 1982.

Downs, F., and Fitzpatrick, J. J., Preliminary investigation of the reliability and validity of a tool for the assessment of body position and motor activity, *Nursing Research,* 1976, *25:*404–408.

Drury, C. G., The use of archival data. In J. R. Wilson and E. N. Corlett, (eds.), *Evaluation of human work: A practical ergonomics methodology,* London: Taylor & Francis, 1990, pp. 89–100.

Dunn, M. A., Development of an instrument to measure nursing performance, *Nursing Research,* 1970, *19,* 502–510.

Ellen, R. F., *Ethnographic research: A guide to general conduct,* New York: Academic Press, 1984.

Field, P. A., and Morse, J. M., *Nursing research: The application of qualitative approaches,* Rockville, Md.: Aspen Systems, 1985.

Fink, A., and Koseocoff, J., *How to conduct surveys: A step-by-step guide,* Beverly Hills, Ca.: Sage, 1998.

Franck, L. S., A new method to quantitatively describe pain behavior in infants, *Nursing Research,* 1986, *35*(1) 28–31.

Hunter, D. E., and Foley, M. B., *Doing anthropology: A student centered approach to cultural anthropology,* New York: Harper & Row, 1976.

Jacobsen, B. S. and Meininger, J. C., The designs and methods of published nursing research: 1956–1983, *Nursing Research,* 1985, *34*(5) 306–312.

Killeen, M. B., Secondary analysis: A little-known strategy for nursing research, *Michigan Nurse,* 1992, *65*(2), 9–10.

Kingry, M. J., Tiedje, L. B., and Friedman, L. L., Focus groups: A research technique for nursing, *Nursing Research,* 1990, *39*(2), 124–125.

May, K., Interview techniques in qualitative research: Concerns and challenges. In Janice M. Morse (ed.), *Qualitative nursing research: A contemporary dialogue* (rev. ed.), Newbury Park, Ca.: Sage, 1991, pp. 188–201.

McLaughlin, F. E., and Marascuilo, L. A., *Advanced nursing and health care research: Quantification approaches,* Philadelphia: W. B. Saunders, 1990.

Mishel, M., Adjusting the fit: Development of uncertainty scales for specific clinical populations, *Western Journal of Nursing Research,* 1983, *5*(4) 355–370.

Moreno, J. L. (ed.), *Sociometry and the science of man,* New York: Beacon House, 1956.

Morgan, C. (ed.), *Beyond methods: Strategies for social research,* Beverly Hills, Ca.: Sage, 1983.

Munhall, P. L., and Oiler, C. J., *Nursing research: A qualitative perspective,* Norwalk, Ct.: Appleton-Century-Crofts, 1993.

Oppenheim, A. N., *Questionnaire design and attitude measurement,* New York: Basic Books, 1966.

Osgood, C. E., and Snider, J. G., *Semantic-differential technique: A sourcebook,* Chicago: Aldine, 1969.

Parse, R. R., Coyne, B. A., and Smith, M. J., *Nursing research: Qualitative methods,* Bowie, Md.: Brady Communication Company, 1985.

Payne, S. L., *The art of asking questions,* Princeton, N.J.: Princeton University Press, 1951.

Pearsall, M., Participant observation as role and method in behavioral research, *Nursing Research,* 1965, *14,* 37–42.

Pigors, P., and Pigors, F., The incident process—A method of inquiry, *Nursing Outlook,* October 1966, *14,* 48–50.

Rich, R., and Dent, J. K., Patient rating scale, *Nursing Research,* Summer 1962, *11,* 163–171.

Roberts, C. A., and Burke, S. O., *Nursing research: A quantitative and qualitative approach,* Boston: Jones and Bartlett, 1989.

Salazar, M. K., Interviewer bias: How it affects survey research, *AAOHN Journal,* 1990, *38*(12), 567–572, 588–590.

Sandelowski, M., Telling stories: Narrative approaches in qualitative research, *Image: Journal of Nursing Scholarship,* 1991, *23*(3), 161–166.

Selltiz, C., Wrightsman, L. S., and Cook, S. W., *Research methods in social relations* (3rd ed.), New York: Holt, Rinehart and Winston, 1976, Chap. 8–12, Appendix B.

Smith, P. C., Kendall L. M., and Hulin, C. L., *The measurement of satisfaction in work and retirement,* Chicago: Rand McNally, 1969.

Spradly, J. P., *The ethnographic interview,* New York, Holt, Rinehart and Winston, 1979.

Spradly, J. P., *Participant observation,* New York, Holt, Rinehart and Winston, 1980.

Stewart, D. W., Secondary research: Information sources and methods. In L. Bickman (ed.), *Applied social research methods series,* Vol. 4, Beverly Hills, Ca.: Sage, 1984.

Sullivan, K., Managing the 'sensitive' research interview: A personal account, *Nurse Researcher,* 1988/1999, *6*(2), 72–85.

Van Maanen, J. (ed.), *Qualitative methodology,* Beverly Hills, Ca.: Sage, 1983.

Van Maanen, J., Dabbs, J. M., Jr., and Faulkner, R. R., *Varieties of qualitative research,* Beverly Hills, Ca.: Sage, 1982.

Waltz, C., and Bausell, R. B., *Nursing research: Design, statistics and the computer.* Philadelphia: F. A. Davis, 1981, Chap. 4, 5.

Waltz, C. F., Strickland, O. L., and Lenz, E. R., *Measurement in nursing research,* Philadelphia: F. A. Davis, 1991.

Ward, M. F., and Felter, M. E., *Instruments for use in nursing education research,* Boulder, Co.: Western Interstate Commission for Higher Education in Nursing, 1979.

Ward, M. F., and Lindeman, C. A. (eds.), *Instruments for measuring nursing practice and other health variables,* Washington: U.S. Government Printing Office, 1978.

Weiss, S. J., and Davis, H. P., Validity and reliability of the Collaborative Practice Scales, *Nursing Research,* 1986, *34:* 299–305.

Whyte, W. F., *Learning from the field: A guide from experience,* Beverly Hills, Ca.: Sage, 1984.

Williams, M. A., Entrapment in method . . . Methods are tools to be used in the generation of knowledge, not ends in themselves, *Research in Nursing and Health,* 1989, *12*(5), iii, iv.

Woods, N. F., The health diary as an instrument for nursing research, *Western Journal of Nursing Research,* 1981, *5:* 76–92.

Yin, R. K., Case study research: Design and methods. In L. Bickman (ed.), *Applied social research methods series,* Vol. 5, Beverly Hills, Ca.: Sage, 1984.

Reliability and Validity of Measurement

$\mathbf{E}$ach step of the research process depends on the preceding steps. If a step is missing or inaccurate, then the succeeding steps will fail. When developing your research plan, be aware that this principle critically affects your progress. For instance, if you asked your question correctly, you can perform an adequate literature review. A good literature review is basic to the purpose of the study. The purpose of the study is basic to the operational definitions. Once you have operationalized your terms, you can proceed with the design, sample selection, and method of data collection. The concepts of reliability and validity will be discussed now, as they ultimately will influence the data analysis and the outcome of the final report.

Reliability and validity, in research, refer specifically to the measurement of data as they will be used to answer the research question. In most cases, the instrument that measures your variables is the central issue in determining the reliability and validity of the data.

Whatever data collection method is used, the intent must be accuracy. How much you can rely on the results depends on the consistency, stability, and repeatability of your data collection instrument—in other words, its reliability. If you were to measure the same variable in the same person again, would your result be the same?

In addition to reliability, you need to know if the measurement technique used to collect data actually measures what it is supposed to measure; in other words, is it *valid?* If you use a questionnaire to measure an individual's moral values, did the questionnaire, in fact, measure that concept or something else? The degree to which answers actually reflect the individual's moral values represents the validity of the questionnaire.

Data collection in nursing research is not a precise science, and there are many factors that can affect the reliability and validity of the results. Estimating the degree to which an instrument is valid and reliable is a critical step in the research process.[1]

This chapter deals with the concepts of reliability and validity of the instruments used to measure variables. The issues related to the validity of the research result are covered under the discussion of internal and external validity in Chapter 7.

ERRORS IN DATA COLLECTION PROCEDURES

The whole point in doing research is to measure differences among the subjects in the sample. When you are looking at nursing interventions, you want to know whether the intervention really made a difference in the patient outcome or if the result was based on some error in the data collection process. What you are looking for are the true differences that occur among patients as a result of the nursing intervention. These true differences are the research objective. Any other differences are errors in the measurement process. Some errors may be due to the way data were collected; others, to the characteristics of the subjects.

When we are measuring or testing a variable, we want to be sure that what we are measuring reflects the true differences in the subjects and not an error either in relation to the characteristic we are measuring or to the measurement process itself. The process of measurement, however, is easily affected by error, particularly when we are measuring abstract concepts that may not be fully understood at the present time.

Errors in the measurement process can be either *constant* or *random*. A *constant error* will consistently affect the measurement of the variable in the same way each time measurement is done.[2] It will provide an incorrect measure of the variable, and the error will be the same for all subjects. An example is a weight scale that consistently weights two grams over the actual weight. The measurement will appear to be reliable, as repeated measures of the same item

1. The basic concepts and their descriptions have been taken from Selltiz, C., Wrightsman, L. S., and Cook, S.W. *Research methods in social relations* (3rd ed.), New York: Holt, Rinehart and Winston, 1976, Chap. 6.

2. Selltiz, C., et al., *Research methods in social relations* (3rd ed.), New York: Holt, Rinehart and Winston, 1976, 168.

will result in the same weight. The measurement, however, will not be a valid weight, as it is always two grams over the actual weight of any item.

The two most stable and problematic "constant errors" in social science research are *social desirability* (where the research subjects respond with what they believe is the positive social response whether or not it is true) and *acquiescent response set* (consistently agreeing or disagreeing with the questions). These two sources of error are examples of constant error in that they are always present in some people, and those people will consistently bias their responses to any questionnaire or interview. For this reason, in any personal interaction with human subjects for the purpose of obtaining information, the researcher is very careful to present questions in such a way as to avoid either of these sources of error. Constant error affects the validity of the measurement or its ability to arrive at "true differences" among subjects. Other traits of individuals can also produce constant error in the measurement of other traits. Intelligence and test-taking skill are two examples. Both characteristics can influence a subject's performance on a paper-and-pencil test, and thereby contaminate the true differences that the researcher is looking for on the trait actually being measured. When developing questionnaires, it is up to the researcher to demonstrate that the tool is not being affected by traits such as these, and because we are unable to know directly an individual's "true position" on many of the variables that we measure, we judge the validity of the instrument by the extent to which its results are comparable with other evidence. Because there are differences in the type of evidence that is available to establish the validity of an instrument, there are different levels and types of validation.

Constant error can be introduced with the independent variable in a Level III study. This problem is a result of the two-group design, in which one group receives the nursing intervention and the other group does not. The validity of the independent variable can be questioned any time there are only two groups, one of which receives "no treatment." For example, a special technique of crisis intervention is being tested for its efficiency in decreasing anxiety. In this study, the experimental group receives one hour of intensive crisis intervention, and the control group receives no special intervention. The two groups do not achieve a valid measurement of crisis intervention in this design, because what is really being measured is "something versus nothing." There is no way of truly isolating the effect of the crisis intervention. This creates a constant error in applying the independent variable and affects the outcome of the study. The error is built into the design controlling the application of the independent variable. The design can be corrected easily by including more variation in the independent variable. For instance, adding one other form of counseling in the form of a second experimental group will improve the validity of the measurement of crisis intervention in the original group.

Random error, in contrast, is unpredictable error that varies from one measurement to the next even though the characteristic being measured has not changed. Random errors are *transient in nature* and *result in inconsistent data.*[3] If measurements are repeated on the same subjects, the results will not be the same. *Random errors directly affect reliability,* but because valid measures must also be reliable, random errors also indirectly affect the validity of the measurement technique.

Random errors can result from many factors related to the research situation, such as an unreliable measurement of variables. The subjects' mood, attention span, state of health, whether or not they are in pain, are all examples of transient personal factors that can cause unreliable responses to measurement and can result in different measurement scores from one time to another. The researcher's general state of well-being may also contribute to random error, in that situations where the data collector is feeling fatigued, impatient, bored, ill, or distracted can affect the subjects' responses to measurement. These possibilities for random error need to be considered in planning the process of measurement in any study, as the goal is to maximize the reliability of the results.

Other transient factors that cause random error in measurement can stem from the physical environment in which the research occurs, such as weather, temperature, lighting, noise, and interruptions. Privacy may be a factor in some studies when subjects may hesitate to answer accurately if they fear they may be overheard by family members or others in the environment. Care must be taken in planning the procedures for data collection so that random error is kept to a minimum.

The wording of the questions can affect both the reliability and the validity of the tool used for an interview or questionnaire. Unclear questions can affect reliability if they lead the subject to answer part of the questionnaire differently. They can affect validity if they lead to systematic misinterpretation of the whole idea. Either way, they produce both constant and random errors in measurement.

When you develop a research instrument, there is no way you can possibly ask every conceivable question about the concept you are trying to measure. You must include some questions and exclude others. In effect, you are sampling the universe of possible data about your variable, thus choosing to collect some data and not others. The sample you select must be representative of the universe of what is known about your variable. Ensuring this representativeness is a difficult process. You can never be completely sure that you have selected a truly representative sample of content for your tool. This type of error affects the validity of your instrument because it will provide a source of constant error for all your subjects.

A final source of error comes not from the process of data collection, but rather from the process of data analysis. Here, you may introduce error in cod-

---

3. Selltiz, C., et al., *Research methods in social relations* (3rd ed.), New York: Holt, Rinehart and Winston, 1976, 169.

ing answers when you transpose from one page to another. Or, you might make a mathematical error in calculating the results of the answers. These are random errors and will affect the reliability of the final data.

Error can be permanently damaging to the research project and very serious or it can be superficial and easily corrected. Error can be obvious to any external reader or it can be hidden from everyone. Error can be a problem or a minor irritant. In any case, every researcher attempts to remove as much error as possible from the research study during the planning phase to increase the credibility of the results.

Bailey presents a table showing the type of error that is likely to occur during different phases of the research process. The serious researcher looks for sources of error during the planning phase, accepting critique from peers and supervisors early in the process in order to produce as valid and reliable a study as is possible under the circumstances. (See Table 10.1.)

The concepts of reliability and validity being presented here are the theoretical underpinnings for the standard tests. This chapter is not intended to provide the mechanisms for testing reliability and validity but rather to present

TABLE 10-1	*Error in the Research Process*
Phase of the Research Process	**Type of Error**
1. The research question The research problem Operational definitions	1. Lack of face validity
2. Construction of measurement instrument (questionnaire)	2. Faulty or ambiguous wording of questions Categories not mutually exclusive Not representative of content
3. Sampling	3. Lack of external validity a. Sampling error b. Not representative
4. Data collection (failure to control)	4. Reliability issues: a. Environment (lighting, heat) b. Personal characteristics of respondent (fatigue) c. Relationship between researcher and respondent d. Mechanical defects (faulty recording, equipment failure)
5. Coding	5. Coding errors such as missing data, incorrect recording, illegible coding
6. Data analysis	6. Incorrect statistics Faulty interpretation of data

Adapted from Bailey, K. D., *Methods of social research*, New York: The Free Press, 1978.

the rationale for these measures in research projects. What kinds of tests to use and why, what kinds of situations require what kind of procedure and why will be discussed in subsequent pages. For in-depth information on how to test for reliability and validity, see Waltz, Strickland, and Lenz, 1991.[4]

VALIDITY

There are three major methods of estimating the validity of a data collection instrument or of the investigator as a valid participant observer. The greater the degree of validity of the data collection device, the more confident you will be that the results you achieve reflect true differences in the scores of your subjects and not some random or constant error. As our concern with validity is primarily one of constant error, the degree of validity will reflect the degree to which we are controlling or accounting for *constant error.*

The degree to which valid measurements can be achieved is directly related to the level of the study design. Exploratory descriptive designs, by nature, have a low level of validation and must rely heavily on estimates of reliability. Level II descriptive survey designs can achieve a greater degree of validity but still rely heavily on reliability estimates. Level III demands the highest degree of validity testing and uses reliability testing only to account for gaps in the attainment of validity. Just as control over the independent variable must increase with the level of design, so must control for error in data collection. Methods of establishing validity of the measurement technique fall into one of three categories: *self-evident measures, pragmatic measures,* and *construct validity.*

Self-evident Measures

These methods of establishing validity deal with basic levels of knowledge about the variable and look at an instrument's apparent value as a measurement technique rather than at its actual value. In other words, self-evident measures refer to the fact that the instrument appears to measure what it is supposed to measure.

FACE VALIDITY. At the most basic level, when little or nothing is known about the variable being measured, the level of validity obtainable is called *face validity.* "On the face of it . . ." merely establishes that the tool seems an appropriate way to find out what you want to know. Looking at the questions you have developed to ask your subjects, you can say, "I think I will find out what I

---

4. Waltz, C. F., Strickland, O. L., and Lenz, E. R., *Measurement in nursing research* (2nd ed.), Philadelphia: F.A. Davis Company, 1991.

want to know by asking these questions. It looks all right to me." This is the extent of face validity. It is the lowest level of validation and is used only when you are beginning to study a particular variable and have no prior research literature to refer to. If there is literature on the variable, either theory or research, then face validity is not sufficient. If you have chosen to study a variable that has not been studied before, you usually will start with face validity, as it is the beginning step of the validation process.

Let's say that you are interested in discovering patient's attitudes toward the labels they are given, and you want to know just what patients would like to be called.[5] There are no previous studies that relate to this area and no questionnaires previously developed. You plan to develop your own tool—a questionnaire or interview schedule. The first step is to write down some questions. For example, you might decide to ask these questions:

What are the different ways that nurses address patients?

Which of these have been used by nurses addressing you?

How do you prefer to be addressed by nurses?

After writing your questions, you look them over and you think they make sense. Next, you give the questions to your family and friends, and they agree that the questions make sense. You now have established face validity. You might also give the questions to some staff nurses and some patients. You are developing more confidence in your questions as these groups also agree that they make sense, but you still have only face validity.

CONTENT VALIDITY. Content validity is also a self-evident measure but involves comparing the content of the measurement technique to the known literature on the topic and validating the fact that the tool does represent the literature accurately. You want to obtain an adequate sampling of the content area being studied. Content validity is frequently estimated from the review of the literature on the topic or through consultation with experts in the field who have become experts by having done unpublished research in the area. After you have critically reviewed the literature, you construct your questions or instruments to cover the known content represented in the literature.

Content validity is a self-evident measure because it relies on the assurance that you can demonstrate an adequate coverage of the known field. An expert should be able to judge whether or not the tool adequately samples the known content. Researchers, therefore, frequently call on experts in the field to verify content validity for newly developed tools.

---

5. This research question was asked by Bernice Tolliver, Clinical Nurse Coordinator, Brentwood VA Medical Center, Los Angeles, and was the basis for a small nursing research project in which she was involved in 1981.

In exploratory descriptive studies using participant observation, you may be in situations where you do not know either the setting or the population. You assume that the persons you select to represent the population are knowledgeable about the content you are trying to elicit. In this case, you assume that the members of a group or population have face validity as experts in their culture or social roles, and you try to further validate each person's report by talking with as many experts as possible. The more people you question, the more content you will gain and the more depth of data you will have at your disposal. "On the face of it" means your informants appear to have face validity; you establish content validity of the data by cross-checking the answers with several informants until you are satisfied that the content is accurate.

USE OF JUDGE PANELS. There are times when you want validation from others that, "on the face of it," your data collection instrument is collecting what it is supposed to, or that your categories for discriminating data in content analysis seem appropriate. You are not concerned that your questions cover or represent the universe of content as in content validity, but rather that people other than yourself think you have a valid instrument. In this case, you put together a group of people that you believe are knowledgeable about the content you are testing or knowledgeable about the process of developing questions. These people are called a *Panel of Experts* who are asked to judge whether or not, "on the face of it," your work appears to be sound, that it will do what you want it to do. This is your judge panel.

Students can use classmates, thesis committee, clinical staff (if it is a clinical study), and so on. Faculty use each other, students in their courses, as well as clinical and administrative staff where appropriate. Clinical agency personnel use each other, visiting faculty, and students. The point is to get opinions other than your own. We become so close to our own studies we tend to lose sight of alternative responses. The use of a judge panel, and taking its advice if it is asked for, is a first step in the development of the validity of your data collection instrument(s). Even if you are using someone else's instrument, the use of the judge panel will assist you in determining its appropriateness to your study.

One use of a judge panel is more closely allied with content validity than face validity. In this instance, the panel of experts is drawn together because it is familiar with the content area or theoretical formulation of your study. The judges are usually researchers in the field. You ask them to look over your questionnaire, interview schedule, or observational tool to judge whether or not your instrument adequately represents the known universe of content you want to cover. Their responses are reported in your proposal according to the percentage of agreement among the judge panel members with the items you have developed.

Pragmatic Measures

Pragmatic measures of validity essentially test the practical value of a particular research instrument or tool and focus on the questions, "Does it work?" "Does it do what it is supposed to do?" Pragmatic validation procedures attempt to answer these questions. The two types of pragmatic measures are called *concurrent validity* and *predictive validity.*

CONCURRENT VALIDITY. Instruments that attempt to test a research subject on some current characteristic have concurrent validity if the results are compared and have a high correlation with an established (tested) measurement. Suppose you had developed a behavioral checklist to measure nurses' job satisfaction. To validate this test, you would need to compare it with the results of an established job satisfaction instrument shown to be valid for nurses. A high correlation between the results of the two dissimilar tests would indicate concurrent validity for your checklist.

A recent study by Walbek and Gordon assessed the concurrent validity of three self-report measures of assertiveness by comparing them with trait ratings of experts in assertiveness behavior.[6] They found that although the three self-reports correlated highly with one another, there was not a high correlation between any of them and the trait ratings. Therefore, concurrent validity was not established for the self-report measures. This example points out the necessity of requiring either a test for which validity has been established or a measure that approaches the concept differently as a criterion for concurrent validity.

PREDICTIVE VALIDITY. Instruments that accurately predict some future occurrence have predictive validity. Measures designed to predict success in educational programs fall into this category, as do aptitude tests. They are designed to measure some current characteristic that is expected to predict something that will occur sometime in the future. Predictive validity is established by measuring the trait now and waiting to see if the event occurs as predicted. Once predictive validity has been established, the instrument can be used with confidence to discriminate between people on the basis of expected outcome.

Both concurrent and predictive validity can be used for the same instrument, as in the example by Selltiz, Wrightsman, and Cook.[7] A test was designed for insurance salespeople that attempted to predict their ability to sell

6. Walbek, N. H., and Gordon, V. C., Concurrent validity of three self-report measures of assertiveness, *Research in Nursing and Health,* 1980, *3*, 159–162.

7. Selltiz, C., et al., *Research methods in social relations* (4th ed.), New York: Holt, Rinehart and Winston, 1981.

insurance. To be validated, the test was first given to a sales force currently selling insurance. Scores were compared with the amount of insurance each person sold in the prior year. This established the concurrent validity of the test. The next step was to follow a new sales force for five years, giving them the test initially and then keeping track of their sales records and noting those who stopped selling insurance. The extent to which the test was able to predict the ability to sell insurance was determined by the accuracy with which it differentiated between successful and unsuccessful sales-people at the end of a five-year period.

This two-step process can be used to develop many instruments intended to predict success. First, concurrent validity is tested by giving the test to groups who are currently demonstrating the characteristic being measured: selling insurance, practicing nursing, and recovering from surgery. If it discriminates between degree of success and failure in a population currently demonstrating the characteristic, then it has some concurrent validity and can be tested further on other groups to determine its value as a predictor. The second step, predictive validation, involves a longitudinal approach, following a sample of people over time to validate the prediction.

In exploratory descriptive studies with no structured tests available and little knowledge of the characteristics held by people in your sample, you must depend on others in the society to point out this information. As a participant observer in a new setting, you often do not know who is a "good nurse" or who does the "best" nursing care plans, so you must ask other people in the setting to point out the person to whom you should speak. This is the most fundamental step in concurrent validation—the discovery of who possesses the particular trait or characteristic that you want to find. When you are in a foreign country or culture and you don't know the rules of the social system, you will rely on pragmatic validation procedures.

In participant observation you can use predictive validity also. Here, you ask your informants to predict what will occur in a given situation and then actually observe the event with the informant. Then, if something happens that was not predicted or happens differently from prediction, you can ask for clarification at that time. This is a beginning level of predictive validation prior to the development of a standardized and structured test or measuring instrument.

Construct Validity

Construct validity is useful mainly for measures of traits or feelings, such as generosity, grief, or satisfaction. The theoretical base for the concept is tested by determining the extent to which the instrument actually measures that concept. Construct validity can be determined using one of three approaches:

(1) contrasted groups; (2) experimental manipulation; or (3) the multitrait-multimethod approach.[8]

The contrasted groups approach is carried out by comparing two groups, one of which is known to be very. high on the concept being measured by the tool, and the other very low on that concept. For example, a group of recently bereaved individuals would be expected to score very high on a measure of grief, whereas a group of people who have not suffered any losses should score very low. The tool can be given to both groups and the scores compared. If the tool is valid, the mean scores of these two groups will be significantly different.

Experimental manipulation requires that an experiment be designed to test the theory or conceptual framework underlying the instrument. Such an experiment would have hypotheses that predict the behavior of people who score at various levels on the tool. Data will then be collected, testing the hypotheses to determine whether the theory underlying the tool is adequate to explain the data collected.[9]

The third method, the multitrait-multimethod approach, was proposed by Campbell and Fiske in 1956 to evaluate of the validity of measurement tools. This is the preferred method of establishing construct validity whenever it is possible to use it. The multimethod approach is based on the premise that different measures of the same construct should produce very similar results and that measures of different constructs should produce very different results. To perform this type of validity, you must have access to more than one method of measuring the construct under study, and you must be able to measure another construct at the same time. Thus, you have data from two or more tools designed to measure the construct you are studying *and* one or more measures of a different construct. If there is good construct validity, you will see a high correlation between the tools that are measuring the same construct. In addition, the measurement of the different construct will allow you to discriminate between the two constructs, and it will be clear that the tools are measuring different traits.[10]

For example, Galassi and others[11] have reported extensive construct validity testing on a *College Self-Expression Scale (CSES)*. This scale measures general assertiveness. The key concepts were determined to be assertiveness, self-expression, and self-denial. The authors correlated the scores of their CSES

8. Waltz, C. F., Strickland, O. L., and Lenz, E. R., *Measurement in nursing research* (2nd ed.), Philadelphia: F. A. Davis, 1991.

9. Waltz, C. F., Strickland, O. L., and Lenz, E. R., *Measurement in nursing research* (2nd ed.), Philadelphia: F. A. Davis, 1991.

10. Waltz, C. F., Strickland, O. L., and Lenz, E. R., *Measurement in nursing research* (2nd ed.), Philadelphia: F. A. Davis, 1991.

11. Galassi, J., Delo, J., Galassi, M., and Bastien, S., College self-expression scale (CSES). In M. J. Ward and M. E. Felter (eds.), *Instruments for use in nursing education research*, Boulder, Co.: Western Interstate Commission for Higher Education, 1979, 108–112.

with the twenty-four scales of Gough and Heilbrun's[12] *Adjective Checklist.* The two scales were found to correlate highly on defensiveness, self-confidence, achievement, dominance, exhibition, and autonomy. The new scale was shown to correlate highly with an existing measure on some of the concepts falling within the construct of assertiveness. Next, the CSES scale was determined to be different from similar constructs such as aggressiveness. Each step increased the construct validity of the instrument. Each step actually tested the theoretical construct of assertiveness, as defined by the authors.

RELIABILITY

Reliability refers to the consistency, stability, and repeatability of a data collection instrument. A reliable instrument does not respond to chance factors or environmental conditions; it will have consistent results if repeated over time on the same person, or if used by two different investigators. The reliability of an instrument says nothing about its validity. It can be measuring the wrong concept in a consistent, stable fashion. Reliability only means that the instrument provides consistent, stable, and repeatable results.

Even if you plan to carry out construct validation procedures on your measuring instrument, you still need to be concerned about its reliability. If an instrument could be proven to have *absolute* validity, there would be no need to test for reliability, as the instrument would automatically have perfect reliability. But because no measurement instrument can have absolute validity, we test for reliability of all instruments, and you will need to include reliability testing in your research design.

There are three methods of testing the reliability of research instruments: tests for the *stability* of the instrument (how stable it is over time), tests for *equivalence* (consistency of the results by different investigators or similar tests at the same time), and *internal consistency* (the measurement of the concept is consistent in all parts of the test). Each test of reliability looks at a different aspect of the instrument. When developing, adapting, or utilizing someone else's research instrument, you need to use one or more of these tests to establish the level of reliability of the instrument for your own use.

Tests of Stability

Stability is undoubtedly the best indicator of an instrument's reliability. *A stable research instrument is one that can be repeated over and over on the same research subject and will produce the same results.* Testing for stability, however, has one major

---

12. Gough, G. H., and Heilbrun, A. B., *The adjective checklist: Manual*, Boulder, Co.: Western Interstate Commission for Higher Education, 1979, 108–111.

limitation—it can be done only when you can assume that the trait being measured will remain constant over time. An example of a stable concept is intelligence. It should be possible to measure intelligence repeatedly, at regular intervals, and to obtain the same score. An unstable concept such as pain, on the other hand, is changeable and subject to frequent fluctuations even in persons with chronic pain. Repeated measures of pain in a subject would result in widely different scores. These differences would not mean that the instrument was unstable, but rather that the individual's pain was changing. This reflects expected differences due to changes in the variable being measured. Tests of stability will not be able to make this distinction. Thus, although stability is a good indicator of reliability when the variable being measured remains constant, it is not useful in the measurement of changeable or transient states. Tests of stability are in two categories: test/retest and repeated observations.

TEST/RETEST. The classic test of stability is test/retest. *Repeated measurements over time using the same instrument on the same subjects is expected to produce the same results.* It is easiest to visualize in the field of education for the development of reliable tests of knowledge. For example, a test is developed to measure knowledge of mathematics. The test is given to a group of students and repeated two weeks later. Assuming that the students have had no additional instruction in mathematics during the two-week period between tests, their scores will be very similar at both testings if the test measures reliably. Knowledge of mathematics is not a trait that is expected to change significantly according to the day of the week or the weather. Results from the first testing can be correlated with results of the second testing and a high correlation should result (+0.8 or higher). Any time you are measuring a relatively stable trait or characteristic, you should be able to ask the same questions and get the same answers every time, regardless of the individual's mood or frame of mind. A reliable questionnaire will give you consistent results over time. If the results are not consistent, the test is not considered reliable and will need to be revised until it does measure consistently. Test/retest is used primarily with questionnaires, but the concept of repeated measurement to establish stability can also be used with such tools as thermometers and hemodynamic monitors and in instances where the variable being measured is not expected to fluctuate.

Test/retest is used in interviewing as well as in examinations and questionnaires. Here the investigator interviews the research subject over time on the same topic. Assuming that the topic of the interview is a stable one, the answers to the same questions should be equivalent. The only allowable differentiation is that frequently subjects will remember more about a topic once interviewed and will expand on all subsequent interviews. Subsequent interviews will incorporate questions on the new material and be asked about as a test/retest. Test/retest would be an inappropriate test of reliability if you were interviewing subjects on "What did you have for dinner last night?" Dinner menus are expected to change. But if the question was, "What did you have for dinner last Thanksgiving?" the answers should be consistent from interview to interview with the addition of recalled food items between interviews. Then, these added items also should be recalled over time.

REPEATED OBSERVATIONS. When using observational methods of data collection, the test of stability of the instrument is called "repeated observations." This method has the same basic elements as test/retest. The measurement of the variable or trait is repeated over time, and the results at each measurement time are expected to be very similar. If you have developed an observational scale to rate nurses' behavior during the process of counting narcotics, you would expect that the same nurse counting narcotics three days in a row would have a similar rating each day. If you get different ratings each day, you will question (1) whether or not you have a reliable rating, (2) whether or not you are measuring a stable trait or characteristic, or (3) whether or not you are observing the same way each day (that is, whether you are a consistent observer). This last point is not a problem when your instrument is a questionnaire, but when you are using observation as your method of collecting data, an evaluation of your reliability as a data collector is part of the testing of the instrument.

Tests of Equivalence

When the concept or trait being measured is not a stable one, the reliability of an instrument cannot be tested by repeated measures. When a group of subjects is collected to test an instrument's reliability on a trait that is known to fluctuate over time, any testing will have to be done within a short enough time so that the trait will not have changed and an estimate of the consistency of the instrument to measure the trait can be obtained. *Tests of equivalence attempt to determine if similar tests given at the same time yield the same results,* or if the same results can be obtained using different observers at the same time. Equivalence is based on the idea of using alternate forms of measurement of the same trait at the same time and comparing the results.

ALTERNATE FORM. A test of equivalence using alternate forms of paper-and-pencil tests consisting of two sets of similar questions designed to measure the same trait is called *alternate form* testing. The two tests are based on the same content but the individual items are different. When these two tests are administered to subjects at the same time, the results can be compared just as with the test/retest method, only this time it is the equivalence of the two measures that is tested rather than the stability of one instrument. Obtaining similar results on the two alternate forms of the instrument gives support for the reliability of both forms of the instrument.

A number of alternative forms of objective tests are used daily in education. One form developed early was for midterm and final examinations for courses in the public school system. Here the instructor, using the same content but different questions, developed two tests for use in the same course. At examination time, two sets of examinations were passed out alternately to the class at the same time. In this way, if a student looked over another student's shoulder he or she would see a different test. In this case, the alternate form of the test is to prevent dishonesty among the students rather than to measure the reliability of the test, but the principle is the same. If one student were to take two forms of the test, the results should reflect the same level of knowledge if the tests are reliable.

Alternate form is used in interview situations in very much the same way as it is used in questionnaires. Because interviews generally take much longer to complete than questionnaires, the interviewer will not repeat all of the content in an alternate form, but rather will incorporate into the interview schedule a few questions that ask the same content in a different way. The way in which the subject answers the questions provides a measure of the consistency or reliability of the subject.

The major problem with alternate form questions is that they tend to be boring for the subject. When the questionnaire or interview is already very long, the addition of another questionnaire of the same length or even the addition of a few extra interview questions may be too tiring for the subjects, and you may actually be introducing new sources of error through subject fatigue and boredom. This is the major factor to consider when deciding whether you can use the alternate form method to test for reliability.

INTER-RATER RELIABILITY. This is the method of testing for equivalence when the design calls for observation and is used to determine whether two observers using the same instrument at the same time will obtain similar results. A reliable instrument should produce the same results if both observers are using it the same way. An observational tool designed to measure assertiveness in social interactions is an example of an appropriate use of inter-rater reliability. Two researchers observe an interaction together, and each one separately rates the assertiveness of the participants using the same scale. These ratings are then compared for equivalence. The extent to which they agree serves as a measure of the reliability of the tool.

Inter-rater reliability is the most common method of testing observational tools for reliability because it can be used with situations that are changeable. Most social interaction situations are not repeated, and so you will rarely get to do repeated observations to test the reliability of your observational tool. However, you can usually find another observer to work with you in testing the tool.

This method is also very useful to test the reliability of interpreting physiological tools. For example, you might expect that every nurse who reads a glass thermometer will read it in the same way and come up with the same results. Nothing is further from the truth. In actuality, thermometer reading can be quite unreliable unless the data collectors are all trained to read the thermometer exactly the same way specifically for the research project. Although the thermometer being used for the research may have been shown to be reliable on test/retest when read by one individual, when two different individuals read the same thermometer they may not arrive at the same numerical score. To test for the equivalence of their thermometer readings, inter-rater reliability testing is used prior to the onset of the actual data collection.

Blood pressure readings using a stethoscope and sphygmomanometer will also appear to provide unreliable data on test/retest when the reading is done with less than ten minutes between tests. This is because blood pressure readings change before and after the use of a tourniquet—a blood pressure cuff—so sphygmomanometers are known to result in different readings on a test/retest procedure. To test the inter-rater reliability of a blood pressure reading, a double stethoscope is used which enables two people to listen and agree on blood pressure readings at the same time.

The concepts basic to equivalence are the use of two measures using alternate form questions or two observers comparing their ratings of the same event using the same data collection tool. Equivalence is used in situations where the characteristic being measured is changeable and is not expected to remain stable over time.

Tests of Internal Consistency

Internal consistency refers to the extent to which all parts of the measurement technique are measuring the same concept. For example, when developing a questionnaire to measure depression, each question should provide a measure of depression consistent with the overall results of the test. In laboratory tests, this concept includes the idea that the results obtained from counting the red blood cells in one drop of blood from a specimen should be the same as those obtained from another drop of blood from the same specimen.

All structured questionnaires designed to measure single concepts, traits, or phenomena on a quantitative scale are tested for internal consistency to ensure that all items on the questionnaire are contributing consistently to the overall measure of the concept. Internal consistency is usually established in addition to tests of stability or equivalence that may be used as measures of reliability. Sometimes, however, internal consistency may be the only measure of reliability that can used with a particular instrument. If the trait being measured is a changeable one, test/retest cannot be used. If alternate form questions are not possible because the length of the questionnaires would prohibit asking subjects to complete two at the same time, then equivalence is not an option. Internal consistency will provide a useful measure of reliability in these cases.

Tests of internal consistency are based on the idea of *split-half correlations* in which scores on one half of a subject's responses are compared to scores on the other half. If all items are consistently measuring the overall concept, then the scores on the two halves of the test should be highly correlated. To provide a good measure of reliability, the division of the test into halves must be done in an unbiased manner. Random division is best since all choice will be removed from the researcher. Special statistical tests have been developed to provide measures of internal consistency for questionnaires. Cronbach's alpha coefficient[13] is the test most frequently used to establish internal consistency. Alpha correlates each individual item with each other item and the overall score, thus giving an overall measure of the consistency with which the score on an item can be used to predict the overall attribute being measured. In addition to providing a measure of reliability, it also assists the researcher in identifying individual problem questions. Internal consistency must be established before an instrument can be used for research purposes. Any new instrument that you might develop will require pilot testing before using it in your research project. If you revise an existing tool, you should treat it as a new tool for purposes of reliability testing, and even an established instrument should be tested for internal consistency each time it is used with a new population.

Internal consistency is a useful device for establishing reliability in a highly structured quantitative data collection instrument. It is not particularly useful in open-ended questionnaires or interviews, unstructured observations, projective tests, available data, or other qualitative data collection methods and instruments.

RELIABILITY AND VALIDITY ISSUES IN FIELD RESEARCH USING PARTICIPANT OBSERVATION

When research is conducted in naturalistic or "field" settings using qualitative or predominantly unstructured data collection instruments, repeatability of the research procedures and reliability of outcomes is difficult to achieve. The reasons are inherent in the setting itself. Field settings are in the process of change all the time. Social interactions between the same participants will differ from one hour to the next. What was studied one year will probably not be the same the next year in the same setting. The people have changed, the setting has changed, and possibly even the problem has changed—sometimes perceptibly, sometimes imperceptibly. For this reason, a second researcher

---

13. Cronbach, L. J., *Essentials of psychological testing* (5th ed.), New York: Harper & Row, 1990.

entering the field to study the same phenomena using the same data-collection procedures will be unlikely to replicate the original study and produce the same results.[14] Many quantitative researchers question the validity of qualitative field research, particularly when participant observation is the major method of data collection. In nursing, however, these types of studies are gaining more acceptance as we are able to see the wealth of data they produce about the behavior of people and to gain an appreciation for the value of this research.

Due to the problem with replication and control over the field situation, field researchers, of necessity, have developed strategies for ascertaining the validity and reliability of their research using slight modifications of the concepts discussed previously.

A significant difference between field and laboratory research is that in field research it is the researcher, particularly as a participant observer, that is the primary research instrument. It is the researcher, not a mechanical research instrument or measurement device, that collects and measures the data through observations and talking to people. The researcher, using participant observation as the major data collection method, is the principal research instrument.

Field research was developed by anthropologists and sociologists to study human behavior *over time* in natural settings. The researcher, as participant observer, either "lives with" the subjects as anthropologists do, or spends time collecting data by visiting the research site regularly over a long period of time. Fieldwork consists of a combination of the following data collection methods: participant observation, in-depth interviewing of "key informants," life histories, census taking, kinship charts (geneologies or genograms), collection of written and unwritten available data, photography (stills, movies, and videos), audio recording of events and interviews, observation of special and repetitive events, and participation with informants in all social events. The purpose of the researcher is to live the life of the subjects as much as possible, to learn the "rules" of behavior as well as possible by living them, and eventually to describe the social life of the people being studied from their perspective. Because data are collected using many instruments or data collection devices; because data collection occurs over long periods of time; because the researcher's training in field methods, objectivity as an observer, ability to record with clarity and precision, sensitivity to the nuances of behavior, and ability to ask relevant and clear questions are critical to the outcome of the research, the issues of reliability and validity and sources of error become very complex.

---

14. This was the famous case of Tepotzlan, where Oscar Lewis and Robert Redfield arrived at totally different ethnographic accounts of the same Mexican town. The fact that they talked to different people at a different time period and asked different questions yielded a different "picture" of the same place.

Issues of reliability are concerned with the consistency, stability, and repeatability of the informant's accounts and the investigator's ability to collect and record information accurately. When key informants are interviewed over time, their responses to the same questions on the same topic should be answered with essentially the same information. This is a type of test/retest of the same informant on the same material. To further test the reliability of the informant, the researcher tape records interviews, transcribes them, then presents the informants with literal transcriptions of the interviews for verification of what was said. Frequently these *verification sessions* will clarify the content as well as the verbatim terminology, expand on the information by clarifying unclear or incomplete materials, and essentially validate that this material is correct. Over time, this procedure is repeated with the same informant, until by the end of the fieldwork period, the material is considered both valid and reliable.

When the field researcher is interviewing an informant for a single time only, the use of alternate form questions within the interview itself is a standard test of the reliability of that particular informant. The same question will be asked in the same way two to three times during the interview as a test/retest. In addition, the subject will be asked two to three different types of questions on the same topic for alternate form reliability.

Several methods are used in the field situation to establish the reliability of the investigator. Because participant observers are often alone in the field and cannot use equivalence with another researcher, equivalence is developed by working with informants. Early in the fieldwork situation when the investigator is a stranger and unfamiliar with the rules of behavior and the setting, establishing equivalence of observation of events is critical. The investigator usually "hires" an informant, who observes the occasion also. The investigator then records the activity on the spot, either taking field notes, taping a running documentary of the events, or photographing events in stills or on film. (A written record along with photographic evidence has greater validity.) The written record is then reviewed with the informant for completeness and comprehensiveness of the coverage. Any conclusions or inferences drawn are also verified with the informant. This is also an excellent time for the informant to explain what has occurred and why (this discussion/interview is, of course, tape recorded). Taking along an informant during these observations is critical to the fieldwork, as questions about the event can be asked and answered at the time it is being observed so that discrepancies between what is observed and what is explained can be clarified. Also, the informant is more interested and involved at the time of the activity and so is more willing to discuss it. The researcher does not have to rely on anyone's memory of the event and thus avoids distortion caused by selective memory.

Validity issues are of greatest concern in field studies. Social desirability and acquiescent response set are as much a factor in field studies as in studies totally based on interviews, thus the fieldworker needs to try to minimize these sources of error. Although all field researchers usually give their final reports to their informants for verification, many informants will not critique the material. They may not want to hurt the investigator who worked so hard and still got it wrong; or they may deliberately want to keep their world a secret and want falsehoods to be published. Final reports are often shared with other researchers in the area as well as with several key informants, not just one. All comments are recorded to find discrepancies between comments and the final report.

A major method of verification of the truth of the data lies in the use of multiple methods itself. Here we are relying on pragmatic validation procedures. Interview materials are always verified by direct observation of the event, interaction, or person. Any discrepancy can be examined more closely. If you are studying mother-infant interaction, it is not sufficient to ask mothers what they do in particular situations; the field researcher knows that what one says is not always what one does. Therefore, observations of mother-infant interactions are critical validation procedures. It is insufficient to interview informants about birth customs without also validating those reports by observing birthing. Both the observation and the interview (verbatim to the degree possible) are reported. This establishes the reporter's verification procedures and assures the reader that the results are reliable.

The fieldworker always looks for written reports on the groups being studied whether they are reports of colonial officers, prior research reports, letters, diaries, newspapers, or historical documents; all are sought for verification purposes. The use of photography validates observational notes (concurrent validity) and also provides a means for repeated observations of the same event (stability). Tape recordings of interviews and social events not only allow for repeated replay (stability) but also can be used as the basis for further interviewing, for clarification of previous interviews, or to elicit new material.

These methods are all critical for an anthropologist working in a field setting such as an African village, particularly when the researcher is not facile with the language and the customs. When the researcher enters the field as a "stranger," everything is new and unfamiliar. Validation of learning is essential while you are becoming familiar with the setting. For the participant observer, fortunately, many social events and interactions are patterned and repetitive; through repeated observations many social rules of behavior are learned early. The observer then uses this knowledge (content validity) and through trial and error discovers what is being done correctly and what is being done incorrectly and why (pragmatic validation). Over time and with greater familiarity with the culture, more and more observations and interview data (both formal and informal) are collected and verified, providing—simply by weight of evidence—that the material is correct. Intensive interpersonal contact with research subjects over long periods of time provides repetitive, and sometimes overwhelming, amounts of data on the topic. The degree to which the field researcher has collected and transcribed data verbatim (in the subject's own words), has verified each transcription with the original informant, and has cross-checked all data against all forms of data collection, establishes the validity of the collected data.

RELIABILITY AND VALIDITY IN THE RESEARCH PLAN

In exploratory descriptive studies, validation procedures frequently reflect self-evident measures or, at most, pragmatic measures; they rely heavily on reliability tests. If you were interested in developing a research program designed to describe and eventually test certain types of nursing interventions, you might begin your program at the exploratory descriptive level by observing nurses intervening with patients in particular settings. You might be interested in specific nursing diagnoses found in the nursing care plans and observe each nurse at planned intervals as care relative to those diagnoses is given. You then interview these nurses to see what nursing interventions they said were used. Your observations are repeated over time as you observe the same nurse with the same patient. In addition, you observe different nurses with the same patient and the same nurse with different patients. To test for equivalence, you would need another person observing with you in certain selected situations, thus determining your reliability as an observer. By virtue of the in-depth study, you have utilized both self-evident and pragmatic measures of validity, as well as stability and equivalence as measures of reliability.

At the descriptive survey level of design, you need to be concerned with the reliability of your measurements, as accuracy in measurement is the key to a reliable Level II study. Instruments must be tested for reliability and validity, and frequently this is done in a pilot study. Even if the instrument has been previously tested in another study, it should be retested as part of your study because it has been shown that both reliability and validity can change over time. Neither is constant.

Level III experimental designs ideally require instruments that have construct validity. Only in this way can there be true confidence in the results of experiments. So few instruments in nursing research have reached the construct validity level of sophistication that studies often are carried out without the validation. This factor must be considered in interpreting the results of these studies.

Each level of research requires some facet of reliability and validity testing of the measurements, whether the research tool is you, the observer, a questionnaire, or a mechanical device. The point is that the results obtained from your measurement should be true results and not due to some error in your instrument. These critical concepts of reliability and validity can make the difference between good research and poor research.

SELF-TEST

The following is a series of examples of research measures used commonly in nursing studies. We first give you the item and ask you what kind of reliability or validity test you would want to use to detect either constant or random errors. Then we give you some answers. You may find other answers just as appropriate.

Test Measures

1. A 40-item questionnaire to measure knowledge of diabetes to be used in a before-after experimental design.
2. An observational scale to measure a nurse's assertiveness in role-playing situations. Responses to be rated as passive, assertive, or aggressive.
3. Blood pressure readings using a sphygmomanometer and stethoscope.
4. Twenty-four-hour urinalysis for sodium, potassium, and catecolamines as a measure of stress.
5. Unstructured interview designed to elicit patients' understanding of their diagnoses or surgery, to be subjected to content analysis.

Answers

1. You can use a test of internal consistency, Cronbach's alpha or Kuder-Richardson, and you can use a test/retest procedure on the control group as part of your before-after design. In addition you may build in alternate form questions as a test of equivalence. If the test was based on the literature on diabetes, and you have subjected it to a panel of expert judges confirming that it covered the material necessary for diabetics to know, then you have self-evident validity. You may use a different test in conjunction with this one as a test of concurrent validity. You also may use a test with construct validity.
2. If the observational scale is being used for the first time, ask two observers to use it and compare their results—a test of equivalence. If their results are discrepant, train them to use the scale, then give them another assignment and compare those results. If their results continue to be discrepant, either the tool needs revision or you need two new observers. The validity of the tool should reflect content validity—the items have been developed from the literature. Document the source of each item and write a rationale for inclusion.

3. The test of blood pressure has a physiological explanatory base, so the use of the instrument has construct validity. We must, however, check to be sure that the particular instrument we are using in our research is both valid (measures accurately) and reliable (is consistent). We can check its accuracy by comparing the results of our blood pressure equipment to another kind of blood pressure equipment. We can check the reliability of our observers by training two observers to use the equipment (equivalence) and providing a stethoscope with two sets of earphones so they can listen simultaneously and compare readings. We can check the reliability of the cuff by using it on a subject in a test-retest situation allowing enough time to elapse for the pressure in the arm to return to baseline.

4. These measures of stress must be validated and justified by the literature. If you are looking at stress as a short-term phenomenon (10-minute stress), is a 24-hour urine specimen appropriate to test the theory? To test your assumption, use a different measure of stress while collecting the 24-hour urine specimen. Compare results (concurrent validity). Urine is easily tested for internal consistency by sending two specimens from the same collection to the same laboratory and the same technician. If the results are identical, both the technician and the sample are reliable on test/retest. Two samples of urine can be sent to two different technicians for a test of equivalence of the technicians.

5. In unstructured interviews the subject has face validity—you assume the subject is telling the truth. You can build in a few alternate form questions for equivalence to see if they answer with the same information. The questions also may have face validity if they glean what the researcher wants to know. The questions also may have content validity if they are based on relevant literature. The interview can be pretested prior to the study in order to determine whether the subjects understand the question, if the interviewer asks questions consistently. Using a tape recorder to review interviewing techniques is a useful test of both reliability and validity.

RECOMMENDED READINGS

Appleton, J. V., Analysing qualitative interview data: Addressing issues of validity and reliability, *Journal of Advanced Nursing*, 1995, *22*, 993–997.

Atwood, J. R., and Hinds, P., Heuristic heresy: Application of reliability and validity criteria to products of grounded theory, *Western Journal of Nursing Research*, 1986, *8*(2), 135–154.

Beck, C. T., Content validity exercises for nursing students, *Journal of Nursing Education*, 1999, *38*(3), 133–135.

Brennan, F., and Hays, B. J., The kappa statistic for establishing inter-rater reliability in the secondary analysis of qualitative clinical data, *Research in Nursing and Health,* 1992, *15*(2), 153–158.

Brinberrg, D., and McGrath, J. E., *Validity and the research process,* Beverly Hills: Sage, 1985.

Brink, P. J., Issues of reliability and validity. In J. M. Morse (ed.), *Qualitative nursing research: A contemporary dialogue* (rev. ed.), Newbury Park, Ca.: Sage, 1991, 164–186.

Brink, P. J., Validity in field research, *Western Journal of Nursing Research,* 1990, *12*(3), 279–281.

Campbell, D. T., and Fiske, D. W., Convergent and discriminant validation by the multi-trait-multimethod matrix, *Psychological Bulletin,* 1959, *56*(2), 81–104.

Cline, M. E., Herman, J., Shaw, E. R., and Morton, R. D., Standardization of the Visual Analog Scale, *Nursing Research,* 1992, *41*(6), 378–380.

Cronbach, L. J. *Essentials of psychological testing* (5th ed.), New York: Harper & Row, 1990.

Cutcliffe, J. R., and McKenna, H. P., Establishing the credibility of qualitative research findings: The plot thickens, *Journal of Advanced Nursing,* 1999, *30*(2), 374–380.

de Monterice, D., Meier, P. P., Engstrom, J. L., Crichton, C. L., and Mangurten, H. H., Concurrent validity of a new instrument for measuring nutritive sucking in preterm infants, *Nursing Research,* 1992, *41*(6), 342–346.

Dobbert, M. L., *Ethnographic research: Theory and application for modern schools and societies,* New York: Praeger, 1982.

Duli, L. S., Measurement issues, *Orthopedic Nursing,* 1989, *8*(4), 56–57, 68.

Dunn, G., *Design and analysis of reliability studies: The statistical evaluation of measurement errors,* Oxford: Oxford University Press; London: Edward Arnold, 1989, viii.

Ferketich, S. L., and Mercer, R. T., Focus on psychometrics, Aggregating family data, *Research in Nursing and Health,* 1992, *15*(4), 313–317.

Ferketich, S., Internal consistency estimates of reliability, *Research in Nursing and Health,* 1990, *13*(6), 437–440.

Field, P. A., and Morse, J. M., *Nursing research: The application of qualitative approaches,* Rockville, Md.: Aspen Systems, 1985.

Froman, R. D., Owen, S. V., and Daisy, C., Development of a measure of attitudes toward persons with AIDS, *Image: Journal of Nursing Scholarship,* 1992, *24*(2), 149–152.

Fullerton, J. T., Evaluation of research studies: Part IV: Validity and reliability—concepts and application, *Journal of Nurse Midwifery,* 1993, *38*(2), 121–125.

Gibson, B., Selecting healthcare assessment tools: Putting issues of validity and reliability into a wider context, *Nurse Researcher,* 1998, *5*(3), 5–15.

Hinds, P. S., Scandrett Hibden, S., and McAulay, L. S., Further assessment of a method to estimate reliability and validity of qualitative research findings, *Journal of Advanced Nursing,* 1990, *15*(4), 430–435.

Hutchinson, S., and Wilson, H. S., Validity threats in scheduled semistructured research interviews, *Nursing Research,* 1992, *41*(2), 117–119.

Jalowiec, A., Murphy, S. P., and Powers, M. J., Psychometric assessment of the Jalowiec Coping Scale, *Nursing Research,* 1984, *33*(3), 157–161.

Kahn, D. L., Ways of discussing validity in qualitative nursing research, *Western Journal of Nursing Research,* 1993, *15*(1), 122–126.

Kerr, M. E., How reliable are your reliability measures? In R. M. Carroll-Johnson and M. Paquette (eds.), *Classification of nursing diagnosis: Proceedings of the tenth conference.* Philadelphia: J. B. Lippincott Company, 1994, 291–293.

Kirk, J., and Miller, M. L., *Reliability and validity in qualitative research,* Beverly Hills: Sage, 1986.

Lynn, M. R., Reliability estimates: Use and disuse, *Nursing Research,* 1985, *34*(4), 254–256.

Mishel, M. H., The measurement of uncertainty in illness, *Nursing Research,* 1981, *30,* 258–263.

Mishel, M., Methodological studies: Instrument development. In P. J. Brink and M. J. Wood (eds.), *Advanced design nursing research* (2nd ed.), Newbury Park, Ca.: Sage, 1998, 235–282.

Nolan, M., and Ruhi, B., Alternative approaches to establishing reliability and validity, *British Journal of Nursing,* 1995, *4*(1), 587–590.

Nolan, M., and Ruhi, B., Validity: A concept at the heart of research, *British Journal of Nursing,* 1995, *4*(9), 530–533.

Norbeck, J. S., Lindsey, A. M., and Carrieri, V. L., Further development of the Norbeck social support questionnaire: Normative data and validity testing, *Nursing Research,* 1983, *32*(1), 4–9.

Pelto, J., *Anthropological research: The structure of inquiry,* New York: Harper & Row, 1970.

Polit, D., and Hungler, B., *Nursing research: Principles and methods* (6th ed.), Philadelphia: Lippincott, 1991.

Thomas, S. D., Hathaway, D. K., and Arheart, K. L., Face validity, *Western Journal of Nursing Research,* 1992, *14*(1), 109–112.

Waltz, C. F. and Bausell, R. B., *Nursing research: Design, statistics and computer analysis.* Philadelphia: F. A. Davis, 1981.

Waltz, C. F., Strickland, O. L., and Lenz, E. R., *Measurement in nursing research,* Philadelphia: F. A. Davis, 1991.

Williamson, Y. M., *Research methodology and its application to nursing,* New York: Wiley, 1981, 154–168.

Ethics in Nursing Research

What happens to people who take part in research? Who is concerned with their welfare? Until recently, these questions received little attention. In the past, some researchers involved their subjects in research without obtaining their permission, gave false information about the subjects' role in the study, or involved people in physically and psychologically harmful experiments. Little attention was paid to the rights of subjects. The scientific contribution of the research was all-important.

Today, the rights of research subjects in all disciplines must be protected to the fullest possible extent. When subjects are vulnerable (as is true of patients), the research proposal must explain how subjects' rights will be protected.

As a result of the Nuremberg trials after World War II, a movement to protect human rights in research began. The world was so appalled by the biomedical experiments conducted on concentration-camp prisoners that a code of behavior for researchers was drafted. The Nuremberg Code was the first set of guidelines drawn up to protect the rights of research subjects. It was an excellent beginning but left out two major classes of research subjects: children and the mentally incompetent. The Helsinki Code (written in 1965 and rewritten in 1975 by the World Health Organization) remedied that omission by making provision for including children if parental permission was obtained and for including the mentally incompetent if proxy consents were obtained. In 1966, the Surgeon General of the United States issued guidelines to protect the rights and welfare of research subjects based on the Nuremberg Code. These guidelines initiated a system of review of research proposals at the local level (Institutional Review Boards) and accepted the notion of proxy consents.

Problems resulting from biomedical research were the subject of Senate hearings in 1973. Two of the most famous were the Tuskegee case and the Willowbrook case.[1] The Willowbrook case concerned an experimental design in which children living in an institution for the mentally retarded were injected with hepatitis virus. In the Tuskegee case, black male prisoners were used for a classic experimental design for treatment of syphilis. One group of infected men received no treatment, and their disease progressed to third-stage syphilis. These cases, among others, raised several ethical issues requiring a set of guidelines and principles on which to judge the ethical nature of research.

In 1974, Congress established the National Commission for the Protection of Human Subjects of Biomedical and Behavioral Research. This commission explored basic ethical issues of human subjects in research and identified principles to assist with the planning and conducting of ethical research. The 1979 Belmont Report summarizes the basic ethical principles developed by the commission over a period of four years. The principles address the major ethical issues found in health-related research and apply to nursing studies as well as to other fields.

As nurses become more involved in research, the issue of protection of human subjects becomes critical. The profession is responsible for establishing guidelines for ethical practices in nursing research. The International Council of Nurses developed a "Code for Nurses: Ethical Concepts Applied to Nursing"; unfortunately, however, none of the clauses within the code related to research.

But you may ask "Why do we need to bother about ethical guidelines for research? Aren't people protected by law?" The law is a written mandate for behavior, based on what people believe is good and bad behavior—their ethics. Before writing down laws, people must decide what they believe in. Frequently, laws are a set of instructions on what you are not allowed to do rather than a set of instructions on what you should do. Ethics is a set of moral behaviors, principles, and rules that determine which actions are right and which are wrong. Ethical judgments are the decisions a person makes on whether a particular act is right or wrong. Ethical rules for behavior classify certain events or actions as right or wrong. Ethical principles are even broader, serving as the basis for the ethical rules. Finally, ethical theory is the rationale that explains the principles and rules in a relatively cohesive fashion. Bioethics is the application of general

---

1. Veach, Robert M., *Case studies in medical ethics*, Cambridge, Mass.: Harvard University Press, 1977, 295–299.

TABLE 11-1	Legal/Ethical Matrix		
		Legal	**Illegal**
Ethical		Marriage	Rosa Parks
Unethical		Cheating on examinations	Murder

Source: Judith M. Saunders, RN, DNS, FAAN.

moral principles to the area of health/illness action and events.[2] When an ethical rule becomes law, people can be punished for immoral behavior. But not all laws are based on ethical rules and principles. You need to distinguish for yourself between an ethical issue and a legal issue. To help you do this, draw a 2 x 2 matrix like the one in Table 11.1, with "legal/illegal" on one axis and "ethical/unethical" on the other. Then fill in examples. Some things are both legal and ethical, such as R.N. licensure and marriage. However, the famous case of Rosa Parks illustrates the difference between a legal and an unethical rule. Rosa Parks, a black woman, sat in the front of a bus and refused to move. As a consequence of her action, she was taken to jail. At the time, it was illegal, in the area where she lived, for blacks to sit at the front of the bus. Rosa Parks's illegal but ethical behavior dramatized the civil rights movement in the United States. (We do not intend to make a statement about when an individual can or cannot break the law; we are only trying to show the difference between legal and ethical behavior.) Cheating on examinations is unethical but not illegal. There are no laws against it, but everyone knows that it should not be done. Murder is, of course, both illegal and unethical.

These are some examples of the difference between legal and ethical behavior. Because the law is frequently twenty years behind the moral codes of conduct, you cannot rely on it to set guidelines for ethical behavior. Therefore, you often need to establish your own guidelines.

PROBLEMS INVOLVING ETHICS

Anything that violates an individual's basic rights becomes an ethical issue. There are many such occurrences in research. Most violations arise from the difficulty of obtaining truly informed consent, whether this stems from the

---

2. Beauchamp, T. L., and Childress, J. E., *Principles of biomedical ethics,* New York: Oxford, 1979, 7–19.

subject's lack of understanding or the researcher's failure to inform the subject adequately. Expert views on the topic of informed consent vary widely, from those who believe that everyone has a moral obligation to participate in biomedical research for the good of humanity[3] to those who think that no one but another researcher in the same field can truly give "informed" consent.[4] The chances that the subject has complete understanding of the research and feels totally free to make a choice are remote, as most subjects are motivated by hopes of earning some ego rewards. If the subject is a patient in the health care system, however, there are additional constraints to free choice. The patient may feel it is necessary to please those on whom he or she is dependent, such as the physician or nurse. In nursing, as in other professions, the state of the art cannot move forward without research; therefore, human subjects must be solicited in order to test ideas and answer questions. The protection of the subject is the obligation of every nurse researcher.

In some cases, consent willingly given to participate in a research project is not informed because the subject is not aware of the true nature of the research. There are two methods of obtaining an uninformed consent. One is to give only partial information about the study, usually in general terms; the other is to give false information about the purpose of the study or the procedures to be followed. Both methods of obtaining consent are questionable in that both inhibit the right of free choice. The use of deception is considered more unethical than the withholding of information, although the line separating the two may be undistinguishable. Withholding of information is widely used in studies where it is believed that complete information about the purpose of the study will influence the subject's response. Thus, patients are told they will be participating in a study to "improve nursing care," when the actual question could be, "What are patients' attitudes toward male nurses?" or "What is the relationship between ethnic background and perception of pain?"

Another instance of withholding information is found in the use of placebos to compare the effect of the "real" treatment. Participants are not informed whether they are receiving the placebo or the real treatment. For example, when testing the effect of a new teaching method on diabetic patients' ability to control blood sugar, patients might not be told whether they are receiving the new or the old teaching method in an attempt to prevent this knowledge from influencing the results. These practices are so widely accepted that the patient's right to complete knowledge before consenting is rarely considered.

The President's Commission for the Protection of Human Subjects has considered the problem of withholding information from subjects. The report states strongly that such research can be justified only if the researcher can

---

3. Visscher, M. B., Medical research on human subjects as a moral imperative. In T. A. Mapes and J. S. Zembaty (eds.), *Biomedical ethics*, New York: McGraw-Hill, 1981, 148–150.

4. Ingelfinger, F. J., Informed (but uneducated) consent, *The New England Journal of Medicine*, 1981, *287*(9), 465–466.

demonstrate that informing the subjects would truly invalidate the research and not just cause the researcher inconvenience. In addition, there can be no undisclosed risks to the subjects. If these criteria are met, the research might be approved, but there must also be a plan for giving the subjects complete information *after the study is over.* Under no circumstances may the investigator lie to the subject, even though a direct answer may make that particular subject ineligible for the study.

Professionals use a number of rationalizations for withholding information from participants. One is that informed consent is necessary only when there is some risk for the participant. If the researcher determines that no risk factor exists, he or she concludes that the subjects do not need complete information about the study. Another rationalization is that researchers are obligated to give only the information that the subject requests about the study and that the responsibility for informed consent, therefore, belongs to the subjects. An assumption that often underlies this rationalization is that people are not really interested in the research question but only in what will happen to them as subjects. None of these positions can override the subject's basic right to autonomy and respect, and, therefore, none are acceptable practices.

Deliberate deception of human subjects was a common practice among researchers at one time. A number of outstanding studies based on deception produced far-reaching results and provided previously unavailable information about human behavior. This practice was based on the belief that the data would not have been obtainable if the subject knew the true nature of the research. For that reason, subjects were deliberately misled about the study or the experiment. In some cases, subjects received the results of the study after it was completed. In others, the subjects never knew.

Examples of deceiving research subjects include telling subjects that they are being tested for one thing when they are being tested for something else, not telling control subjects that they have received a placebo when they have come for the experimental item (such as birth-control methods), telling subjects that someone else is being observed and not they as subjects, and not telling subjects that they are involved in a research project even when they ask. As a general rule, the deception of research subjects should be avoided.

Coercion of Subjects to Participate

The assumption behind the concept of informed consent is that, given sufficient information on which to base a decision, the subject's consent to participate is made freely. However, there are various ways in which consent may be partly, or even wholly, coerced by the circumstances under which it is obtained.

Many times, the researcher is in a position to influence subjects' participation in the study. For instance, the researcher may be the subject's employer or teacher and thus may exert considerable control. An employer or a teacher may require that individuals participate as a condition of remaining employed or passing a course. Without question, this is coercion.

Another type of coercion occurs when patients are required to give consent to participate in research in order to be accepted as patients in a particular institution. This might happen in medical centers and specialty hospitals such as those specializing in the treatment of catastrophic illnesses. The patient is likely to feel that his or her "last chance" rests with that institution and, therefore, feels compelled to consent to anything.

Coercion also occurs when people are given the option to refuse but with the sense that refusal will not go unpunished. For instance, when a nursing supervisor brings questionnaires to a nursing unit, distributes them, and says she will be back to pick them up in an hour, at least some of the nurses are likely to feel that a refusal will offend their supervisor, even though they are given the option, perhaps thinking it will have an effect on their days off or their shift rotation.

Patients are particularly vulnerable to requests to participate in research when the person making the request is someone the patient must depend on for critical needs. The physician and the primary nurse can easily take advantage of a patient's vulnerability.

The ethical position is to recognize that people are never obligated to assist with research. Many times it may seem obvious that it will be to the advantage of the individual to participate in the research. Perhaps the individual will benefit from extra nursing care or a special teaching program. Perhaps employees will reap the benefits of shorter working hours, less shift rotation, or improved supervision. While this may be true, it is still the individual's right to decide; thus, although the advantages of participation can be mentioned as part of the information needed for informed consent, the decision should never be made for that person.

Withholding Benefits from Control Subjects

This issue is particularly critical for studies in which the new treatment would be of value to all the subjects, including the control group, or when a control group is deprived of something they had access to earlier in order to obtain a more accurate assessment of the new treatment. Both instances provide ethical dilemmas for researchers. Remember, however, the majority of control groups suffer no deprivation.

Sometimes problems with control-group deprivation occur because of the overzealousness of an inexperienced researcher, when, in fact, they are not necessary. For example, in a study to test the effectiveness of a preoperative teaching program on postoperative anxiety, the nursing staff was told not to answer any questions from the patients and families in the control group. This overzealousness deprived the control group of their expected privileges and introduced a new variable—withholding of information—which was not part of the research question. This kind of mistake can easily be identified in the proposal if the researcher addresses the topic of human rights for all subjects, including the control group.

In some experimental studies, the benefit of the experimental variable is so obvious that those who are cooperating with the researcher in carrying out the study will refuse to deprive the control group of the benefit. This kind of study is particularly difficult for nurses to carry out, as their primary responsibility is the care of patients and not experimentation. Dedicated nurses would find it difficult to deprive a group of patients of an obvious beneficial treatment, such as a simple relaxation exercise that relieves postoperative pain. If this difficulty could be predicted, perhaps control data should be collected before introducing the experimental variable, thus avoiding the problem for the attending nurse.

Sometimes, withholding benefits from the control group can be rectified at the end of the experiment by making the benefits available at that time. A method of teaching diabetics that has proved immensely successful could be provided for the control patients after the data have been collected. Remember, however, that this effort must be planned in advance along with the actual experiment, so that time and money are budgeted for carrying it out.

Invasion of Privacy

All research has the potential of being invasive, whether it is simple observation and recording of behavior or an experimental design. If you, the researcher, decide to take movies of persons leaving a bar, a church, or a jail, you may unintentionally be taking movies of people who don't want others to know where they were. When you show these movies publicly, you are invading the privacy of the persons you have photographed. When you go to people's homes for interviews, particularly when the topic is sensitive, you are again invading individuals' privacy; these persons have a right to refuse to participate in your research or to have all identifying data about themselves removed from your study.

Another violation of privacy is observing patients on wards when they are living in the institution. Patients have as much right to privacy in the hospital as you do in your home. Because their privacy is limited, it must be protected even more. Hospital records are private documents—not to be shared for the sake of curiosity. As private citizens, we have the right not to have our private lives spread all over the front page of a newspaper or be placed on TV for the purpose of research. Without our permission, researchers simply don't have the right to violate that principle.

INFORMED CONSENT

Just as all patients entering the health care delivery system have the right to know what will happen to them and to sign a consent form for any procedures, so do the participants in a research project. The protection of the rights of the research subject revolves around the concept of informed consent.

Informed consent has three major elements: the type of *information* needed by the research subject; the degree of *understanding* required of the subject in order to give consent; and, finally, the fact that the subject has a *free choice* in giving consent.

Information

All research subjects need to know in full detail what will happen to them during the research project. In order to receive consent, the researcher must explain the study and the subject's participation in the study. Therefore, the "informed" portion refers to the amount and type of information that should be given so that the research subject is thoroughly oriented. The information needed by research subjects includes: the nature, duration, and purpose of the study; the methods and procedures by which data will be collected; how the data will be used; all the inconveniences, potential harm, or possible discomforts that may reasonably be expected from the research protocol; the benefits to be gained from the study; the results, effects, and side effects that may come from participation in the study; and the alternatives available to the subjects. In addition, the researcher must inform the subjects that they may withdraw from the study at any time without prejudice. Subjects should also be told if they will receive any compensation for being in the study and, if so, what, and how any injuries resulting from participation will be treated.[5] In an experimental design in which the researcher manipulates the independent variable (such as in a clinical trial or clinical experiment), subjects must be told about the entire experiment, including the risks and benefits, and that they may be assigned to either the control or the experimental group. In order to give consent as informed, knowledgeable subjects, participants need as much data as possible to make a decision. Just imagine how you would feel if you were a research subject and found out about the hazards of the research later!

---

5. Code of Federal Regulations, 45 CFR 46 Protection of Human Subjects, PRR Reports, November 1978.

Understanding

The information given to the research subject must be presented in such a way that the subject can understand the study in its entirety. The researcher, therefore, is obligated to inform the potential research subject about the research so that the subject fully understands all the ramifications of the study. In order to do this, subjects must be informed in their own language, at their own level of understanding, and in their own common vocabulary. When health care professionals explain to patients that they must "void" or have an "EMG" right after they have been "prepped," they are not communicating in terms that most patients will understand unless the patient, too, is a health care professional. Therefore, all research or medical jargon should be eliminated from the information given to the potential subject. In experimental designs especially, language that is "loaded" in favor of consenting to participate in the study should be avoided as much as possible, as biased language does not provide the balanced explanation needed for full comprehension. Lay terminology rather than professional jargon must be used to describe the study.

Free Choice

This last aspect of informed consent implies that the subject should not be coerced, in any way, to participate in the study. Coercion in this sense ranges from mild coercion such as the offering of remuneration that may be irresistible to severe coercion such as threat of failure in school, refusal of treatment, physical punishments, and so on. When an individual feels coerced or threatened, choice is not free. Similarly, excessive rewards limit freedom of choice. The subject may feel constrained to act in one way or another. For this reason, subjects must be told that they are free to withdraw at any time before or during the study. In this way, the subject is ensured freedom of choice.

When you plan your research project, consider the issue of informed consent in your research proposal. Write down exactly how you intend to tell the research subject about the study. Write out what you will say in simple language and look up synonyms for words you think may not be clearly understood. As you write your explanation, make sure that the nature and amount of information your subjects will be given, as well as the steps you intend to take to ensure freedom of choice, are present in the informed consent portion of your proposal.

Obviously, not all research meets the criteria for informed consent. Many studies fail in one or more of these areas to protect the subject's rights fully, often because completely informed consent is impossible. The reasons vary— from using data from deceased subjects to giving subjects incomplete information so as not to bias the data. Whatever the reason and however sound, just, and reasonable it may be, all violations of the basic right of subjects to informed consent result in ethical problems for the researcher. These problems must be attacked in the proposal and may be so pervasive that the researcher should consider abandoning the study.

Proxy Consents for Research

Ethical guidelines for research demand that the subject's informed consent be based on enough information, comprehension of that information, and freedom to choose. There are certain groups in society who do not meet these basic criteria for informed consent. Those who are mentally retarded may lack the ability to comprehend; children, because of their parents' legal rights, may lack the right to make a free choice. Other groups who cannot meet one or more of these essential criteria are the comatose and the unborn. The researcher who wishes to study any of these groups has an additional burden to assume—that of assuring that the human rights of the subjects will be protected and obtaining legal permission (usually by proxy from the parent or guardian). Federal guidelines require that consent be obtained from the subject and permission be obtained from the guardian, if possible. If the subjects are children, the researcher must explain the study, at the appropriate level so that the child understands the explanation, and obtain consent from the child as well. Similar guidelines apply to the mentally retarded. If the subject cannot understand either the spoken or the written word, then only the permission of the guardian is required.

BALANCING POTENTIAL BENEFIT AGAINST ACTUAL COST

In all disciplines, scientists must develop new knowledge through research. In any research proposal, the researcher is obligated to weigh the potential contribution of the research, both to the discipline and to society, against the costs to participants in the study. In some cases there is no problem. Full, informed consent can be obtained from the participants; they can make a free choice based on sufficient information. In other cases, because of the nature of the question and the procedures necessary to elicit the required data, there is some violation of the rights of the subjects. The benefits of the research must be carefully examined in light of the cost of these subjects.

The process of weighing the costs and benefits is always a subjective one. The investigator will always be slanted in favor of the research. To reduce subjectivity, three areas should be addressed: *potential contribution to knowledge, practical value to society,* and *benefit to the subject.* The first includes the development of theory to explain nursing practice and an improvement in the consumer's understanding of health care delivery. The second involves improvement in the delivery of health care to the public and improved assessment of the health care needs of ethnic minorities. The third might be more rapid recovery from illness because of improved nursing care or increased understanding of preventive health measures. Addressing one or more of these three areas should produce substantial evidence to balance the potential cost to the subject.

The process of balancing potential benefits and costs requires analysis of degree as well as benefit or cost. How important is the problem under study? It is frequently difficult to say. Questions about current issues in nursing will assume more relevance and importance than those of interest only to the researcher. The same question can be asked of the potential cost to the subject. How serious is the potential infringement on the subject's rights? How much harm might it do? Is it likely to be fleeting or lasting? Answers to both questions will meet with considerable disagreement among colleagues. Once again, the researcher is likely to be biased in favor of the research; therefore, all possible resources should be used to help make the decision to go ahead possible.

Consultation can be obtained from a number of sources to evaluate the protection of the rights of subjects in the proposal. People who are interested in the same or similar research area are a valuable resource. You may obtain helpful advice on how to proceed from other researchers who have faced the same dilemma. There is one shortcoming to using colleagues: they may be as biased as you are in favor of the proposed research. It is difficult for one closely involved in the field to be objective about balancing pluses and minuses, and the tendency might be to view the potential contribution as much more valuable than someone not involved in the research subject would.

Persons with different backgrounds, from other disciplines, and even laypeople can help to assess the importance of both the contribution of the study to society and the potential effect on the subjects. Many nursing studies would also benefit from consultation with patients regarding their view of the dilemma.

Medical centers, schools, universities, and many hospitals have formed committees to review research proposals for the purpose of monitoring the protection of subjects' rights. These committees must approve proposals before research can be carried out. They do not relieve the researcher of the responsibility for protecting the rights of subjects, but they can provide consultation. Accustomed to reviewing proposals, these committees can sometimes help to put the study in proper ethical perspective for the researcher.

There are no easy rules for solving the ethical issues in planning research. The major consideration must always be the safety and well-being of the participants. After this, the research question should be looked at in relation to the rights of the subjects. When there is a conflict, priority must be given to protection of the subjects. If questionable practices are used in lieu of informed consent, they should be such that when subjects are told about them at the end of the study, the subjects will find the practices reasonable and express a willingness to participate again.

MAINTAINING ANONYMITY AND CONFIDENTIALITY

As a research investigator, you may find yourself in the position of having to promise confidentiality and anonymity to your subjects before they sign a consent form. The meaning of these terms is important. "Confidentiality" implies that you will keep all records closed and that only persons involved in the research will have access to them. Therefore, only you, the investigator, your research committee, and other researchers who wish to replicate your findings can have access to the raw data. Thus, your promise of confidentiality implies that you will screen individuals before they have access to the data. "Anonymity" means that you will not publish the names and addresses of your data sources and that you will make every attempt to group your data so that personal characteristics will not become known. Basically, you promise to publish or report your findings in such a way that the subjects will remain anonymous.

When promising subjects anonymity and confidentiality, it is wise to plan ahead for problems that might prevent you from keeping these promises. For instance, the institution where you plan to collect the data may expect you to share them with their administration. Parents may expect to have access to research data involving their children. Other researchers may request your data to use in their own research. None of these possibilities becomes a problem if you have planned ahead. The institution must understand and agree that it will have access only to the summarized results and not to the raw data. If this is not acceptable, either do not promise anonymity to the subjects or select another institution. Whatever the request for access to the data might be and however innocuous, no information should be released without the subject's permission.

All researchers should be aware that confidentiality of research data is not recognized by law. This means that research data can be subpoenaed for use in court and that a researcher may be required to testify about people who have been research subjects. When your subjects are heroin addicts, child abusers, and others who may have broken the law, you need to consider the possibility that you may be required to surrender your records or to testify against your subjects.

Before they consent to participate, your subjects need to be told that you intend to publish the results of your study. In studies of groups of people, it is frequently impossible to maintain anonymity of the group when publishing your findings. It may be the only group of its kind, so that, even disguising names and location, it is possible to identify the members. This possibility can prove embarrasing to the individual members, and they need to be aware of it before they can give full consent to be studied.

Your method of data analysis can cause loss of anonymity for your subjects if you are not careful. If, for instance, you are reporting findings in an attitude study of staff nurses, and you cross-tabulate them by shift, unit, and position, you may find that there is only one R.N. on the night shift of a particular unit, and her responses will be easily identified. To maintain anonymity, you may be required to omit some of your data analysis from the published report.

These potential difficulties in maintaining confidentiality can be avoided by planning ahead. It is not enough just to avoid promising what you "can't deliver." The onus is on the research to inform the subject that some or all of the data will become public knowledge or that some individuals other than the researcher will have access to them. Otherwise, the subject has the right to assume that all data will be kept confidential.

FEDERAL GUIDELINES ON THE SUBMISSION OF PROPOSALS FOR REVIEW

When you have written your research proposal, you probably will be asked to submit it to the Institutional Review Board (IRB) at your institution. If you plan to collect data in a hospital setting, or in the community, you will have to submit your proposal to those IRBs as well. All review boards have the same general guidelines, based on the federal guidelines; you need to be aware of these guidelines and how to incorporate them into your research plan.

The Code of Federal Regulations[6] was revised as of November 1978, and again on January 26, 1981. The code governs the development of IRBs, the function of IRBs, and their record keeping. You are responsible only for submitting your proposals to the IRBs according to their requirements for submission. From now on, the Health and Human Services regulations and those of the Food and Drug Administration will be nearly identical. In this way, research that crosses the two areas can have one format for the protection of human rights rather than two. The new regulations unequivocally state that only proposals funded by a federal agency must be reviewed. In the past, all research conducted in a setting funded by federal grants was reviewed, whether directly funded or not. Second, broad categories of certain behavioral and social science research have been exempted from review. These studies "normally present little or no risk or harm to subjects."[7] The exempted categories include research on normal educational practices and surveys, inter-

---

6. Code of Federal Regulations, 45 CFR 46 Protection of Human Subjects, PRR Reports, November 1978.

7. New Human Subjects Research Regulations Effective in July, Hastings Center Report, Vol. 11, No. 2, 1981, p. 3.

views, or observation of public behavior that does not in any way identify the subjects or place them at risk if their participation becomes known or that does not involve some sensitive aspect of behavior. The collection of available data such as documents, records, pathology reports, and diagnostic specimens is exempted if the information recorded maintains the privacy of the subject.

Certain categories of research that can be processed via an expedited review process include the collection of nail clippings or human hair, excreta, dental plaque, records of routine noninvasive clinical procedures, moderate exercises on normal, healthy subjects, as well as individual or group behavior or characteristics of individuals such as studies of perception, cognition, game theory, or test development.[8]

The new regulations place the burden of protecting human rights on the investigator rather than on the IRB, thus reopening the question of "who is to decide" whether a research proposal is ethical.[9]

If there is an IRB at your institution, ask for their guidelines on protection of human subjects and incorporate the relevant guidelines to protect your research subjects. If you are using animals in your research, you need to know how they are protected, and your institution will also have those federal regulations.

ETHICAL PRINCIPLES UNDERLYING PROTECTION OF HUMAN SUBJECTS

Three major ethical principles guide researchers: autonomy, beneficence, and nonmaleficence. Each is important, and each must be valued by the researcher. Different researchers, however, will emphasize one principle over the others or will rank order them according to their importance in a particular piece of research. Below, three principles are defined, then examples are given as to their use by different researchers.

Autonomy refers to the individual having the right to self-determination. People are considered individuals and not just members of a group. Individuals are not interchangeable. Each has worth, and each has the freedom to decide whether to participate in a research project.

Beneficence is the principle of "doing good" for another. Doing good for another person requires that someone make the decision that the act will be good for that individual. Someone needs to decide. The principle is fairly clear in a simple description of parent-child interaction. The parent teaches the child about dental hygiene to prevent tooth decay. The parent is "doing good" for the child despite the child's attempts to avoid the daily scrub. Our society also

---

8. Ibid, p. 3.
9. Hastings Center Report, Vol. 11, No. 3, 1981, pp. 9–14.

has decided that it is good for its citizens to be protected from infectious diseases. Some individuals, however, are allergic to the vaccine. In medical research, beneficence includes developing new treatment procedures as well as preventive interventions. These are all intended to benefit the patient.

The corollary concept is *nonmaleficence* or "do no harm." Both concepts are fairly obvious on initial reading but are never completely clear-cut. Nonmaleficence requires that the researcher do no direct harm although indirect and unanticipated harm may occur. This concept is specific to experimental designs in which the experimenter cannot intend harm to either the experimental or the control group. The Willowbrook and the Tuskegee studies described earlier are examples of maleficence—the experimenter directly harmed the research subjects to see what would happen to them. In the Willowbrook case, the children were infected with hepatitis, and in the Tuskegee case, the patients with syphilis were untreated. In both cases, there was direct harm to the subjects. At the same time, the researchers sincerely believed that they were acting on the principle of beneficence—doing good— by studying the effects of these diseases in a controlled experiment. Today, studies like the Tuskegee case are not allowed because we know the outcome of untreated syphilis.

The question posed by human subjects review committees is, "Can the information be found from any other source or with any other research methods than the one in which there is direct, anticipated harm to the subjects?"

These three ethical principles form the basis of ethical review of research proposals. Each is weighed against the other two. Assuming that the research protocol is sound, approval of the research will depend on the degree to which the investigator plans to protect the rights of subjects.

In an analysis of all professional codes of conduct, Veatch[10] concluded that the nursing code of ethics was heavily influenced by the principle of autonomy whereas medicine and dentistry were more influenced by nonmaleficence. Just as our professional codes of conduct emphasize one ethical principle over another, so do our research review committees.

From these three ethical principles, the following research issues are derived (see Table 11.2). The ethical principle of *autonomy* underlies several research issues. First is the issue of obtaining informed consent from the research subject by: (1) providing adequate information so the subject is able to judge whether to participate, and (2) providing that information in a form that is clearly understandable to the subject. The second research issue is that the subject must feel free to make the decision—there must be no known coercion to participate either overtly or covertly. There is an ordinal scale of pressure to participate, however, from mild pressure to extreme coercion. The

---

10. Veatch, R. M., Medical ethics: An introduction. In R. M. Veatch (ed.), *Medical ethics*, Boston: Jones and Bartlett, 1989, 1–26.

TABLE 11-2	Ethical Issues in Research

Ethical Principle	Research Issue

Autonomy	Informed consent
	   Information
	   Understanding
	   Free choice/proxy; no coercion
	   Anonymity/confidentiality

Beneficence	Benefit to: research subject; society; or to knowledge
Nonmaleficence	Avoidance of harm to research subject; reduce risks to subjects Weigh risks versus benefits
Social justice	Right to be represented in the sample; right to equal access to knowledge Right not to be discriminated against according to class or category

committee needs to establish where on that ordinal scale the particular proposal lies. Finally, issues of confidentiality and anonymity also are based on the principle of autonomy. A person has the right to privacy. Persons need to be told, if or when they lose their privacy, how this loss will be handled by the researcher.

The principle of *beneficence* underlies the determination of what good this study is going to do anyone. Is it going to benefit the research subject directly? If not, will anyone else benefit from the research findings? This determination is very important as, if there is any harm at all to the research subject, the good must outweigh the harm. In medical research particularly, the risk–benefit ratio is critical.

The principle of *nonmaleficence* simply reaffirms that no research shall be undertaken that has direct harm to the research subject as its primary goal. Although this may sound somewhat silly, an article in the *Western Journal of Nursing Research* by Hilda Steppe[11] poignantly describes what happens to the ethics of nurses when they live and work in a totalitarian environment. There are oppressive environments in which nurses work every day. They may not be as blatant or as maleficent as the one described by Steppe, but they may be just as harmful to the patient.

Finally, the principle of *social justice* is beginning to be discussed in research circles. Feminists argue from this principle when they protest the lack of

---

11. Steppe, H., Nursing in Nazi Germany, *Western Journal of Nursing Research*, 1992, *16*(6): 744–753.

women in samples ostensibly on human beings. For years, drug companies have avoided including women subjects on their drug trials on the assumption that they would "skew the data." Many drug studies, therefore, were done on male-only samples and the findings generalized to females. Feminists assert, and rightly, that women have as much right to know what will happen in their bodies when they take a certain drug as men do. This is the principle of social justice. The operationalization of this principle is to include both men and women in any study of human beings.

RECOMMENDED READINGS

American Nurses Association, *The nurse in research: ANA guidelines on ethical values,* 1968.

Anema, M. G., Ethical considerations in conducting clinical research, *DCCN: Dimensions of Critical Care Nursing,* 1989, *8*(5), 288–296.

Beauchamp, T. L., and Childress, J. F., *Principles of biomedical ethics,* New York: Oxford, 1994.

Beauchamp, T. L., and Walters, L. (eds.), *Contemporary issues in bioethics,* Belmont, Ca.: Wadsworth Publishing, 1999.

Belmont report: Ethical principles and guidelines for the protection of human subjects of research, Report of the National Commission for the Protection of Human Subjects of Biomedical and Behavioral Research, Department of Health, Education and Welfare, Office of the Secretary, Federal Register 44(76): 23192–23197.

Capron, A. M., Human experimentation. In R. M. Veatch (ed.), *Medical ethics,* Boston: Jones and Bartlett, 1991, pp. 125–172.

Cook, S. W., Ethical issues in the conduct of research in social relations. In C. Selltiz, L. S. Wrightsman, and S. Cook (eds.), *Research methods in social relations* (3rd ed.), New York: Holt, Rinehart and Winston, 1976, Chap. 7.

Creighton, H., and Armington, C., Legal concerns of research and nurse researchers, *Issues in Research: Social, Professional, and Methodological.* Selected papers from the ANA Council of Nurse Researchers Program Meeting, August 22–24, 1973, 18–30.

Davis, A. J., and Aroskar, M. A., *Ethical dilemmas and nursing practice,* New York: Appleton-Century-Crofts, 1978.

Davis, A. J., Informed consent process in research protocols: Dilemmas for clinical nurses, *Western Journal of Nursing Research,* 1989, *11*(4), 448–457.

Diers, D., *Research in nursing practice,* Philadelphia: Lippincott, 1979, Chap. 11.

Fleming, J., Human rights and ethical concerns of scientists, *Issues in research: Social, professional, and methodological.* Selected papers from the ANA Council of Nurse Researchers Program Meeting, August 22–24, 1973, 36–49.

Guidelines for conduct of research involving human subjects at the National Institutes of Health, 1995, http://helix.nih.gov.8001/ohsv/guidelines.html

Kite, K., Anonymising the subject: What are the implications? *Nurse Researcher,* 1999, *6*(3), 77–84.

Mapes, T. A., and Zembaty, J. S. (eds.), *Biomedical ethics,* New York: McGraw-Hill, 1996.

Noble-Adams, R., Ethics and nursing research 1: Development, theories and principles, *British Journal of Nursing,* 1999, *8*(13), 888–892.

Northrup, C., Data collection: Human research and the law. In S. D. Kramptiz and N. Pavlovich (eds.), *Readings for nursing research,* St. Louis: Mosby, 1981, Chap. 10.

Ramos, M. C., Some ethical implications of qualitative research, *Research in Nursing and Health,* 1989, *12*(1), 57–63.

Rankin, M., and Esteves, M. D., Perceptions of scientific misconduct in nursing, *Nursing Research, 46*(5), 270–276.

Smith, L., (1992), Ethical issues in interviewing, *Journal of Advanced Nursing, 17,* 98–103.

CHAPTER 12

Planning for Analysis of Data

The goal of data analysis is to provide answers to the research questions. The plan for data analysis comes directly from the question, the design, the method of data collection, and the level of measurement of the data. The choices you have made in these areas will both direct and limit what you can do to analyze your data.

The basic differentiation in plans for analysis is between *descriptive* and *inferential analysis.* Descriptive analysis provides description of the data from your particular sample; therefore, your conclusions must refer only to your sample. Inferential analysis, on the other hand, provides statistical support for the answer to your research question, allowing you to draw inferences about the larger population from your sample data.

Descriptive analysis includes content analysis of unstructed data, which results in summarizing the data into categories. It also includes presenting categories of data in tables or graphs that provide a pictorial description of the sample, the use of descriptive statistics to further describe individual variables, and the use of statistical analysis for the purpose of looking for relationships among categories or variables.

Inferential analysis always involves the use of statistical tests, either to test for significant relationships among variables or to find statistical support for the hypotheses. In either case, your purpose is to support your explanation of

217

the relationships among your variables, thus testing the conceptual or theoretical framework behind your study.

The data analysis is intended to provide the answer to your research question. Thus, it must be planned ahead along with the rest of your study. Too often, researchers stop planning after they complete their plans for data collection, thinking that the analysis can be done later. "Later" may bring a rude awakening when you suddenly discover that the data collected will not provide the answers needed. Then it is too late to plan the analysis. Keep in mind that you want to answer your question. Critically examine your data analysis plan with this thought in mind, and you will not become bogged down in a mass of irrelevant statistics.

This chapter will present descriptive analysis, followed by a discussion of inferential analysis. Because there are many excellent references for the actual performance of statistical tests, the tests will be discussed here only as they relate to answering the research question, and then only in general terms.

DESCRIPTIVE ANALYSIS

Within descriptive analysis there is a wide range of choices for planning the analysis of the data, from simple to complex. But descriptive methods all have one thing in common—they summarize the data. Summarization ranges from the use of content analysis to organize the data into categories to the use of descriptive statistics such as frequency distributions and measures of central tendency. A descriptive analysis might also include looking for statistical relationships among categories or variables.

The type of analysis you choose depends on how precisely you were able to measure your variables, the level of question you asked, and the number of subjects in the sample. Very imprecise, crude measurement is apt to be non-quantifiable or quantifiable only at the nominal level. Therefore, the analysis is limited to depicting the data summary in charts or graphs. You can categorize, list, and describe your findings, giving a graphic representation of how your sample might fall in each category. Then all that is left for you to do when you have collected your data is to describe how each case was different from or similar to each other case and on what dimension.

For some studies, this analysis technique is sufficient, particularly if you are using a new or different way of categorizing and describing your variable, or if you are describing something for the first time. On the other hand, you might want to investigate which categories are most frequently associated with others, which always stand alone, and which seem to vary depending on the interaction with one or more factors. Because you are exploring relationships, all possible combinations of these relationships need to be described and given some kind of rationale. Exploratory studies require the most time-consuming and detailed analysis of data of any research. Do not be fooled by the simplicity of the design; the analysis is the hardest part of this type of study simply because you know so little about what you are studying. And, obviously, from the literature review, neither does anyone else. Therefore, it is up to you, the one who asked the question, to describe in detail everything you observed so that your study is informative and capable of being replicated.

The time and effort involved in the analysis of exploratory studies cannot be overemphasized. The simplicity and flexibility of the design lead many novice researchers to think that exploratory studies are the easiest to conduct. These people obviously have not considered the analysis of data. Take, for instance, an exploratory study of stress reactions of hospitalized children. This study can be likened to a series of in-depth case studies of individuals undergoing the stress of hospitalization. Initially, the subjects are chosen for their similarity to one another: they are all children, and they are all hospitalized patients. Perhaps they even have similar diagnoses. However, as soon as you begin to observe them in depth, differences begin to emerge. The more you observe, the more differences you see. When you have finished data collection, there will be a tremendous volume of material describing a lot of different children and their reactions to a stressful situation. These data could be reported as a series of case studies in story form with no analysis on your part. But as an exploratory researcher, you are obligated to organize the data from these individual children in such a way that the similarities and trends can be examined as well as any differences. Further, when differences are described, they must be looked at in terms of other descriptive characteristics of the children so that tentative hypotheses can be formulated for further study.

In descriptive analysis, the process is very similar in all types of studies, but more precise measurement enables you to use more techniques in your analysis. The choice always depends first on your question and then on the type of measurement you plan to use.

Structured versus Unstructured Data

When you plan your data collection procedures, you choose one of the major methods of data collection: questionnaires, interviews, physiological measures, available data, or observation. Your plan for data collection becomes more structured at each level of design, so that no matter which method you choose, the level of design influences the structure of your data. At Level I, when you are doing exploratory descriptive studies, your data are predominantly descriptive and unstructured. At Level II, when you are comparing and contrasting two or more variables, your data must be far more structured, although you might have some unstructured data as well. At Level III, the experimental design calls for highly structured data collection techniques; if any unstructured data are collected, they will not be central to the hypotheses. The degree of structure of the collected data influences the ease and rapidity of data analysis. The more structured the data, the more likely it is that there will be a statistical program that is just right to answer your question. The less structured your data, the more likely it is that you will have to spend time introducing order to the data so that they make sense. Unfortunately, no one will be willing to read all your field notes, diaries, and interviews in order to find out what you studied. You must condense all that unstructured material into a summarized form so that it can be communicated to others.

Content Analysis: Structuring Unstructured Data

One of the most difficult steps in data analysis is to structure "unstructured" data. Whether the data are a result of participant observation techniques, projective tests such as Draw-a-Man, or open-ended interviews, the process is the same—to develop categories of answers and either describe those categories or make frequency tabulations of them. Structuring unstructured data takes both an extremely creative mind and an extremely analytical one. The fields of biology and anthropology have been based on this type of research. Sometimes, there is no preset structure into which to place the data; sometimes there is. When you categorize unstructured data, you are following in Darwin's footsteps. Darwin compiled an extensive collection of observations of the plants and animals he saw around the world. The categories developed from these observations formed the basis for the science of biology, provided the basic biological taxonomies used today, and represented the beginning of his theory of evolution. Collecting unstructured data still has a place in scientific circles, but knowing what to do with them is what separates the scientific, analytical mind from the simple observer.

The process of structuring unstructured data is called *content analysis.* Because all unstructured data are subject to content analysis, you need to be aware of the complexity of this process when you are planning your study. If the process of content analysis does not appeal to you, then plan your data collection procedures so that you do not need to collect unstructured data. Whether your unstructured data are the result of participant observation, interviews, or available data, the process of analysis takes the same form.

The first step in the process is to look for "themes" in the data. What are the groupings of similar data that fall into mutually exclusive categories? The term "theme" is used to denote the fact that the data are grouped around a central theme or issue. When you are looking over your data, sometimes these themes arise naturally out of the data themselves. Other times, you must make some decisions about how to organize the content.

A study on nurses' attitudes toward heroin addicts[1] resulted from an open-ended questionnaire of the nursing staff who were working with heroin addicts being detoxified at an inpatient psychiatric unit. One of the questions asked was, "People turn to heroin because . . .," and the nurses were asked to

---

1. Brink, P. J., Nurses' attitudes toward heroin addicts, *Journal of Psychiatric Nursing and Mental Health Services,* 1973, *11* (2), 7–12.

complete the sentence in their own words. The answers ranged from one or two words to an entire paragraph. To make some sense out of the answers, categories were developed that seemed to fit the answers. For example, one person said that people became addicts because there were people in their families who were addicts, or that they came from an environment where other people were addicts, or that they were psychologically "predisposed" to addiction. These three different responses came from the same person. Each was placed in a different category. If there were answers that presented some similarities and were different from others, they were grouped together. The final result was several major categories of answers that explained why nurses believe people turn to heroin and that accounted for all the answers given by the staff nurses. In other words, they were mutually exclusive, nominal scale categories. Some examples of the categories were social deficit, environmental causes, and "kicks" or excitement. Interestingly enough, the actual categories developed from unstructured data are dependent on the point of view and personality of the researcher. Another person could group the data in an entirely different way.

In a study of widow bereavement, Saunders[2] condensed each taped interview into 8 × 5 cards that reflected the major topic discussed during that interview. Each interview was then coded according to the month after death and the type of death. From the perusal of these cards, Saunders derived several concepts about widow bereavement. One of these she termed "uncoupled identity," which she saw as part of the transition from the married state to an independent state. This concept has provided new insight into the transitions that follow loss.

The last step in structuring unstructured data is to develop frequency tabulations for the categories you have developed. Frequencies indicate for each category how often that response occurred, how many subjects gave that response, and how many times each subject gave that response. Now you have completed the circle—from reams of data to a few categories. Your data can now be described in terms of how many times each response occurred. These frequencies can then be looked at in relation to the characteristics of the subjects.

One of the reasons this discussion on data reduction has been extensive is that many beginning researchers feel that qualitative research is the easiest form of research. So, they set out to ask open-ended questions of many people. But they don't know what to do with the reams of data they collect. To prevent you from making the same mistake, we may have provided an overly detailed description of the difficulties involved in content analysis. However, if you limit your sample size to fewer than twenty and limit the number of open-ended questions to fewer than fifteen, then you have a manageable first study. This type of study is exciting and fun to do if it

2. Saunders, J. M., Uncoupled identity: Process of widow bereavement, *Western Journal of Nursing Research*, 1981, 3(4), 319–336.

remains of manageable size. When it becomes unmanageable, it is less likely you will finish the analysis.

Reliability and Validity in Content Analysis

The subjective nature of developing categories for the data underscores the need for reliability as the responses are placed in the categories. The definition of each category should be clearly different from those of all other categories, and the results should be mutually exclusive. The simplest measure of reliability of this process is to ensure agreement between two or more persons analyzing the same data. These persons should agree which category best describes each response. It is up to you to develop the categories and to define them, after which anyone should be able to categorize the data. To establish the reliability of the content analysis, you need to have a random sample of your data analyzed by one or more people. This procedure is a type of equivalency similar to that used in estimating the reliability of instruments.

Validity in content analysis refers to the extent to which the categories represent the theme or concept on which they are based. In studies where the categories come from a theoretical or conceptual framework, their content validity must be established. This is done by explaining where they came from, why they fit the theory or concept, and how they measure a single theme or concept. If you are classifying nurses' responses to physicians as "assertive," "passive," and "aggressive," you must first relate the three categories to your conceptual framework and then show that they are on a continuum measuring one dimension of the theme and not three independent concepts.

Most exploratory studies do not have theoretical or conceptual frameworks; therefore, it is not possible to establish more than face validity for the categories. This is done by developing a rationale for the categories and their definitions and by showing that they are appropriate to the data. Face validity is further supported by the ease with which the responses can be classified into the categories and the apparent relevance of the categories to the research question. Further studies using these categories add support to their validity.

Structured Data: Statistical Analysis

A major concept in statistical analysis of data is the use of a frequency distribution to predict the probability that a specific event will occur. Descriptive statistics are used to communicate the results when there is no intent to generalize beyond the study sample. Inferential statistics are intended to determine the likelihood that the results of the study could have happened by chance (Streiner, 1986).[3]

---

3. Noman, G. R., and Streiner, D. L., *PDQ statistics* (3rd ed.), Hamilton, Ontario: B. C. Decker, 1999.

DESCRIPTIVE STATISTICS. The various methods of summarizing numerical data for descriptive purposes are only briefly discussed here, as they can readily be found in any statistics text.

Measures of central tendency—mean, median, and mode—isolate one response that is representative of the sample. Each requires a specific level of measurement. To have a meaningful measure of central tendency, the appropriate one must be used. The mean requires interval or ratio data; the median, ordinal data; and the mode, nominal data.

To arrive at a mean, the scores of the sample are totaled and the sum is divided by the number of scores. The mean represents the "average" score of the sample. You can use the mean with physiological variables such as blood pressure, pulse, and blood volume or with age, income, time, and other interval data.

The median is meant to be used with ordinal data, although you can certainly use it with interval and ratio data, as well. The median is simply a point on a scale where half of the scores fall above and half fall below. You can use the median with any rating scale.

When the measurement scale is nominal, the mode is the only appropriate measure of central tendency. The mode indicates the category that occurs with greatest frequency. In Table 12.1 the categories of "anesthetic" and "no anesthetic" were nominal data. The measure of central tendency from the data in that table indicates that "no anesthetic" is the modal category, as the majority of subjects fall in that category.

Measures of variation describe how widely the individuals in the sample vary. Are your subjects quite similar to one another, or is there a great diversity among them? The most often-used measures of variation are the range, the quartile range, and the standard deviation.

The range shows the highest and lowest scores in the group, or the extremes of variation. The range can be used with ordinal, interval, or ratio data. As an example, you might say, "The ages of the subjects ranged from 3

TABLE 12-1	Frequencies of Nonverbal Indicators of Stress and Use of Local Anesthetic		
	Anesthetic	*No Anesthetic*	*Total*
Relaxed	47	35	82
Tense	5	21	26
Total	52	56	108
	Chi-square = 11.5, d.f. = 1, p = .01		

months to 97 years." As you can see, the range is affected by extreme cases and gives no indication of what lies between the highest and lowest scores.

The quartile range gives the middle points between which half of the subjects fall. For instance, if the ages of subjects range from 3 months to 97 years, the quartile range might be from 45 to 60 years. That tells you that one-fourth of the sample is below 45, one-fourth is above 60, and the remaining half is between 45 and 60. Now you have a much better picture of the age range than you did before.

The standard deviation, on the other hand, is a measure of the average distance of each subject from the group mean. Like the mean, the standard deviation requires interval or ratio data. The standard deviation derives from the normal curve, so you know that approximately 75% of the sample falls within two standard deviations above or below the mean. Thus, if the mean age is 52 years and the standard deviation is 4 years, you know that 75% of the sample is between 44 and 60 years of age (8 years, or two standard deviations, above and below the mean age of 52).

If you have nominal data, the number of categories needed to represent a theme or concept indicates how much variation there is in the sample. If two diagnostic categories are sufficient to represent the range of diagnoses in the sample, that indicates less variation in diagnosis than if several are required.

Table 12.2 clarifies the different types of statistics used in descriptive studies and relates them to the level of measurement of the data. It will help you choose the appropriate methods of describing your data in Level I and Level II studies.

CROSS-TABULATION. The old saying that a "picture is worth a thousand words" describes the reason for developing tables. A cross-tabulation is simply a tabular presentation of data, either in frequency or in percentage form, or both, in which variables can be examined for any relationships among them. Cross-tabulations enable the researcher not only to look at the relations among variables but also to organize the data into a convenient form for statistical analysis.

The variables used to cross-tabulate the data are either the categories resulting from content analysis or the variables found in the purpose of the study. Although cross-tabulations are used mainly with nominal data, they can also be used as a first step in more complex analysis.

Imagine a descriptive study of stress in which the purpose is to describe patients' reactions to stress while in the dental chair. Data will be collected by observing nonverbal behavior and by measuring blood pressure, pulse, and palmar sweat volume. Data will be compiled on the procedures and instruments used by the dentist, the length of the procedures, and demographic variables from the patients. In this descriptive study, you know in advance what you will observe, how, and what instruments you will use to collect data. Most of the data will be in numerical form. In developing a plan to analyze the data from this study, you would start by cross-tabulating the variables.

TABLE 12-2	Selecting the Appropriate Descriptive Statistic	
Type of Statistic	**Level of Measurement**	**Statistic**
Measures of central tendency	Nominal scale	Mode
	Ordinal scale	Median
	Interval/ratio scale	Mean
Measures of variation	Nominal scale	Number of categories
	Ordinal scale	Range
	Interval/ratio scale	Standard deviation
Tests of relationships	Nominal data	Chi-square (X^2)
	Ordinal data	Spearman rank
	Interval/ratio data	Pearson r

The simplest cross-tabulation is a 2 × 2 table. In the dental patient study, look at nonverbal behavior ("relaxed" or "tense") according to whether or not the dentist used an anesthetic. (See Table 12.1.)

In this example, the categories are set up using variables found in the purpose of the study. In another study, they could just as easily be the categories that result from content analysis. The categories used in cross-tabulation must meet the same criteria as those developed in content analysis: they must be independent, mutually exclusive, and constructed so that there is a category for all observations. (In Table 12.1 there is no category for general anesthetic, so it is possible that it does not meet all the criteria.)

Cross-tabulations can be used to describe three or four variables, each one of which has multiple categories. Theoretically, it is possible to cross-tabulate any number of variables, but when more than three are used, the table becomes confusing to read and loses its major value, simplification of the data.

Table 12.3 illustrates the cross-tabulation of three variables. In this case, increase in apical pulse is used as a measure of patient stress during dental work and is examined in relation to the age and sex of the patients.

It is now possible to compare males and females in each of the age groups on apical pulse increase. This can be done for any number of sets of variables you wish to examine. Statistical analyses of data, including descriptive statistics, are almost always done on a computer. Most researchers now have access to a personal computer capable of using appropriate statistical software, and making the data analysis process readily accessible to all researchers.

TABLE 12-3	Relationships among Age, Sex, and Average Increase in Apical Pulse during Dental Work					
	Males			**Females**		
	20–30	*31–40*	*41–50*	*20–30*	*31–40*	*41–50*
Apical pulse increase						
>10/min.	25	60	10	30	40	25
<10/min.	75	40	90	70	60	75

If cross-tabulation is appropriate to your study, it must be planned in advance. As pointed out in the discussion on sample size, the number of variables you plan to cross-tabulate can affect your sample size. Therefore, it is wise to plot out your tables ahead of time. Make up some fictitious data while you are planning your tables. This will give you a good idea of what your results will look like; you can then be sure they will provide the answer to your research question.

PARAMETRIC AND NONPARAMETRIC STATISTICAL TESTS. Every statistical test is based on certain assumptions that tell under what conditions the test is valid. The line between parametric and nonparametric statistics is fuzzy. Parametric tests generally are based on strong assumptions about the population from which the observations (measurements of the variable) were drawn. If the population meets these assumptions, the parametric test is very powerful and, hence, the most likely one to reject a null hypothesis when it is, in fact, false. Nonparametric tests are based on fewer assumptions and are less powerful. They can be used to analyze data from populations about which very little is known. Since the nonparametric test is less powerful, it is sometimes safer to use with data from unknown populations because the risk of error will be smaller. This is particularly true when the sample size is small.

The parametric test can be used if the population meets the following assumption of parametric statistics:

Known Distribution
The distribution of the variable in the population is known. For many tests, the variable must be normally distributed in the population. The sample must be randomly selected so that its distribution is the same as that for the population.

Equal Variances

When two or more groups are being compared on some variable, variances of scores are assumed to be the same among the groups. In other words, the variances are homogeneous from group to group.

Equal Intervals

Because of the arithmetic operations used in computing parametric tests, the variables are usually measured on an interval or ratio scale. Ordinal scales are also acceptable under certain conditions.

Since the 1940s, researchers have insisted that measurement should be on an interval or ratio scale in order to use parametric tests. However, use of these tests with ordinal scales has not made a significant difference to the results of data analysis (that is, it has not increased the likelihood of a Type II error) and so it is now considered quite acceptable to use parametric statistics for ordinal data as well.[4] In previous editions of this text, we advocated the use of nonparametric statistics for ordinal data. We have, however, been convinced that the only time this is necessary is in the case of a small sample (less than 30). We still, however, discuss the equivalent nonparametric test whenever appropriate, so that in the event that you are working with ordinal data but a small sample, you will know which test to choose.

Nonparametric tests do not specify conditions about the parameters of the population from which the sample was drawn. They are sometimes said to be "distribution-free" and thus can be used when you do not know the distribution of the population. Also, there are nonparametric tests for use with nominal data. In behavioral research, we frequently measure variables on nominal scales. Therefore, nonparametric tests assume a prominent role in data analysis.

LOOKING FOR RELATIONSHIPS. In descriptive studies, the plan is to describe the variables and also to look for significant relationships among them. For instance, you may wish to know if patients' ethnic backgrounds are related to their responses to group therapy. Or you may wonder if education and income level are associated with career choice in high-school students. You may have a long list of demographic variables, and you want to know if any one or a combination of these variables is related to a student's success in nursing school.

There are several statistical methods of showing the relationships between variables, and some of the more commonly used ones will be discussed. Remember, however, that in descriptive studies, no attempt is made to draw conclusions about causal relationships from the data. Rather, hypotheses are

---

4. Armstrong, G., Parametric statistics and ordinal data: A pervasive misconception, *Nursing Research*, 1981, *30*(1), 60–62.

formulated from statistically significant relationships, and these relationships are later tested in more controlled studies from which causal relationships might be developed.

Chi-square analysis is designed for analyzing categories of nominal data that have been set up in cross-tabulation form. The Chi-square test is based on the assumption that if there is no relationship between two or more variables, then the likelihood of the individuals in your sample falling into the various categories of each variable is a chance occurrence. For example, in Table 12.1 if there is no relationship between stress (as measured by "relaxed" or "tense") and use of local anesthetic, then the 52 subjects who received local anesthetic should have an equal chance of falling into either category of stress; this chance would be the same for the "no anesthetic" group. The Chi-square test picks up the significance of any true departures from the frequencies that would be expected by chance. When you find significantly more subjects in one category than would be expected by chance, you can interpret this finding as an association between the two variables being tested.

In Table 12.1, a Chi-square analysis was done using the method described by Siegel.[5] The results indicate that there is a significant relationship between local anesthetic and nonverbal indicators of stress. The probability of the sample falling into the categories of "relaxed" and "tense" as they would simply by chance was less than .05 (the actual probability was .01); therefore, the results are considered to be statistically significant.

If your data consist of pairs of numbers (that is, two variables have been measured for each subject in your sample), then a measure of correlation can be used to tell if these variables are related to each other. For example, you might be planning to measure IQ and attitude toward women's rights, blood pressure and temperature, or self-image and body weight. A correlational test will tell you whether these pairs of variables have a tendency to vary together. Does blood pressure increase (or decrease) as the body temperature goes up? Is a negative self-image related to being overweight, and, therefore, does self-image go down as weight goes up? If the direction of the relationship is *positive* (both variables increase or decrease together), the numerical value of the correlation will be positive (somewhere between 0 and +1). If the direction of the relationship is *negative* (as one variable increases, the other decreases), the correlation will be negative (somewhere between 0 and −1). The strength of the relationship between the two variables is greater as the correlation approaches +1 or −1, so that a correlation of .9 is much stronger than a correlation of .3.

All measures of correlation require at least ordinal data. If you plan to have nominal data for one or both of your variables, use a Chi-square analysis instead. Ordinal measurements require at least a three-point scale to qualify as

5. Siegel, S., *Nonparametric statistics for the behavioral sciences*, New York: McGraw-Hill, 1956, 104–110.

an ordinal scale for statistical testing. A scale that measures "old/young" or "pass/fail," therefore, must be used as a nominal scale even though it has some degree of quality or quantity to its measurement.

If your variables are measured on ordinal, interval, or ratio scales, you will be able to test for correlation between your variables. The usual parametric test of correlation is the Pearson Product Moment Correlation (r). The correlation coefficient (r) obtained with this test tells us the extent and type of relationship that exists between two variables (that is, somewhere between $+1$ and -1, and either positive or negative). When you have obtained the correlation coefficient, a further test can demonstrate whether or not the coefficient you obtained is significantly different from what you would find from chance alone. If you use a packaged statistical computer program, the level of statistical significance will be given to you automatically. If not, you will find tables in most statistics books in which you can look up the "Critical Values of the Correlation Coefficient."[6] A rule of thumb to keep in mind to clarify the meaning of correlation coefficients is that the coefficient squared (r^2) is a measure of the *shared variance* between your two variables. Thus if $r = .5$, $r^2 = .25$. You can interpret that to mean that one of your variables accounts for 25% of the variance of the other. This is a considerable amount, but still leaves 75% variance unaccounted for. This illustration demonstrates why relationships between variables, even when statistically significant, do not support cause and effect. There are still other factors influencing these variables that are not part of your study.

If you wanted to do a nonparametric test of correlation, the Spearman Rho or the Kendall Tau would give you a correlation coefficient similar to that of Pearson r. If you are hand calculating your own statistics, you will find Spearman Rho easy to do by hand. Kendall's Tau, on the other hand, is available as an SPSS program for the computer.

INFERENTIAL ANALYSIS

In Level III studies, it is not enough to describe the data; you are expected to draw conclusions from those data. Statistical inference, based on probability theory, is the process of generalizing from samples to whole populations. The tools of statistics help identify valid generalizations and those that are likely to stand up under further study.

Statistical techniques are designed to objectively evaluate the outcome of a study and help the researcher to decide whether or not the results occurred by chance. Probability theory is the basis for this evaluation. Look at the following example:

---

6. Munro, B. H., *Statistical methods for health care research* (3rd ed.), Philadelphia: Lippincott, 1997.

Each research subject is seated in a room with two doors, one blue and one yellow. For ten minutes, loud music is played over the intercom. Then a voice tells the subject to leave the room. The researcher notes which door each subject chooses. When this experiment was done with ten subjects, seven subjects chose the blue door. The researcher concluded that loud music causes people to choose a blue door over a yellow one.

Is this a valid generalization? Of course not. The fact is that those results could be purely chance happenings.

Now consider another experiment. A drug was injected into ten healthy subjects. Within five minutes, seven were vomiting and the other three apparently were fine. The researcher concluded that the drug causes vomiting. Recalling the previous experiment with the blue and yellow doors, would you argue that the results of this experiment could also easily have occurred by chance? Let's examine the probabilities.

In the first experiment each person had a 50–50 chance of choosing the blue door, without the music being a factor in the choice. Seven out of ten is not enough to show a relationship between music and the color of the door when five of the ten are expected to choose either door by chance. In the drug experiment, however, the chance that seven out of ten persons would have started to vomit without exposure to the drug is extremely slim. Therefore, seven out of ten in this case may be conclusive evidence that the vomiting was caused by the drug. The results of these two experiments must be measured against different probabilities. Statistical analysis provides the means of eliminating most of the subjectivity that goes into the researcher's conclusions, thus separating science from opinion. This is done by using statistical models against which the results of research can be compared.

Because statistical procedures dictate some of the conditions for collecting the evidence, they must be part of the research plan. If planning data analysis is left until after the data are collected, often the optimal statistical technique cannot be used because some necessary condition of data collection was overlooked.

The basic steps in planning data analysis are summarized in Table 12.4.

Testing Hypotheses

The overall aim of experimental research is to determine the acceptability of hypotheses. The outcome of the study may be to retain, revise, or reject the hypothesis and the theory from which it was derived. To reach an objective conclusion, there must be an objective procedure for either rejecting or accepting that hypothesis. This procedure is based on the data to be collected and on the amount of risk the researcher is willing to take that the decision to accept or reject the hypothesis will not be correct.

TABLE 12-4	*Basic Steps in Planning Data Analysis*

Level I

Step 1: Content analysis of unstructured data.

Step 2: Descriptive summaries of data categories.

Step 3: Placing the data in charts, graphs, and tables.

Step 4: Tests of association between sample characteristics and data categories.

Level II

Step 1: Placing the data in charts, graphs, and tables.

Step 2: Correlational analysis of relationship among the variables.

Level III

Step 1: Placing data into charts, graphs, and tables.

Step 2: Analysis of the differences among the groups on the dependent variable.

THE NULL HYPOTHESIS. The first step in planning a decision-making statistical procedure is to state the null hypothesis. Null hypotheses usually state the opposite of what you expect to find, which means stating that there will be no relationship between the variables. The reason for using null hypotheses is that statistical tests are designed to reject rather than accept hypotheses. In this sense, rejection is an action word, whereas acceptance is a passive one. Active rejection of the null hypothesis is as close as you can come to proving your hypothesis. You never actively reject your research hypothesis, as it is never directly tested; only the null hypothesis is directly tested. Your goal in statistical analysis is to reject the null hypothesis, thus giving support to your research hypothesis as the alternative. Failure to reject the null hypothesis means only that you failed to support your research hypothesis with this particular study, leaving the door open for you to test it again under other circumstances.

If your hypothesis states, "During dental procedures, those patients given a local anesthetic will exhibit less stress than those not given a local anesthetic," the null hypothesis would be written as: "There will be no difference between the stress exhibited by patients receiving local anesthetic and the stress exhibited by patients not receiving local anesthetic during dental procedures." There are two possible alternatives to this null hypothesis:

1. Patients given a local anesthetic will exhibit *more* stress than those not given a local anesthetic; and

2. Patients given a local anesthetic will exhibit *less* stress than those not given a local anesthetic.

Since this latter alternative is the one predicted by your research hypothesis, you will apply a "one-tailed" test, which will reject the null hypothesis only if there is less stress among the local-anesthetic group.

Two types of error can be made when testing the null hypothesis. The first, called Type I error, is to reject the null hypothesis when it is actually true. The level of significance that you select for your statistical analysis is the probability that Type I error may occur. If the level of significance is .05, the researcher runs the risk that five times out of a hundred the null hypothesis may be rejected when it is actually true. You always determine the level of significance in advance so that the decision to reject or accept the null hypothesis remains objective.

The second type of error (Type II) is to accept the null hypothesis when it is actually false and should have been rejected. The probability of committing a Type II error can be decreased by increasing the sample size (which is another reason for having as large a sample as possible).

CHOOSING A STATISTICAL TEST: WHAT DOES YOUR HYPOTHESIS ASK?

Although the field of statistical analysis is quite complex, you can use some simple guidelines to help you choose the appropriate technique. The best indication of what general technique to use can be found in your own hypothesis. Look at what it says. Are you looking for a significant difference between two groups or among several groups? Are you interested in significant correlations between (or among) variables? Or are you trying to estimate what the population is like from findings in your sample? The technique you choose will depend on which of these questions your hypothesis is asking. Let's look at each one individually.

Difference between Two Groups

In some studies the subjects are randomly assigned to two groups, one of which is subjected to an experimental independent variable. In other studies, the sample is selected from two populations—for example, two ethnic groups or two educational groups. Both types of studies are interested in the same kind of data analysis. They ask, "Is there a difference between the two groups?"

The *t* test is the classic technique for analyzing the differences between the means of two groups. It is a powerful parametric test; thus, the data must meet these four assumptions.

1. The dependent variable is normally distributed in the population.
2. There are equal variances between the two groups (that is, they represent a single population).
3. You are using interval data.
4. The two groups are independent (that is, a single subject will not be in more than one group).

If your data do not meet these assumptions, a nonparametric test such as the *Fisher exact probability* test or the *Mann-Whitney U* test can be used to test for a significant difference between the two groups.

Sometimes you have two sets of scores from the same group, such as "before-and-after" measurements of some variable. In this case, you are looking for a change in scores from one measurement time to another, and you want to know if the change is statistically significant. Often a difference score will be obtained for each subject by subtracting one measurement from the other. The *t* test can be used to test for the significance of the difference if the assumptions are met. When the *t* test cannot be used, nonparametric tests for ordinal data include the *sign* test and the *Wilcoxin* test. The *McNemar* Chi-square test can be used with nominal data. These tests are all designed to analyze the significance of the difference in two sets of scores from the same group of subjects.

Difference among Multiple Groups

In reality, there are few studies that compare only two groups. A study is more likely to involve several groups, particularly if it is an experimental design. Your study may be comparing several groups on a particular measure and determining whether the groups vary from one another in the way they score on that measure. For example, you might include four groups receiving different patient teaching strategies and compare their postoperative anxiety levels. This could be tested using several *t* tests, but running multiple tests increases the possibility of a Type I error. To avoid this possibility, you can examine the differences among the groups through an analysis that looks at variation across all groups at once. This test is the Analysis of Variance (ANOVA). The resulting *F* test indicates whether any of the groups are significantly different from the others. It does not, however, tell us which of the groups being compared is different from the others. For that, further analysis is required, and several tests are available to clarify the source of the difference for example, the Tukey test for multiple comparisons or the Scheffé test.[7] ANOVA can be used for groups numbering from two upward (for two groups it will provide the same results as a *t* test). The ANOVA tests whether group means differ from one another. It requires that the independent variable be at the nominal level and the dependent variable be interval or ratio level. The null hypothesis assumes that all groups are equal, that is, drawn from the same population.

The usual assumptions for parametric tests are required for analysis of variance. If these do not hold, there are several nonparametric tests from which to choose. For nominal data, the Chi-square test can be used with multiple groups. Table 12.5 gives an example of what the Chi-square table might look like. The Chi-square test tells you whether certain ethnic groups choose any of the health care systems more often than would be expected by chance.

If the data are on ordinal scales, and you have small groups (<15 subjects per group), the *Kruskal-Wallis one-way analysis of variance by ranks* can be used. This technique tests the null hypothesis that the groups come from the same population or from identical populations with respect to the variable being measured. It is the most powerful of the nonparametric tests for independent groups.

Correlation between Variables

In Level II studies, the purpose is usually to find out if a significant relationship exists between two or more variables. The Pearson Product Moment Correlation Coefficient (*r*) is used when two or more variables have been measured on each subject and the goal is to test for a significant relationship among them. For example, in a study of obesity, you might be interested in the relationship between body mass index (BMI) and amount of daily exercise in your subjects. It is possible to use any level of data when calculating *r*. Even nominal data can be coded for use with *r*. Meeting the assumptions of the test, however, will ensure that the results can be generalized beyond the sample, which, after all, is the main purpose of a survey design.

The assumptions are first that the sample be representative of the population from which it was selected. Next, the variables (e.g., BMI and amount of exercise) must each have a normal distribution, and their scores must have equal variability. Thus, for every possible BMI score, the distribution of exercise scores must have approximately equal variability. Lastly, the relationship

7. Munro, B. H., *Statistical methods for health care research* (3rd ed.), Philadelphia: Lippincott, 1997.

TABLE 12-5	*Frequency of Selecting a Private Physician, Government System, or Health Maintenance Organization by Subjects from Five Ethnic Groups*					
Health Care System	**WASP**	**Asian**	**Black**	**Native American**	**Latin**	**Total**
Private physician	14	12	10	2	6	44
Government system	1	2	11	25	4	43
Health maintenance organization	3	14	20	20	1	58
Total	18	28	41	47	11	145

between the variables must be linear, so that when they are entered into a graph they would tend to form a line, rather than a clump or a curve.

The results of the Pearson *r* will provide you with indicators of the direction (+ or −) and the strength of the relationship between the two variables, along with a measure of the exact probability of this *r* occurring by chance. The significance of a correlation coefficient increases dramatically with the sample size, so that in a very large sample, a small correlation may well be statistically significant. The correlation itself may not be meaningful, as it may not explain much of the variance in the two variables. To counteract this possibility, the coefficient of determination *(r2)* is calculated to provide a measure of the meaningfulness of *r*, as it approximates the shared variance between the two variables. If the correlation between BMI and exercise were 0.7, for example, *r2* would be 0.49, and we could say that exercise accounts for half of the variance in BMI. The other half would presumably be explained by many other factors, such as genetics, age, or diet, making the relationship between BMI and exercise a powerful one.[8]

In addition to testing the relationship between two variables, one independent and one dependent, correlation can be extended to measure the relationship between one dependent variable and several independent variables, simultaneously. In Multiple Correlation, the statistic *R* can range from 0 to 1, and *R2* represents the amount of variance accounted for in the dependent variable by all the independent variables together. These tests of correlation are among the most commonly used techniques for the analysis of data in nursing research. With ordinal data and small samples, the nonparametric test

---

8. Munro, B. H., *Statistical methods for health care research* (3rd ed.), Philadelphia: Lippincott, 1986.

called Spearman *Rho* will provide a good test of correlation, and Chi Square is often used for nominal data to establish whether or not the observations could have occurred by chance.

Estimation of Population Parameters from Sample Data

Your hypothesis may predict a population parameter (such as the mean or variance) from the sample statistic. For instance, you might plan to use the mean IQ from a sample of registered nurses to predict the IQ of the whole population of registered nurses. An ideal estimator provides an unbiased estimate of the unknown population parameter. As such, it will correspond closely to the population value when a large number of sample estimates are averaged.

All the descriptive statistics discussed in the previous section are examples of sample statistics that can be used to predict population parameters (such as means, medians, and standard deviations). An individual estimate obtained from one sample, however, will not necessarily be an accurate estimate of the population parameter. It usually is necessary to take the average mean from a large number of samples to get an accurate estimate of the population mean. Because you will not generally use a large number of samples, you must establish the accuracy with which your sample statistic predicts the population parameter. This is done by the use of a confidence interval.

A confidence interval gives you a range of values within which the true value of the population parameter is estimated to fall. You decide in advance how confident you would like to be in your estimate (say, 95% or 99%). Then, instead of saying that the population mean is 80, you will say that you estimate the population mean to be somewhere between 75 and 83 and that you are 99% certain your estimate is correct. The range between 75 and 83 is your confidence interval.

Confidence intervals for the mean and standard deviation can be obtained using the versatile *t* test, provided that the observations come from a normally distributed population with equal variances and are measured on an interval scale. Nonparametric tests for establishing confidence intervals include *Tukey's confidence interval* for the median and the *binomial* test for the confidence intervals of quartiles.

Be Sure You Can Answer Your Question

The brief discussion of statistical analysis presented here has been for the sole purpose of guiding you to plan a simple analysis for a simple question. The major criterion for analysis technique is that the results provide the answer to the question. It follows from this that you must understand the technique. If you choose a technique that is beyond your understanding, it will be difficult to interpret the results of your study. It is better to be simple and sure than complex and incomprehensible.

THE ANSWER IS IN THE QUESTION

The plan for data analysis is intended to provide support for one answer to your research question rather than another. As we have emphasized throughout this book, the type of answer you require depends on how you asked the question. Look again at the table in the front of the book that outlines the three levels of studies. Now is the time to review your plan to make sure that it logically follows one of the three levels and that the answer you have planned will be the answer to your original question. If your plan is consistent and logical, the data analysis plan will help you distinguish the best answer among possible alternatives. So look now at your stem question, because it specifies the answer you need.

Level I Questions

As you have seen, Level I questions lead to exploratory descriptive research designs that, in turn, dictate primarily unstructured data obtained from small convenience samples. The quality of the answer you obtain depends on how successfully you have mastered the steps in data analysis.

You will have masses of data, both structured and unstructured, and your primary task will be to order those data into some form that can be described, tabulated, and perhaps even subjected to tests of association. Therefore, unlike the other two levels of research, Level I studies have at least two (and sometimes three) steps to the process of data analysis.

The two basic steps in the analysis of data at Level I are those of content analysis and frequency tabulations. You must make some sense out of the data and subject them to categorization of some sort. These categories usually will be scaled on a nominal scale, although occasionally an ordinal scale might be developed. As you develop the categories, you must define them carefully so that you know they are mutually exclusive.

After development of the categories, your content analysis will not be complete until you have verbally described what you found. This is called a descriptive summary of the data. You may want to go on to the next step and develop charts and graphs that further describe what you found. These charts usually include a summary of the characteristics of your sample as well as frequency tabulations based on your categories. These visual pictures of your results can help clarify your description of the data. These charts and graphs can include descriptive statistics so that the reader will have an even better idea of the sample characteristics (such as mean age and education level). To do this, you must have collected some structured, demographic data on your sample, so be sure to plan for this information even if the rest of your data are unstructured.

When you have completed these two steps, structured your data into categories, and compiled frequencies and descriptive statistics, you may attempt to do some tests of association if you feel this will enhance the answer to your question. (See Table 12.2 for the appropriate test of association for your level of data.)

Level II Questions

Questions at Level II ask about the relationship between (or among) variables and lead to descriptive survey designs and to structured or quantitative data. Answers at Level II require statistical analysis to determine the significance of the relationship between the variables.

The first step in the analysis of Level II data involves placing the results into tables, charts, and graphs. It is the same process as the second step of the analysis of unstructured data. At Level II, you always present a cross-tabulation of your variables, which would look somewhat like the following chart for the relationship between anxiety and pulse rate in preoperative patients.

	Pulse Rate	
	Low	High
Anxiety Low		
Anxiety High		

In this cross-tabulation, you need only fill in the number of patients who were highly anxious and had high pulse rate and those with low anxiety and high pulse rate. Then fill in those with high anxiety and low pulse rate and those with low anxiety and low pulse rate. Now you have a complete picture of the relationship between these two variables. A test of association will tell you if the relationship is significant. The tests of correlation in Level II studies involve both parametric and nonparametric tests, depending on the level of measurement of the variables.

At Level II, you have two steps in the data analysis. The first is to put the data into tables for descriptive statistics; the second is to test for the significance of the relationships.

Level III Questions

At Level III, your original "why" question leads to an experimental design for which you have developed hypotheses. Data analysis at Level III focuses on testing the hypotheses.

An experimental design provides at least two groups of subjects, and the hypotheses predict how these groups will respond in the experimental situation. The data analysis must test for the difference between (or among) groups. No matter what the original question asked, the analysis at this level will always examine the difference between/among groups, and this difference will relate only to the dependent variable. The independent variable has been manipulated by you, in that you have applied it, in its various forms, to the experimental and control groups. You have controlled extraneous variables through sample selection. Now you are ready to test your hypothesis: are the measurements of the dependent variable significantly different among the groups in the design?

The type of statistical test you will choose at Level III, as at Level II, depends on the level of measurement of the dependent variable and whether or not you can assume a normal distribution from your sample. These factors affect your choice of a parametric or nonparametric test. Table 12.6 will help you to select the best technique for data analysis.

TABLE 12-6	Selecting the Appropriate Test for Statistical Analysis	
Parametric tests	**Nonparametric tests**	
Assumptions: The distribution of the variable in the population is known.	Assumptions: Thought to be "distribution-free." Parameters of the population are unknown.	
Variables are measured on either interval or ratio scales.	Used with nominal and ordinal data, as well as with interval scales.	
Difference between Two Groups		
t test	Fisher exact test (small groups) (nominal data)	
	Mann-Whitney *U* test (ordinal data)	
Two Sets of Scores for the Same Group (Before and After)		
t test	McNemar Chi-square test for nominal data	
	Sign test or Wilcoxin test for ordinal data	
Differences among Multiple Groups		
One-way analysis of variance (*F* test)	Chi-square test for nominal data	
	Kruskall-Wallis one-way analysis of variance for ordinal data	
Correlations between Variables		
Pearson *r*	Chi-square test (nominal data)	
	Spearman rank correlation (ordinal data)	

RECOMMENDED READINGS

Abdellah, F. G., and Levine, E., *Better patient care through nursing research* (3rd ed.), New York: Macmillan 1986.

Abraham, I. L., Nadzam, D. M., and Fitzpatrick, J. J., *Statistics and quantitative methods in nursing: Issues and strategies for research and education,* Philadelphia: W. B. Saunders, 1989.

Brogan, D., Choosing an appropriate statistical test of significance for a nursing research hypothesis or question, *Western Journal of Nursing Research,* 1981, *3*(4), 337–369.

Eaton, N., Parametric data analysis, *Nurse Researcher,* 1997, *4*(4), 17–27.

Ferketich, S. L. and Verran, J. A., Technical notes: Exploratory data analysis—introduction, *Western Journal of Nursing Research,* 1986, *8*(4), 464–466.

Fielding, N. G., and Fielding, J. L., Linking data (Qualitative Research Methods Series 4: University Paper), Beverly Hills: Sage, 1986.

Krippendorf, K., *Content analysis: An introduction to its methodology,* Beverly Hills: Sage, 1980.

Kviz, F. J., and Knafl, K. A., *Statistics for nurses: An introductory text,* Boston: Little, Brown, 1980.

Lewthwaite, B., and Klassen, F., The cycle of life: An experience with qualitative data analysis, *The Canadian Nurse,* 1997, 24–26.

Miles, M. B., and Huberman, A. M., *Qualitative data analysis: An expanded sourcebook,* Beverly Hills: Sage, 1994.

Munro, B. H., *Statistical methods for health care research* (3rd ed.), Philadelphia: Lippincott, 1997.

Norman, G. R., and Streiner, D. L., *PDQ statistics* (3rd ed.), Hamilton, Ontario: B. C. Decker, 1999.

Notter, L., and Hott, J. R., *Essentials of nursing research* (2nd ed.), New York: Springer, 1994.

Pagano, R. R., *Understanding statistics in the behavioral sciences,* Pacific Grove: Brooks/Cole Publishing, 1998.

Rempusheski, V. F., Research data management: Piles into files—locked and secured, *Applied Nursing Research,* 1991, *4*(3), 147–149.

Reid, B., Potential sources of type I error and possible solutions to avoid a "galloping" alpha rate, *Nursing Research,* 1983, *32*(3), 190–191.

Siegel, S., *Nonparametric statistics for the behavioral sciences,* New York: McGraw-Hill, 1956.

Sweeney, M. A., and Olivieri, P., *An introduction to nursing research: Research, measurement and computers in nursing,* Philadelphia: Lippincott, 1981, Part IV.

Verran, J. A. and Ferketich, S. L., Residual analysis for statistical assumptions of regression equations, *Western Journal of Nursing Research,* 1984, *6*(1), 27–40.

Waltz, C. J., and Bausell, R. B., *Nursing research: Design, statistics and computer analysis,* Philadelphia: F. A. Davis, 1981, Chap. 6.

Watson, H., and McFadyen, A., Nonparametric data analysis, *Nurse Researcher,* 1997, *4*(4), 28–40.

CHAPTER 13

Writing the Research Proposal

From the beginning of this book, you have read over and over again that the research plan is the most critical phase of the research process, as it forms the basis for the rest of the process. As you know, it is easier to change a plan than it is to change an almost finished product based on a faulty plan.

Now that all the parts of the research plan have been considered, all that is left is to write a final proposal. Research and word of mouth are not compatible. Every part of research, from the beginning question to the final report, needs to be written down. Therefore, the research plan not written into a proposal is not complete.

You may be asking how we differentiate research plan from research proposal at this late date. In our opinion, the difference between the two is as great as that between your initial working definitions and your final operational definitions. The research plan is the basic outline of your entire research idea, with your bibliography cards, your working definitions, and so on. Your research proposal is your essay that fills in all the gaps of the outline, makes all the logical transitions for the reader, and shows the consistent development of the idea from question to answer.

The art of writing the proposal in such a way that someone else can follow your train of thought requires serious consideration. You don't want your project to be lost at this stage simply because you were inarticulate. This final step is worth the effort.

Every research proposal has a slightly different character, as you will notice when you look over those in the Appendix. The reason is rather basic— a research proposal reflects the personality of the writer. Although the basic parts of a proposal are identical and include every major point in this book, the way that you write each aspect of the proposal is a reflection of you.

There are two major parts of any research plan, whether you write it for yourself, for a class, or for a grant proposal: the introductory matter and the research design. Both parts are always present, though the titles may differ. Each part has its particular components, though they too may have different terms. Both the structure and the components within the structure are derived from the research question.

Chapters 1, 2, and 3 described the process of converting the topic of your research question into the problems of the research proposal. Because the research question is the basis for your research plan, and because the problem is the foundation of the rest of the research proposal, the emphasis on these two areas was quite deliberate.

Your research question is your guide to what you have to do and think and read and plan in order to arrive at your research proposal. Your question is an activity guide; your proposal is the end product. Put another way, your question is the process; your proposal is the content.

The difference between question and proposal is the same difference you found between the planning of patient assessment and the actual assessment in the nursing care plan. When you plan your assessment, you begin by gathering information from the patient, the patient's chart, and textbooks on the pathology and medical intervention and by looking up medications and treatments with which you are not familiar. You then put these data together, analyze them, and arrive at your final formulation of the patient's problems and needs. The culmination of all your questioning, reading, and analysis is written in a final form called an "assessment." You didn't write down your entire step-by-step process; you wrote only the end result.

The same process is used for the research proposal. The question guides and directs your activities; the proposal is your end result.

The basic structure and the components of the research plan are fairly standardized, and each component is based on the previous ones, thus we will discuss each of the basic components in turn. In addition, the concepts of reliability and validity of the research and the protection of human rights for the people involved also will be discussed even though their placement in the proposal is not standardized. Omitting them from the proposal would seriously jeopardize your chances of eventually doing your project.

THE INTRODUCTORY MATTER

You will rarely see the title "Introductory Matter" in any research report or proposal. Usually the titles are "The Problem," "Introduction," "Rationale," "Conceptual (or "Theoretical") Framework," or even "What This Study Is All About." Whatever the title, the purpose of the first section is to introduce the reader to the subject matter of the research. This part of the proposal should always include the "problem," the "purpose" (or "hypotheses"), and "definitions of terms." The order may vary, but not the content. We recommend that you use no title at all. The title of the proposal serves as the title for the introductory matter and is placed at the head of the first page of the proposal. Following the proposal title is the essay about the topic, the format of which is discussed below.

In nursing research, there is a tendency to write what we call "colon-ized titles" or titles with colons. There is no good reason for this practice. A thoughtful researcher can write a straightforward title for a research project that is brief and informative. Novice researchers tend to put everything into a title, which may take up half a page. You can see many examples of colonized titles in the list of references at the end of each chapter. Many of these titles could be a single, brief, descriptive title had the researcher taken a little time and effort. Remember, you can usually follow the title with an abstract if you want your reader to know more about your research.

FORM OF THE FINAL RESEARCH PROBLEM

The first portion of any proposal introduces the subject matter of the research, the rationale for selecting the problem, the literature to substantiate the rationale, and the direction the study will take. As you have seen, the problem derives from the topic of the research question. If you have thought through your problem well, the theory and the literature will substantiate your choice of topic. You don't need to be repetitive to get your point across. You can, however, subhead your problem according to the different theories or concepts that relate to your subject. But a well-written problem should introduce the entire research plan under the one heading.

Whether you end up with one page or twenty-six, the full and final research problem has the same form and shape. Like an essay, article, or term paper, the research problem has an introduction, a middle part, and a conclusion. In fact, your final problem has the same requirements as a good essay: you introduce your question, you point out the pros and cons for your argument, and you end with the statement of what you are going to study and why. The rest of the research plan is an expansion, an explication of your problem.

Your nursing research plan is only as good as your research problem. If you have a strong method but a weak problem, you will have a weak piece of research. Although the reverse is just as true, it's easier to salvage a weak method than a weak problem. There is nothing worse than using a sophisticated method to answer a trifling question. If anyone reads it, few will use it, and all your work is wasted. And because usability is a keynote for nursing research, you don't want your efforts to be considered irrelevant. So, for now, concentrate on writing the best possible problem. Not only will you have a sense of satisfaction, but your credibility will increase enormously.

The Introduction

Regardless of the length of your problem, you need to introduce your topic to your reader. All introductions follow the same pattern and include the same kinds of information. Your introduction does not need to be any longer than one paragraph—and a short one at that—but if it isn't there, it's like being pushed into a swimming pool with all your clothes on. The introduction is the preparation for the rest of your discussion.

Introductions are exactly what you think they are: they introduce the subject under discussion.

The first sentence in the introduction sets the general tone and direction for the subject matter. The middle sentence (or sentences) narrows the focus. The last sentence begins with such words as "Therefore" or "Finally."

We recommend that you use your original question as the first sentence of your introduction. This immediately sets the tone for the paper and lets the reader know exactly what your proposal is all about. You can rephrase your question or use it as written, but if you begin your paper with your question no one needs to hunt for your topic. Follow your question with a few brief statements about what your study is about and then state your intention to answer this question in your study.

One function of the introductory paragraph is that it tells the reader what the rest of the research problem will discuss; it is the abstract of your problem. The rest of the problem is an expansion of the introductory paragraph in which each sentence will be substantiated, argued, and supported. When you are writing your research problem, write the body first, then go back and write the introduction.

The Body

The body of the research problem is where you present arguments for your project, supported by your cited literature. Subtitle your problem according to the concepts you are discussing, or have one long uninterrupted series of arguments from general to specific. Whether you use subheads or not is up to you. But use descriptive labels for the content. Avoid terms such as "conceptual framework" and "theoretical framework" as your headings or subheadings. They are simply labels and do not describe the content you are using. Your problem could be headed with the terms you used for your topic in your original question and your subheadings can reflect the different areas you have looked up in the literature to support your choice of topic. Look at the way other students have headed their content areas in the proposals at the end of the book. Build up to your major point. Be sure that you account for the three major elements of the problem: rationale, literature review, and theoretical/conceptual framework.

Use your theory or concept outline and your references here. This is not the place to describe your sample or your methods of data collection. Both topics are dealt with elsewhere in the proposal, under their own headings, so do not waste this precious space detailing the method of data collection used by someone else. You may introduce it, of course, along with methods used by others, but the full exposition of your methods, the specific instruments, who developed them and what they found, is left to the design section. Fill in the outline with your reading. Paraphrase as much as possible. There is nothing more boring than reading a series of quotes. The readers want to know what you think, what your argument is; if they want other opinions, they can check the sources you have cited. So write this section as much as possible in your own words. When you cannot improve or paraphrase an author's statement, then quote, but only sparingly. When you are quoting (copying work verbatim) from one published source or document, you are allowed to quote up to 300 words, total, throughout your paper, without requesting permission, but for anything over that you must ask permission to reprint from the publisher. Once received, the permission is then cited as an acknowledgement at the beginning of the paper or at the end.

Use repetition only for emphasis. If you want to emphasize a point, paraphrase several authors who make the same statement. Or quote one, paraphrase another, and list several others who have said essentially the same thing. But use this technique only to emphasize major points. Otherwise, quote or paraphrase the originator of an idea or research and then simply list the authors who agree. You can type pages and pages of everyone's position on the same idea, but all that work will go unread.

Because you are using references to substantiate your points, you may find yourself beginning each statement with "Jones said," or "Maxwell stated," or "According to Pinchpenny." Don't worry about it as you are working on the first draft of your problem. But *never* let it stand that way. After you have finished writing the body and have exhausted every single argument for every part of your question, go back and rewrite every sentence that begins with "Jones stated" or "A comment by Jones et al." Reference Jones at the end of the quote or at the end of your paraphrased paragraph. The whole point in the body of your problem is to maintain the flow of ideas, not to list sources. When you introduce each sentence with a source, you are essentially writing a

Who's Who in the literature, not a statement of your argument. And the difference is critical.

This section of the proposal is also called an integrated literature review. All of the relevant literature is integrated into an interesting explanation of why this project is necessary and appropriate.

The Rationale for your Research

Every research proposal, whether for a student thesis or dissertation or for a major national grant, has an explanation of why the research is being conducted. Grant funding agencies entitle this section of the proposal "Significance." Student theses and dissertations have two sections: "The Problem" in Chapter 1 and "The Literature Review" in Chapter 2. Both sections are required in the traditional format. Whatever the label, this section supports the entire research process. This section explains why the research is being conducted in the way it is being conducted; why the variables were chosen for study; why the variables are expected to vary; and why the research instruments, the sample, and the data analysis are right for the study. In other words, the researcher's decision on what and how to do this piece of research is supported by relevant literature. The researcher writes what is known as an "integrated" literature review to support the rest of the proposal.

An integrated literature review is really an essay about the topic chosen for the research supported by the relevant literature. The title for this section is not "The Integrated Literature Review," rather the title should reflect the major conceptual topic(s) dealt with in the project. Look at the proposals at the end of the book. Notice how the titles of the proposals reflect the topic of the research. The titles are not all "Proposal." The same idea applies to the problem segment of the proposal. Label it by the content area and give the reader an idea of what is to come. Jennifer Medves' proposal is on Neonatal Cord Healing. Her problem statement, supported by an integrated literature review, should have that heading or something that reflects that content. When the reader sees this heading, assumptions are made about what the literature will cover. We can assume that Jennifer will discuss all the known forms of neonatal cord healing, all the research that has been done on those forms, and the pros and cons of the different methods that have been used to facilitate healing. Had she simply entitled this section "Literature Review," we would have no clear idea of what she plans to talk about.

As with an essay, there is a logical flow between paragraphs. The researcher takes us through a chain of thinking demonstrating how the research is an integrated whole. A mistake novice researchers make is to write an annotated bibliography rather than an integrated literature review. An annotated bibliography is a summary of each relevant article, with one article summarized per paragraph, strung together under a single topic heading.

Sometimes the student arranges these summaries by date of publication, sometimes in alphabetical order by author. This is not the correct form to present the literature base for the research.

The integrated literature review should be "representative" of the "body" of literature on the topic, not give the entire bibliography available on the topic. To make the review representative, the researcher has gone through an analytical process of culling literature that is not relevant, is redundant, or is based on secondary sources. You want the strongest argument for the study, so use the strongest literary support for the argument. The strongest literature review uses a variety of sources, not just one journal or medium, and represents the characteristics of the primary research.

One way in which researchers arrive at an integrated review is through the use of a conceptual map. (Some people find mapping the concepts in the research question helps them to visualize the entire process.) They begin by writing the central concepts on large sheets of paper. Then they try to indicate, by arrows, how each concept interacts with the other concepts. The concepts are represented by circles or squares, which are arranged in order of their importance to the project: central variables in the middle of the page, extraneous variables on the edges of the page. Then each variable is connected. Sometimes central variables are represented by large circles, with smaller supportive variables inside the circle. Use whichever way you find easiest to visualize how your concepts and variables work together in your research plan.

Once you have the basic visual map, list the articles dealing with those concepts and variables under that concept. (Some students find that putting these sheets of paper on the walls of their study room is extremely helpful. By doing so, for example, they may find that they have read a great deal on one variable but very little on the others.) The articles can be listed either alphabetically or chronologically. Sometimes the same article will be listed under more than one topic heading.

Another step in the process is to use a spreadsheet format (Table 13.1) with headings such as author, date of publication, source, variables studied, purpose and hypothesis, methods, instruments, sample, data analysis, and major findings and conclusions. As each article on the topic is read, it is entered into the database. When viewed in the spreadsheet format, similarities in certain articles become immediately apparent. Articles can be grouped according to methodologies or designs, sample sizes or characteristics, decade published, list of references, author(s), variables studied, or findings and conclusions. With every rearrangement, you can see more clearly new insights that were not possible when simply reading one article after another. These insights might be explicitly stated in yet another column of the spreadsheet. These rearrangements form the basis for the integrated literature review.

Sometimes a single author or researcher appears to be overly represented. In reading that person's work, you may find that they have quoted themselves extensively. This may be because they are the only person writing on the

TABLE
13-1

Integrated Literature Review Spreadsheet

Author(s)	Journal	Year	Purpose/ Hypothesis	Variables	Design	Sample	Methods	Reliability/ Validity	Analysis	Major Findings

topic, or they coined the term, or they created the area. If, however, you find many other authors writing on the same topic but this one author rarely cites the other authors, you may feel free to question their scholarship and include or not include their work in your review. (These issues become very clear if you have a heading for the major references listed.) When you see this, it is best to read the original work to be sure the author has been correctly cited.

Each of us has a different visualization process. You may have created a conceptual map of the variables and concepts in your research at the very beginning and used this as a basis for your literature review. You may have found that as you read, you had to expand (or contract) your conceptual map. The most complex maps to draw are, of course, the maps for experimental designs. That's because so much research has been done previously. Your independent and dependent variables form the center of the map, with an arrow indicating which variable influences the other. You know you must survey all the literature available on each variable, and the literature on all research that studied the two variables together. From that research, you discovered all the intervening variables that are to be accounted for in your study. You may have a separate column for these in your spreadsheet. You also map them. You need to indicate how and when these variables intervene in the action of the primary variables, and how they influence and counter-influence each other. The intervening variables must also be included in your integrated literature review. The next step is to map the extraneous variables in your study—those that may or may not influence the action of the independent on the dependent variable, but which are not of direct interest to the research design. If you planned ahead, you have a column for these in your spreadsheet. If not, you can always add a column. These variables also need to be discussed in the literature review. (Recall that the extraneous variables often include the research environment or type of sampling.)

Whatever your method of mapping or visualization, this process will help you to see what you need to include in your literature review and how to organize it logically.

As you develop the body of your problem, remember to leave the strongest, most central point for last. You are leading the reader along the path of your logic, and you want to make your strongest point just before the conclusion. You want to leave the impression that there is not one single "i" that has not been dotted, a single comma left out, or a point neglected. You have used and manipulated each point in your outline to its fullest extent, and you have led up to your research question—again.

The Conclusion

Like the introduction, the conclusion should be no more than one paragraph in length. Unlike an essay, in which the conclusion moves from the specific to the general for closure, the conclusion of the research problem serves as the introduction to the rest of the research plan. Your conclusion pulls all the strands of your argument together and ties up loose ends. It ends with your revised research question, written as a statement. Your question is better rewritten as a statement introduced by "Therefore, this study . . .," or "For this reason, this study . . .," or "As a result, this study . . ."

Your conclusion places your rationale, thinking, and arguments into one neat package. You want to leave the reader—and yourself—with the feeling that there is nothing further to be said, explained, or argued about your choice of topic. You have closed the door on this aspect of your proposal.

One way of writing a conclusion is to rephrase the introduction. Because the body of the problem simply expands and explains the introduction, the conclusion can restate the introduction with authority. In this way, the conclusion ties in with both the introduction and the problem, and the sense of completeness is achieved.

At the same time, the conclusion also leaves the reader on a high note, with a sense of anticipation of what is to come. This is achieved through the restatement of the research question that appeared in the introduction. Although this brings the reader full circle from question back to question, the answer and how it is to be reached are yet to come. The reader is fully aware of this if your problem is well written.

So, keeping in mind that you don't need to repeat everything you have already said, use your conclusion to pull together all the major points covered in the body of the problem, and lead directly into the research question. Remember: Keep it brief, keep it to the point, and keep it interesting.

STATEMENT OF THE PURPOSE OF THE STUDY

Once you have written the problem of your study in full detail, you need to state the purpose of the study in a separate section entitled "purpose of the study." Here you simply will head this section and write your purpose as shown in Chapter 5. Don't introduce your statement of purpose. Your problem has already done this, and another introduction will be redundant. So, just state your purpose under its own heading.

This is also the place in which you are required to write the series of hypotheses (if you have more than one) that you intend to test. Write your hypothesis as a research hypothesis, not as a null hypothesis. When you write the data analysis section of the proposal, you may rewrite your hypothesis as a null hypothesis, but under the section entitled "purpose of the study," simply state: "The purpose of this study is to test the following hypothesis . . ."

The statement of the purpose of your study is as simple as that. Set it off and state your purpose as a declarative statement (Level I), as a question (Level II), or as a hypothesis (Level III).

DEFINITION OF TERMS

The next step in your proposal is the section entitled "definition of terms." Here you will list the variables you intend to study (one or more) and operationally define them as you learned to do in Chapter 6. The "definition of terms" always follows the statement of "purpose of the study" so that the reader knows exactly what you mean by the key variables in your purpose. Check and double-check your definitions to be sure that you have included *what you mean* by the term and *how you intend to measure the variable.* Most proposals fall short at the operational definitions.

When you are at a Level I exploratory descriptive study, you will usually have one variable that needs to be defined—the central variable you are studying. You may find that the one variable has several components that also need definition. Go ahead and include all the operational definitions you feel are necessary for the clarity of your proposal. When someone looks over your final proposal for you, he or she will tell you whether you are being unnecessarily exhaustive.

At Levels II and III you need to define each variable completely, particularly at Level III. In fact, this is probably the most precise point of definition in Level III studies, and you will need to concentrate heavily on this aspect of your proposal. The definitions must relate closely to your theoretical framework.

You have now finished all the introductory matter in your proposal. You have introduced your research subject and explained the reasons for your choice; you have described whom you are studying; and you have explained the theoretical basis for your study and how you will measure your terms. You are now ready to proceed to the research design.

THE RESEARCH DESIGN

You may have noticed in the table of contents that the chapter on research design is subtitled "Blueprint for Action." That's exactly what the design is all about. It is your blueprint, or guide, to your activity. If you have ever seen the blueprint or plan for a house, you know that on one page is a master print of the building, which shows the number of stories and their basic outlines. You can see the number of rooms on each floor, the relationship of the rooms to one another, the placement of doors and windows, and so on. Succeeding pages deal with each room separately. The smaller the area being planned, the more specific the detail. Your research design follows the same principle. Your introductory material is your master plan; you are now going to deal with each section separately and in detail.

Although not required, it is often helpful to introduce the design with a general statement about what it will encompass. Frequently, this introduction states the general direction the research will take. When you identify and label your design, give it the appropriate title: exploratory, descriptive, correlational, comparative, quasi-experimental, experimental, historical, and so on. If you are not using all the required elements of a particular design, it is best to use a more generic label for the design. When you say, "This is a Level II design . . ." you are misusing the concept of levels. The level refers to the level of knowledge and/or theory about the topic, which in turn directs and guides the thinking and planning for the research. A level is not a name of a design. This introduction puts the reader in the right frame of reference and also makes you, the researcher, more careful in handling the rest of your proposal.

You should be aware at this point that the level of study you have chosen to do will be reflected in the amount of detail that goes into the research proposal. At Level I, when you may have absolutely no idea what you will find because you are doing an exploratory study, your proposal will not have the detail based on research findings that you will need for Level II. Level III studies are the most highly detailed and exhaustive in the review of literature and in relation to the experiment itself. Therefore, the design discussion of the proposal must be meticulously written and referenced, more so than at either of the other two levels. The reason becomes very clear after you have had some actual research experience. At Level I, most of the work of the research goes into the content analysis of the data and the final write-up of the project. At Level III, most of the work goes into the proposal because everything must be planned in advance. If you keep this in mind as you write your proposal, you will find it easier to understand what you have to do at each level.

THE SAMPLE

Following the introductory statements on the research design, you may describe either the sample or the methods of data collection. You will find it easier to describe the sample next, as it will be easier to discuss methods and procedures of data collection just prior to data analysis.

The heading for this section of the proposal can simply be "the sample." Other headings just as acceptable are: "criteria for sample selection," "sample selection procedures," and "sample selection." You may also find the heading "sample population" in published research reports. This heading is often used when the sample is the entire population. We don't recommend its use because the terms contradict each other.

Target Population

When you describe your sample, begin with a description of the population from which you intend to draw your sample. Describe the population in great detail, discussing who they are, where they are located, and when they can be found. Here is where you will probably mention whether or not there is a listing of your population anywhere and if that listing is available to you.

If you are doing a Level I study, describe your target population in as much detail as you possibly can. Because you may be doing a convenience sampling technique, your reader needs to know what you know about your population and just how representative your sample may or may not be. If you know nothing about your sample except what you have read in the literature, be honest and say so. If anyone knows the population you are referring to, it will be obvious in reading your proposal that you have no first-hand information. Don't try to fake it; just tell what you know. If you know anything at all about the people, describe them as best you can according to age range, gender, educational level, and so on. The demographic characteristics of a population need to be included here—if you have those data. If you are studying burn patients on X hospital ward, say so. If you are investigating runners, dieters in Weight Watchers, heroin addicts, or staff nurses, say exactly who it is you are studying.

Where you intend to study your population is also important information. If you intend to sample from the entire country, you need to let the reader be aware of the population to which you wish to generalize. If you are limiting your target population to a particular city, school, or hospital, say that too, because that is the population to which you generalize.

Give the time frame for your study here, as sometimes you will have to stop a study before you have achieved your ideal sample. You may want to have a certain minimum number of people in your study, but if you cannot get that number in the amount of time you wish to spend collecting the data, say so. Because your proposal will be sent to more than one place, have as much information as possible in it about your population so that you don't have to write several different drafts.

Sample Selection

Once you have exhausted the subject of the population from which you plan to select your sample, you can discuss the sample selection techniques. Because you have been precise about your description of the population, you have little left to do. At Level I, you will mention your sampling technique and specify the number of research subjects or time limits of the study. At Level III, you will have to spend a great deal of time describing precisely your method of assigning your population to groups and how you intend to go about it. Whether you are conducting your experiment in one hospital or several, you will have to describe the procedures explicitly and in detail, clarifying the number of experimental and control groups, how you intend to do the random assignment, how many you need in each group, what you intend to do about replacement, and so on. If you are using a matched sampling technique, you must detail the process of matching and on what variables. Again, precision and clarity are key at Level III.

If you are at Level II, remember that the method of sample selection is critical to generalizing your findings back to the population. The ideal method on which survey designs are based is the probability sample. Be sure when you are describing your sample selection procedures that you identify what type of probability sample you plan to use: simple random, stratified random, multistage, or cluster. Give your reason for the choice, state the sample size you intend to obtain, and identify the percentage of the population it represents. There are statistical programs available for estimating the power of your sample size. Be sure to include all the information you have. Then specify how you intend to go about obtaining the sample. It is not enough to say what the sample will be; you have to describe your "procedures" for getting subjects. Describe the numbering used in your list—and whether you will use those numbers or will assign new numbers—and then tell how you will use a table of random numbers to make your selection. It sounds tedious, but the more detailed your procedures are during the planning, the less error in the end. If you are not using a probability sampling method for your Level II study, you must explain why you are not and point out to your readers that your method is a limitation of your study.

You will need to discuss the concept of replacement at Level II or III. You want to have a specified number of people in your sample. What will you do about "dropouts," "no-shows," and people who refuse permission? Will you replace them, or will you go on without them? Here is where you discuss your method of obtaining an alternate list for dropouts using the same probability sampling technique you used to obtain the original sample. We recommend that you plan to use approximately 10% more subjects than you need as replacements. These problems must be discussed here along with the rationale for your decision.

It is easier to be detailed in the proposal stage than to make these decisions later in the study when the usual disasters occur. If you plan ahead for your sample (for every possible contingency you can think of) and write it down in your proposal, you have a guide for yourself to follow if things go wrong. So be precise, be detailed, and be complete.

METHODS AND INSTRUMENTS

You should now describe the method or methods you intend to use to collect your data. These include anything from questionnaires and interviews to projective tests or laboratory experiments. If you are using more than one method, you will need to explain your rationale for each method, how the methods interrelate, and why they are appropriate in view of your sample selection.

Your methods must be consistent with your sample. On the basis of the method selected, you are now ready to discuss which research instrument you have chosen to collect the data from your sample. You will need to explain why you have chosen this instrument, discuss its strengths and weaknesses, and outline what tests of reliability and validity have been done on the instrument and on what populations it has been used before. If you have decided to develop your own instrument, the same type of rationale must be presented. Always keep in mind that the instruments must be consistent with the methods.

Here again, you will need to have reviewed the literature thoroughly in order to present the arguments for your choice of instruments with an authoritative voice.

RELIABILITY AND VALIDITY

When you are discussing your research instrument or instruments, incorporate your discussion of reliability and validity testing in that section. Entitle that section "procedures for establishing reliability and validity of _____ instrument," and then describe what you will do and how you will do it. If you are planning to do a test of internal consistency by a split-half correlation, describe how you will do it, which test you will use, and what correlation you will accept. The same would be true for an alternate form test or a series of repeated observations or test-retest situations. Establishing face and content validity are discussed by a review of the literature, and the use of a judge panel to determine universe of content. Concurrent validation procedures are described by contrasting your instrument with the research findings from another instrument. If you are using an instrument that only has face validity, you will need to judge its content validity and perhaps test its concurrent validity and establish why the test is as good as the one you used for comparison. If you prefer, you may have a separate section just for these issues, particularly if you are planning to develop your own research instrument. If you are doing participant observation, describe how you will attempt to ensure that your research instrument is reliable, valid, or both. It's easier to discuss reliability and validity of data collection when you are using someone else's instruments. Simply describe how those were tested, if you know, and indicate how you intend to test them for your study.

In Level I studies, you will need to discuss reliability and validity issues in content analysis. You may discuss this subject either under the heading "data analysis" or under a separate heading. The choice is up to you.

Level III experimental designs require detailed testing of the theories underlying the experiments, and a discussion of the reliability and validity of the tests is a major focus of the proposal. You can still decide whether to discuss these concepts separately or in conjunction with the data collection procedures. If you deal with them separately, you may find that you have a more complete discussion of both the instrument and its tests. If you discuss them together, you may overlook certain details critical to your plan. But again, it is up to you.

Remember that reliability and validity refer to the methods used by researchers to attempt to eliminate error or to account for the error that will occur. So when you are writing your proposal, this section is a very important one that needs particular attention.

DATA ANALYSIS

This is probably the easiest part of the research proposal to write, because it usually follows the data collection section as a separate section.

Because data analysis procedures follow directly from sample selection and data collection techniques, you should know precisely which analytical technique you will use. You can either describe the steps in detail or name the analytical tools your will use. So long as you know in advance how you will analyze your data, and say so, you are in fine shape. Although this might be the hardest part of the proposal for you to do, it's probably the easiest to write. Go back to the tables in Chapter 12 on data analysis (Tables 12.4 and 12.6), check how many steps are involved at each level of research design, look up the measurement scale you intend to use, and find the appropriate research data analysis technique. That's really all there is to it.

PROTECTION OF HUMAN SUBJECTS

This last section of your research proposal should describe in detail exactly how you intend to protect the rights of your sample. You need to include statements on how you intend to obtain their informed consent to be research subjects, how you intend to protect their anonymity as research subjects (make sure that no one can possibly know who they are), and how you intend to explain your research to them so that they can understand it. Here you will probably want to write a complete statement of what you will say to them, beginning with "Hello, my name is . . . "

If you are a student, you may be asked to submit your research proposal to your Institutional Review Board (IRB) for the protection of human rights. If you are a staff member, your hospital or agency will have an IRB to which you will be expected to submit your research proposal. Always follow their format to describe the protection of human rights for your sample. You can also submit your entire research proposal, so that they have a complete understanding of your project.

One of the key issues on which IRBs base their decisions is weighing the benefits against the risks of a study. This is an aspect of your statement of the protection of human subjects that you simply cannot neglect. If you can see no possible benefit to humanity from your study (except to yourself because you will get your degree from it), no one will approve it. "No benefit" cannot possibly outweigh even the slightest risk. Remember, every time you do research, you are posing some degree of risk to someone in your sample, as you are intruding in their lives. No matter how slight, it is still a risk. Any kind of risk needs to be counterbalanced by some kind of benefit. So, don't neglect this aspect of your proposal.

You will need to include a copy of the informed consent statement that you are going to ask your subjects to sign or a complete transcription of an oral informed consent statement and an explanation of why you will not have it signed. You will also want to include your rationale for having, or not having, a witness present.

SUMMARY

You now have completed the basic outline for the research design section of the proposal. You will have noticed that each section follows directly from the previous ones. Over and over you keep reading that this must be consistent with that. As each section is based on the previous ones, they must be logically related. But you must show this relationship. You must make the connection, and close any gaps. In other words, don't throw something into a section because it looks sophisticated. If it doesn't fit, don't use it. If it wasn't introduced, it doesn't belong.

And, finally, you will have noticed that from time to time in this book a reference was made to looking up something in the literature. You weren't really finished with your literature review when you wrote your problem. Every item in your proposal should command authority. If you don't know enough about reliability and validity, look them up. If you don't know which method of data analysis to use, look it up. If you don't know anything about your sample or your methods, go to the literature. No one else can do this for you. Because you have to have a rationale for every part of the proposal, make sure your rationale is based on fact, not hearsay. By the end of your proposal you are not just an expert in your content area; you are an expert on the people you are studying, the particular method and design, and a specific form of data analysis. And by becoming an expert, you have developed credibility. You will be sought out by your peers and by employers because of your expertise. And you will have developed self-confidence as a nurse researcher.

VARIATIONS IN THE PROPOSAL FORMAT

The proposal outline you have just read is suitable for a number of functions. It is, first and foremost, the model for every other proposal you will write. If you have access to a word processor, we recommend that you put your proposal on a storage disk for later manipulations.

Second, if you do not deviate substantially from the proposal, you may use it as the basis for the first article you write for publication. All you have to do is change your future tense to past; update and abbreviate your problem essay to four typed pages or less; make changes in the proposal that reflect the changes you had to make in the actual data collection process and data analysis; enter your findings and conclusions; and presto! you have an article for publication in the approved format for a nursing research journal.

Thesis or Dissertation

If you are using this proposal as the basis for a thesis or dissertation proposal, talk to your advisor and find out the approved format at your school. Then alter this proposal to suit that format. For example, at some schools, master's and doctoral students present the first three chapters of their thesis or dissertation to their committee and are orally examined on those chapters prior to entering the data collection phase. In this instance, the first three chapters would include the following information:

Chapter 1
This is the "problem" chapter that includes the introductory materials with a very abbreviated literature review to substantiate the choice of this problem. This follows with a paragraph called "the problem" which is an expanded statement of purpose, followed by hypotheses or a list of research questions that further expand on the problem.

Chapter 2

This chapter is the literature review which is, in essence, an expanded version of your problem essay. More detail is given and more references are cited here than we have recommended in our abbreviated proposal. Your committee may want a justification for not using other theories, concepts, or methods in addition to those you have chosen to support your study. This is an area you should discuss with the chair of your committee.

Chapter 3

This chapter is "design and methodology." Here you simply put everything else in your proposal: design, sample, methods, data analysis, reliability and validity, and protection of human subjects.

References

Here you need to use the style required by your institution and call it a bibliography or a list of references or whatever style your school requires.

Appendixes

These will be presented in the format required by your school. Each appendix will be given a different letter (beginning with A) and grouped by content: human subjects forms, letters of agreement from agencies stating they will let you do research at their institution, maps of the region if needed, copy of the data collection instrument(s), and so on.

A useful guide to writing thesis or dissertation proposals can be found in Elizabeth M. Tornquist, *From Proposal to Publication: An Informal Guide to Writing about Nursing Research.*[1]

Grant Proposals

If you are writing a grant proposal, the granting agency's requirements determine how you will alter your original proposal. If you are submitting to a foundation or private agency, write and ask for their guidelines on how they like to have proposals submitted to them. In other words, ask for their proposal specifications and then follow that format. Sometimes it is a simple matter of abbreviating the proposal you have just written. Foundations frequently want a brief summary of your idea first, and then if they are interested in the study you will be asked to submit a more detailed proposal.

---

1. Tornquist, E. M. *From proposal to publication: An informal guide to writing about nursing research,* Menlo Park, CA: Addison-Wesley, 1986.

If you are planning to write a federal grant, the requirements are fairly standard. The grants office in your college or university will have copies of the guidelines. Other than the budget and personnel, the proposed research protocol is in the following format:

Abstract of Research Plan

A. Specific Aims (1 page)

B. Significance (3 pages)

C. Preliminary Studies (8 pages)

D. Experimental Design and Methods

E. Human Subjects

F. Vertebrate Animals (for animal studies)

G. Consultants

H. Consortium Arrangements

I. Literature Cited

Appendix

This material is to be typed (on a letter-quality printer or typewriter) within the margins specified, on copies of the sample page. We recommend you type in your name and social security number on the example page then make twice as many copies of the blank page as you believe you will need. Then type (or print) onto those copied pages.

Federal grant guidelines are very specific. Section A, specific aims, is a single page of what the study is about specifically. This is the purpose of the study written as hypotheses or specific research questions. Section B, significance, is the literature review, or background information for the project and is limited to three pages, total. Section C, preliminary studies, is limited to eight pages and is a summary of the principal investigator's qualifications to do this particular study. Here you are expected to describe your completed pilot project or feasibility study in detail. If you didn't do one, talk about other research projects you have done to convince the granting board of your ability to do unsupervised research. What is your background? Describe other studies you have done in the same or similar content (or theoretical) area or studies done using this type of methodology.

Section D, design of the research, is where you talk about your sample, design, method(s), procedure(s), reliability and validity testing, and data analysis. Take as many pages as you wish but be specific, do not ramble. You need to substantiate, provide rationale for certain procedures, and define terms in order to assist the reader to understand what you intend to do and why.

Section E, human subjects, is a brief summary on one page and is easily completed from your original proposal. You will submit your proposal to the human subjects review board (IRB) at your school or agency for approval and an approval notice will be forwarded with the grant. Your IRB will tell you what materials it needs to adequately review your proposal.

If you are not using animals in your research, head a blank piece of paper, F. Vertebrate Animals, and then under that state "Not Applicable." If you are using animals, follow the directions specified in the guidelines.

Section G, consultants, is composed of the letters you have obtained from individuals who have agreed to serve as consultants to your grant. If you are a student, this should include a letter from the chairperson of your research committee. Similarly, section H, consortium arrangements, consists of letters from those agencies who have agreed to collaborate with you in the conduct of the research. This is not the area for letters of agreement from agencies who have allowed you to do the research on their premises. That is part of ethical clearance and is not included in your grant proposal.

Section I, literature cited, is the list of references you used in developing your proposal. Whatever form you used in writing the initial proposal is acceptable as long as it is complete.

The appendix section is for whatever illustrative material you feel is necessary to assist the reviewer in understanding your proposed work. One thing many researchers find useful is to include a timetable for the research. But whatever you feel will be helpful can be included.

Even if your grant proposal is not funded, you will receive excellent feedback from the review panel and you may submit your proposal again, provided you have complied with the recommendations for revision. Again, the book by Tornquist provides helpful hints in writing the final grant.

THE FINISHED PROPOSAL

The difference between the first draft of a research proposal and the final, polished version is enormous and generally reflects the amount of time spent on it.

Students usually have a limited amount of time for learning how to write a proposal, performing all the steps involved in the research process, and actually submitting that proposal. As a result, the product submitted is often a first draft—rough, awkward, and almost inarticulate.

To minimize these defects, we suggest that a friend review the first draft before you submit it to the instructor. Have the friend describe the project to you. This will tell you if the proposal is clear and logical. On the basis of this initial critique, changes should be made in the paper prior to submitting it. If your friend doesn't understand what you are doing, it is likely that your instructor won't either.

If possible, put your first draft of the proposal away and let it "sit" for at least two weeks, preferably two months. You will be amazed at what happens to your thinking when you can see what you have written with a critical, analytical eye—not the eye of a fond parent. Your mistakes will loom before you—how your sentences seem muddy, your logic obscure, and your ideas poorly articulated. Now you are ready to polish the first draft. This is simply a matter of rewriting. Now is the time to clarify your ideas, write transition sentences, make the tenses consistent, clean up typographical errors, and so on. You may end up revising the entire proposal, but better that than having it turned down because it failed to communicate your ideas.

Check Your References

When you write a research proposal, you are expected to be accurate in all details, major and minor. But most important is to be accurate in your referencing. Nothing is worse, especially in research, than misquoting, misreferencing, or failing to give proper credit. You never know if the author of a research report on which you based your ideas will be reading your proposal.

Unfortunately, human beings tend to make errors. To be sure that you have listed all the references cited in the body of the paper, reread your entire proposal just for the references, and check each one against your list. Time consuming? Yes. Worth it? Definitely. You never know when the exact, correct reference will be noticed.

One of the most difficult things to remember when writing from your notes is where those notes came from. Your notes may have come from someone else's work that you transcribed verbatim but forgot to reference. They may have come from a lecture, a letter, a book, or a reading, in fact any source for someone else's ideas. We all do this; it's not at all unusual. In fact, that's the way some people do all their writing. But when you do this, you run the risk of being accused of plagiarism. Plagiarism means using someone else's work without acknowledging the source. Using someone else's work refers to using their ideas, literally copying their words, or following their phraseology without acknowledgment. It is insufficient to say, "Some authors . . .," when in fact the idea came from one specific source. So keep your notes as complete as possible at the time you take them. You will be very glad later as you write your finished proposal.

Polishing the Draft

The finished proposal should have a sense of closure and completeness about it. All parts are present and accounted for, including the title page.

Completed proposals look good. They are typed double-spaced and have page numbers. Handwritten proposals simply are not acceptable, nor are proposals that have been edited so much that they are practically handwritten.

Clean, neat proposals are not just pleasing to the eye; they also create a positive impression on the reader. Don't let typographical errors stand uncorrected in the final copy simply to preserve the whiteness of the sheet. By all means, correct your typos. If you have too many, retype the page.

Your finished proposal, ideally less than twenty-five typed pages, is what you will present to your instructor at the end of the course or to a committee for the protection of human subjects, as the basis for any grant proposal you may decide to write later; it also will serve as a guide for the rest of the research process. Because it serves so many functions, make more than one copy of the proposal; consider how you would feel if it were lost. Also, make sure everything you need for your future research is included in the proposal, as that is probably all you will be referring to, rather than your stacks of notes and bibliography cards. If you keep the uses of the proposal in mind, you may consider brevity a virtue—and, indeed, it is. Be as brief as possible without losing your train of though or neglecting an important point.

The final polish includes reviewing the manuscript for grammar, style, and sexist language. Some of us persist in the use of sexist language, forgetting the subtle influence of language in our lives and in our thinking. Sexist language is a bias that needs to be ruthlessly abandoned in our research. Not all humans are "he" and not all nurses are "she." Simply eliminate these pronouns from a sentence by rewriting it. Avoid words such as "should" which is a moralistic judgment and substitute a "could" which indicates possibility. Sentences that either begin with or include a clause such as, "It has been stated that . . . , it is assumed that . . . , or it is clear that . . ." use up a number of words to sound scholarly. Rewrite them to eliminate everything from "it" to "that" and begin with the next word. Or just say, "Clearly, . . . " Other editing hints refer to sentences that use phrases such as: "The findings of this study reveal that . . ." or "the findings state." Cut your sentences to say something like "The findings were" or "the study resulted in" and let it go at that. The more you attempt to sound scholarly, the more ponderous you become.

Type the final proposal on bonded paper that has some rag content so the words will not smudge. If you use "corrasable" bond, the paper not only sticks to your hands but also smudges every time you touch the type; so use durable bond paper and erase with white correction fluid. If you do, your written proposal will last until the end of the project and beyond.

As your write up your proposal, try to remember that what you are writing about is what you intend to do in the future. Therefore, your proposal should be written in future tense. Write clearly, with as little superfluity, pomposity, and garrulousness as possible. Some people believe that a scholarly proposal is unintelligible to the general reader. This does not have to be true. Write it so you can understand it; when you read it a month or two later, you will remember what you were thinking about and can go on from there.

The finished research paper, whether written by one person or a group, is a reflection of the time and thinking that went into the plan from question to proposal. The finished proposal marks the end of one phase of research—it is a mile-stone achieved.

RECOMMENDED READINGS

Artinian, B. M., Conceptual mapping: Development of the strategy, *Western Journal of Nursing Research*, 1982, 4(4), 379–393.

Burns, N. and Groves, S. K., *The practice of nursing research: Conduct, critique and utilization* (2nd ed.), Philadelphia: W. B. Saunders, 1993, Chap. 7, 8.

Campbell, W. G., Ballou, S. V., and Slade, C., *Form and style: Theses, reports, term papers,* New York: Houghton Mifflin, 1990.

Cooper, H. M., *Integrating research: A guide for literature reviews* (2nd ed.), Newbury Park: Sage, 1989.

Ganong, L. H., Integrative reviews of nursing research, *Research in Nursing and Health,* 1987, *10,* 1–11.

Lauffer, A., *Grantsmanship* (2nd ed.), Beverly Hills: Sage, 1983.

Lauffer, A., *Grantsmanship and fundraising,* Beverly Hills: Sage, 1984.

Markman, R. H., Markman, P. T., and Waddell, M. L., *10 steps in writing the research paper,* Woodbury, N.Y.: Barron's, 1994.

Menzel, D. H., Jones, H. M., and Boyd, L. G., *Writing a technical paper,* New York: McGraw-Hill, 1961.

Payne, L. V., *The lively art of writing,* New York: Mentor, 1965.

Publication manual of the American Psychological Association (4th ed.), Washington: The American Psychological Association, 1994.

Reif-Lehrer, L., *Writing a successful grant application* (Science Books International), Boston: Jones and Bartlett, 1989.

Strunk, W., Jr., *The elements of style,* Boston: Allyn and Bacon, 2000.

Sultz, H. A., and Sherwin, F. S., *Grant writing for health professionals,* Boston: Little, Brown, 1981.

Tornquist, E. M., *From proposal to publication: An informal guide to writing about nursing research,* Menlo Park, Calif.: Addison-Wesley, 1986.

Tornquist, E. M., and Funk, S. G., How to write a research grant proposal, *Image: Journal of Nursing Scholarship,* 1990, *22*(1), 44–51.

Turabian, K. L., *A manual for writers of term papers, theses, and dissertations,* Chicago: University of Chicago Press, 1955.

White, V. P., *Grants: How to find out about them and what to do next,* New York: Plenum, 1975.

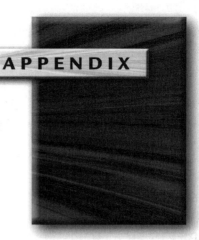

Sample Research Proposals

What Do Edmonton Seniors Say Are the Reasons for Including Herbal Supplements in Their Diet for the Maintenance of Their Health?

BRETT HODSON

What do seniors say are the reasons for including herbal supplements in their diet for the maintenance of their health? This question requires attention as individuals are increasingly demanding more choice regarding health care services and products. The reasons an individual has for choosing a particular type of care service or product are important for the development of good communication and relationships between patients and caregivers, and providing information and programs regarding health care to those in need. Developing an understanding of possible limitations of orthodox care systems, and accepting and supporting an individual's choice for alternatives to traditional medicine by traditional caregivers are also deemed important. The trend of herbal supplement use is particularly interesting in North American-born seniors of European descent. The senior's relative late stage in life, and their upbringing in a social environment where traditional medicine is dominant, would suggest a certain belief pattern regarding health maintenance. Herbal supplements are part of a group of alternative or complementary medicines that are considered outside the mainstream of conventional western medicine. In most cases herbal supplement use is associated with little risk, although information on their efficacy is often not based upon scientific evidence. Therefore, it is important to understand what specific reasons North American-born seniors, of European descent, living in Edmonton give for the use of herbal supplements for health maintenance.

USE OF HERBAL SUPPLEMENTS AS AN ALTERNATIVE THERAPY

In the United States, approximately 61 million individuals, spending approximately 11.7 billion dollars, use some form of alternative therapy treatment exclusively or in addition to traditional medical practices for health maintenance (Eisenberg, Kessler, Foster, Norlock, Calkins, and Delbanco, 1993). Alternative therapies include, but are not limited to, acupuncture, massage, homeopathy, reflexology, iridology, naturopathy, aromatherapy, and herbalism. Herbalism is a therapeutic system based on the curative power of herbal remedies (Fulder, 1984). Herbs when used for disease prevention or health-promoting purposes are plant or plant parts that are taken with therapeutic intent (Fulder, 1984), and may be used to stimulate the body's own natural healing powers or to restore general health (Griggs, 1981). The use of herbs for improving health can be traced to aboriginal, folk, or Chinese historical records. As a result, knowledge about the benefit of herbs as a form of medicine is often based on anecdotal, testimonial, and popular literature, all of which can be considered powerful persuaders (Roe, 1993; Campion, 1993). Very little of what would be considered analytical evidence is available on the efficacy of any specific herb and its effects on a particular disease or its ability to increase health or well being in general.

Limited information is available about the prevalence of alternative medical therapies in any population, let alone seniors' use of herbal supplements. However, general demographic data regarding the population of interest are available. The number of individuals 65 years of age and older residing in Edmonton is approximately 60,638 (City of Edmonton, 1993). Broken down by sex, the number of males is 25,289, while the number of females is 35,349. Very little data are available regarding the education level of seniors living specifically in Edmonton. Of the seniors living in Canada, 76% of individuals older than 85 years, 70% of individuals 75–79 years of age, and 63% of individuals 65–69 years of age do not have a degree of any kind, including trades or high school (Norland and Statistics Canada, 1994).

Herbal supplements are unique in that these products are available off the shelf at health food, supermarket, and chain stores (Roe, 1993). Diagnosis of health conditions and prescription of herbal medications for the treatment and prevention of various illnesses is often completed by a layperson, a self-proclaimed expert, or the self. In fact, up to 75% of individuals treat themselves with nonprescription medicines and home remedies (Furnham and Bhagrath, 1993). Real risks have been identified as a result of readily accessible health foods and herbal supplements and include toxicity of the supplement, supplement contamination, delay in treatment from a conventional physician, and people not taking the appropriate prescription drugs for their condition (Roe, 1993). These risks may or may not be known to potential users, therefore it is important to understand the reasons for the use of herbal supplements. Having knowledge of the reasons for use may provide insight into how and what kind of information regarding the efficacy and the potential risks is delivered.

Knowledge and understanding about the reasons for the use of herbal supplements can provide opportunities to develop an understanding of the health needs and concerns of seniors. This information is invaluable to physicians and other health care providers (including alternative medicine providers) when dealing with patients who use herbal supplements in their diet for health maintenance. Such information can be used in planning and evaluating health promotion initiatives that identify and target seniors' health needs (Levy and Schucker, 1987). Identifying trends in health attitudes and gauging the impact of consumer education efforts can also be based partly on the reasons for herbal supplement and alternative therapy use (Levy and Schucker, 1987).

Skepticism and fear about the efficacy and use of herbal supplements is rampant in physicians practicing traditional medicine. This attitude is so prevalent that many people do not bother to tell their physicians that they have tried or are currently using alternative forms of therapy for health maintenance (Eisenberg et al., 1993; Furnham and Bhagrath, 1993). Physicians need to better understand the use of herbal supplements and be less judgmental and more open to discussion to develop stronger relationships with their patients (Campion, 1993; Hogan and Ebly, 1996). There is widespread concern among health providers regarding the greater potential for disease or ill health in the elderly. As a result, seniors may be easy targets for supplement manufacturers and sales companies. This statement is supported by Read and Graney (1982) when they studied food supplement usage by the elderly, and Roe (1993) in her commentary about health foods. This also reflects fear in the traditional medical community regarding the use of alternative therapies, herbal supplements included.

Outside the assumption that herbal supplements are used for improving health and well being, very little research has gone into determining the reasons or motives for using this type of therapy. Moreover, the research that has been published is typically quantitative and compares users of alternative medicine to users of orthodox medicine in the general population, or studies patients with specific disorders and diseases. This literature, however, is relevant because it may provide some key indicators into the differences in attitudes and beliefs between those seeking traditional medicine and those seeking alternative forms of therapy.

For instance, users of homeopaths over general practitioners are more likely to believe their general resistance to illness can be improved, and are less confident in the treatments of traditional medicine (Furnham and Smith, 1988). Alternative therapy users have also been reported to be firmly dissatisfied with their last visit to a general practitioner compared to clients of orthodox medicine (Furnham and Smith, 1988; Furnham and Bhagrath, 1993). In addition, users of alternative treatments tend to know others who have had some success with an alternative treatment (Furnham and Forey, 1994). Alternative therapy users were also more likely to believe that practitioners should focus treatment on the whole person rather than just the sickness (Furnham and Forey, 1994). Interestingly, the more individuals believe in alternative medicine, the more they believe in controllable or internal causes of health, illness, and recovery regardless of whether they are psychological, environmental, or provided through a medical provider (Furnham, 1994; Furman and Beard, 1995). Positive attitudes toward alternative therapies are negatively correlated with fatalistic or external health beliefs (Furnham, 1994), and complementary medicine patients stress self-medication as a factor that influences future health status (Furman and Beard, 1995).

This research is significant because it may provide some insight into potential beliefs and reasons why seniors use herbal supplements for the maintenance of their health. As herbal supplements are considered to be "alternative" it is quite possible that users may exhibit dissatisfaction with a general practitioner, or have feelings of internal control over health and illness. There is danger in generalizing the results of these studies to the population of interest to this investigator in that these studies do not specifically measure the prevalence of, beliefs about, or reasons for herbal supplement use in seniors.

What may also be of value in understanding herbal supplement use is research that investigates the reasons behind the use of nutritional supplements, specifically vitamin use by the elderly. Even though vitamins are different from herbal supplements in some respects, there are some common issues regarding their use. Promises of prevention and relief with the use of vitamins have been expounded by popular literature. Vitamin supplements may also be unnecessary, expensive, and risky, and may be used to replace traditional medical treatment (Read et al., 1982).

Prevalence of food supplement use in the elderly has been as high as 66% (Read et al., 1982), 13% of which could be classified as herbal supplement use. Reasons cited for food supplement use in the elderly were illness prevention, prescribed by a physician, provided energy, used as a safety measure, and taken for general health (Read et al., 1982). This corroborates other findings of reasons for nutritional supplement use that include opportunities to decrease suspected or actual severity of health problems and increase energy (Bender, Levy, Schuker, and Yetley, 1992). Sources of information regarding food supplements included physicians, family, popular literature, television, and friends (Read et al., 1982). Interestingly, some of the reasons for food supplement use, such as illness prevention and general health, fit with what has been presented by Furnham and associates in their studies of beliefs of users of alternative medicine. The elderly also seem to rely on a large amount of unsubstantiated information regarding supplementation that may be unreliable (Read et al., 1982). Vitamin supplement use has also been correlated with a greater number of health protective habits in the elderly (Gray, Pagnini-Hill, Ross, and Henderson, 1986). Again, this fits with the results presented by Furnham and associates regarding the belief about the control of health being internalized.

Previous research has been identified that relates the use of alternative therapies by patients with specific health problems. For instance, the use of different complementary medicines has been reported among dementia patients for impaired cognition and general health promotion (Hogan and Ebly, 1996). Herbal supplements were among the self-prescribed treatments. The attendance of patients with Alzheimer disease in a support group provided a forum for shared experiences and pressures to experiment with unproven treatments, thus the use of herbal supplements (Hogan et al., 1996). The use of alternative therapies by gastroenterology patients has shown that users are often encouraged by others and cite reasons for use that reflect upon the poor efficacy of traditional treatments and physicians (Verohef, Sutherland, and Brkich, 1990; Sutherland and Verhoef, 1994).

There has been an increase in the number of choices the general public can purchase and receive for health care services and products. Included in these choices are herbal supplements that can be self-prescribed and purchased off the shelf at health food stores, pharmacies, and supermarkets. Outside of the fact that herbal supplements are used for maintaining or improving health, seniors of European descent, born in North America and living in Edmonton, are of specific interest because of their upbringing in a society that has long placed value in orthodox medicine. Developing an understanding for herbal supplement use is important as this knowledge can assist orthodox health providers in building stronger relationships with patients, support individuals in their choice for health care services and products, assist in understanding the need for accurate information regarding alternative forms of medicine, and targeting the health needs of special groups such as seniors. This understanding may also highlight the need for controlled scientific studies to be carried out on herbal supplements to determine their efficacy in maintaining or improving health. Therefore, this study will determine the reasons seniors include herbal supplement in their diet for the maintenance of their health.

PURPOSE OF THE STUDY

The purpose of this research study is to explore and describe the reasons North American-born seniors, of European descent, living in Edmonton have for using herbal supplements for the maintenance of their health.

DEFINITION OF TERMS

Reasons: Statements that explain behaviors or beliefs regarding the use of herbal supplements for maintaining health as elicited through an unstructured interview.

THE RESEARCH DESIGN

This is a descriptive study.

SAMPLE

Participants are to be born in North America, a senior, of European descent, and residing in Edmonton, Canada. In this study a senior is an individual who is 65 years of age or older. For the purposes of this research, participants will have used herbal supplements within the last six months, or are currently using herbal supplements for the maintenance of their health.

This investigator intends to successfully enroll enough participants to develop an understanding about why herbal supplements are used in the population under investigation. Taking into account constraints of time and other resources, the investigator will attempt to enroll a satisfactory number of participants within a six-month time period. The number of participants required to obtain enough relevant data to fulfill the purpose of this research study is believed to be between 6 and 15 subjects.

SAMPLE SELECTION

Network (Brink and Wood, 1994) or "snowball" sampling will be the method of acquiring participants for this research study. The first potential participant, and key informant, has been identified and has agreed to act as a source for other potential participants. Network sampling will provide the best results, and will be the most effective and efficient use of resources for obtaining a sample that fits the selection criteria. Networking provides a means to readily identify and easily contact potential participants. By using the network sampling technique to obtain participants for this research study, subjects will be much more open and honest during the data collection process as participants will be familiar with the individual who has identified them as a potential participant.

Sampling and acquiring participants from the population will also be highly dependent on the analysis of data and concepts or information that may prove to be relevant to the purpose of this research (Strauss and Corbin, 1990). Particular characteristics regarding the potential participants may be sought depending on the repeated presence or absence of concepts that appear significant in the analysis of the data (Strauss et al., 1990).

METHODS AND INSTRUMENTS

Unstructured interviews of each participant enrolled into the study will be the method of data collection of reasons for herbal supplement use in the population for this investigation. The advantages of interviews include direct observation of the responses of the subject, opportunities to clarify questions if misunderstood, and ability to ask questions can be at several levels to get the most information from the subject (Brink and Wood, 1994).

The interview will be guided by one question in an attempt to elicit a response that will provide the necessary information from the participants. The grand tour question for this research investigation is "Could you describe to me your reasons for using herbal supplements?" It is the intention of this investigator to allow the participants to provide as much information with as little encumbrance as possible. Probing questions such as "Where did the idea for the use of the herbs come from?" and "Where did the information about the benefits of the herb come from?" will only be used when it is felt that more complete and detailed information may be available or desired from the participant. The interview guide with potential probes is located in Appendix A.

The grand tour question and probes will be pilot tested using a small sample of one or two seniors who are known to fit the selection criteria. The results of the pretest will provide the opportunity to evaluate the effectiveness of the grand tour question in eliciting the desired information. Adjustments will be made to the question based on suggestions and responses from the pilot sample.

Aside from the grand tour question, interviewing and data collection may become rather indiscriminate in nature (Strauss and Crobin, 1990). Due to the lack of literature that currently exists in this subject area, it is rather unclear what information may be relevant. Again, data collection may depend upon the emergence of concepts and data that may be significant to fulfilling the requirements of the purpose of this research (Morse and Field, 1995).

Each interview will be conducted in the home or primary residence of each participant by the principal investigator. This will provide a comfortable and familiar environment for the participant that will be conducive to the collection of data. If this is unsatisfactory to the participant, a location that will be chosen by the participant and agreed on by the principal investigator will be used. If a participant feels the need to have someone present in addition to the interviewer, this will be accommodated, with the understanding that questions are to be answered solely by the participant and without any prompting or clarification from the third party.

It is unclear at this point how many interviews for each subject will be necessary; however, it is expected that there will be at least two per participant, one for the initial data collection and the second for clarification purposes. The collection of data from the sample may be considered complete when a saturation point (Morse and Field, 1995) has been reached and no new information can be elicited from the sample regarding their reasons for herbal supplement use for the maintenance of their health.

Raw data is to be collected by tape recording the interview and taking field notes. The tape-recorded interview will be immediately transcribed for analysis. Field notes will be kept in a field journal that will provide a medium for the recording of setting and any nonverbal information.

Basic demographic data will also be collected at the end of each interview from every subject. Specifically, information such as age, sex, household and individual income, maximum level of education reached, and occupation or occupation prior to retirement will be asked. This information will be used to describe the sample. The instrument for collecting demographic data is located in Appendix B.

DATA ANALYSIS

Each interview will be immediately analyzed by reviewing field notes and the transcripts as soon as they are available. Data analysis of the transcribed interview tapes will take place initially by content analysis (Brink and Wood, 1994) and open coding to identify conditions, actions, phenomena, consequences, and of course reasons for herbal supplement use (Strauss, 1990; Glaser, 1978). Codes are to be developed based on the participants' own words as much as possible (Morse and Field, 1995; Glaser, 1978) to ensure the participants' experiences are captured and remain unbiased.

After the second participant has been interviewed, an intensive and constant comparative analysis will be conducted with the results of the data analysis of the first participant (Glaser, 1978). This constant comparative analysis will be conducted between the analyzed data of each subsequent interview of every participant. Subjecting the data to second level coding to re-categorize and condense codes will summarize the relationships between the data sets (Morse and Field, 1995). Identifying and linking concepts between the data analyzed of each of the participants will be completed in an attempt to derive an explanatory model of the reasons for herbal supplement use by North American-born seniors of European descent living in Edmonton.

SAMPLE DATA

Interview Number: 01

Subject Number: 01

Date/Time: December 4, 1997/1300h

Setting: Participant's home, South East Edmonton

Interviewer: Could you describe to me your reasons for using herbal supplements?

Participant: Well, I guess, the real reason I started using St. John's Wort is I was feeling a little, um, depressed. My husband passed away, oh, last year and I just couldn't seem to move ahead with things. One of my sons said I should try a herbal remedy for my depression rather than carrying on the way I was. He is really in to those sorts of things. I didn't really like the idea until he brought me a magazine from the health food store in the mall over here that had an article in it about St. John's Wort. I read it and the next time I went to the mall I talked to the girl at the store about it. She had said that there were a number of seniors who were using herbs for all kinds of things. I ended up buying some and used it for about a month. I didn't really notice a difference in how I was feeling until I ran out and didn't buy anymore. I talked about it with a friend of mine and she noticed I just didn't seem the same either. So, I ended up buying some more. I don't use it as regularly as I did before, but it does seem to help me feel a little better when I do use it.

Statements that explain behaviors and beliefs made by the participant could be coded by considering and using words or categories used by the participant herself. For instance, the participant uses herbal supplements to help with *depression* or for *psychological* reasons. The participant's decision to use herbal supplements was influenced by her *son,* a *family member,* a *magazine* or *popular literature,* and a *health food store clerk* or *so-called expert.* All of these influences were *external* in nature. The participant did, however, notice a change in her *behaviors* or *feelings* that was substantiated by a *friend.* These *realizations* of changes, or *perceived effect* of the herbal supplement, prompted the participant to continue her use of herbal supplements. Therefore, codes that have been developed for this particular data set include:

Reasons: depression/psychological

Influence: son/family member, magazine/popular literature, store clerk/so-called expert, realization of perceived effect, friend

This data set would be set aside until data from the second interview had been coded. The two interviews would then be compared and similarities and differences in the data could be recognized and noted. Again, this process would continue with all subsequent interviews until data saturation was reached. Codes would then be summarized, and concepts and codes could be linked together. An explanatory model could then be developed that would describe the reasons for herbal supplements by North American-born seniors, of European descent living in Edmonton, Canada.

RIGOR

The credibility of this research study will be maintained by ensuring the gathering of diverse perspectives, and verifying the data with the key informants (Horne, 1995). The process of theoretical sampling will provide the opportunity to gather data from individual seniors with various experiences using herbal supplements, which may result in a diversity of motivations and reasons for using supplements. Verification of the data collected from interviews by the informants will ensure statements and events are accurate. Sharing conclusions with the informants may also verify patterns of reasoning observed by the evaluator.

Due to the qualitative nature of this research study, the dependability of the evaluation will be ensured through the recognition of the researcher's own subjectivity and ensuring the integrity of the data gathering processes and analysis procedures (Horne, 1995). By recognizing the researcher's own ideas and feelings regarding why seniors use herbal supplements, the influence of this perspective when observing and analyzing data can be taken into account. Ensuring the integrity of the collection and analysis of data through careful documentation of the procedures, the rationale behind code development, the recognition of themes, and the conclusions made will provide an audit trail for others to determine why differences in findings or opinions may result.

PROTECTION OF HUMAN SUBJECTS

Approval for this study will be obtained from the University of Alberta Health Research Ethics Review Board. Interview subjects for this evaluation will have volunteered. All potential informants will be provided an information sheet that outlines the details of the evaluation and specifics related to the interview prior to the informed consent being signed. Participants will be informed that they may terminate the interview, or ask that the tape recorder be turned off, at any time during the interview. The subjects will also be informed of the right to refuse to answer any questions, or to ask any questions of the interviewer at any time.

The anonymity of the subjects will be protected by (1) transcribing the data by code number; (2) storing the interview tapes and transcribed notes in locked cabinets, in a locked room; and (3) storing the consent forms and identifying data in a locked cabinet separate from the interview tapes and transcribed notes. Any place or person names that appear in the transcribed interview or field journal notes will be removed. The interview tapes will be destroyed seven (7) years after the completion of the study. The final report will not include any identifying information about the participants.

Potential risks to the individual participants in this study are not foreseen. This research may not be of any direct benefit to the informants in this study who use or have used herbal supplements. However, as explained above, the benefits may be far reaching if a better understanding about the reasons for herbal supplement use in this population can be developed. The results of the research will only be explained to the informant if the informant makes the request by signing the appropriate area of the information sheet.

REFERENCES

Bender, M. M., Levy, A. S., Schucker, R. E., & Yetley, E. A. (1987). Trends in prevalence and magnitude of vitamin and mineral supplement usage and correlation with health status. *Journal of the American Dietetic Association, 92:*1096–1107.

Brink, P., & Wood, M. S. (1994). *Basic steps in planning nursing research: From question to proposal* (4th ed.), Boston: Jones and Bartlett.

City of Edmonton (1993). *Population figures and trends as compiled in the 1993 census.* Edmonton: Office of the City Clerk.

Campion, E. W. (1993). Why unconventional medicine? *The New England Journal of Medicine, 328:* 282–283.

Eisenberg, D. M., Kessler, R. C., Foster, C., Norlock, F. E., Calkins, D. R., & Delbanco, T. L. (1993). Unconventional medicine in the United States. *The New England Journal of Medicine, 328:* 246–252.

Fulder, S. (1984). Glossary and classification of therapies. In *The handbook of complementary medicine* (p. 20). Great Britain: Coronet Books.

Furnham, A. (1994). Explaining health and illness: Lay perceptions on current and future health, the causes of illness, and the nature of recovery. *Social Science in Medicine, 39:*715–725.

Furnham, A., & Beard, R. (1995). Health, just world beliefs and coping style preferences in patients of complementary and orthodox medicine. *Social Science in Medicine, 40,* 1425–1432.

Furnham, A., & Bhagrath, R. (1993). A comparison of health beliefs and behaviors of clients of orthodox and complementary medicine. *British Journal of Clinical Psychology, 32:*237–246.

Furnham, A., & Forey, J. (1994). The attitudes, behaviors and beliefs of patients of conventional vs complementary (alternative) medicine. *British Journal of Clinical Psychology, 50:*458–469.

Furnham, A., & Smith, C. (1988). Choosing alternative medicine: A comparison of the beliefs of patients visiting a general practitioner and a homeopath. *Social Science in Medicine, 26:*685–689.

Glaser, B. (1978). *Theoretical sensitivity: Advances in the methodology of grounded theory.* Mill Valley, California: Sociology Press.

Gray, G. E., Pagnini-Hill, A., & Ross, R. K. (1986). Vitamin supplements in a southern California retirement community. *Journal of the American Dietetic Association, 86:*800–801.

Griggs, F. (1981). The price of miracles. In *Green pharmacy: A history of herbal medicine* (pp. 284–298). Toronto, Ontario: Methuen Publications.

Hogan, D. B., & Ebly, E. M. (1996). Complementary medicine use in a dementia clinic population. *Alzheimer Disease and Associated Disorders, 10:*63–67.

Horne, T. (1995). *Making a difference: Program evaluation for health promotion.* Edmonton, AB: WellQuest Consulting Ltd.

Levy, A. S., & Schucker, R. E. (1987). Patterns of nutrient intake among dietary supplement users: Attitudinal and behavioral correlates. *Journal of the American Dietetic Association, 87:*754–760.

Morse, J. M., & Field, P. A. (1995). *Qualitative research methods for health professionals, 2nd ed.* Thousand Oaks: Sage Publications.

Norland, J. A., & Statistics Canada. (1994). *Profile of Canada's seniors.* Ottawa: Statistics Canada and Prentice Hall Canada Inc.

Read, M. H., & Graney, A. S. (1989). Food supplement use by the elderly. *Journal of the American Dietetic Association, 80:*250–253.

Roe, D. A. (1993). Health foods and supplements for the elderly: Who can say no? *New York State Journal of Medicine, 93:*109–111.

Strauss, A., & Corbin, J. (1990). *Basics of qualitative research: Grounded theory procedures and techniques.* Newbury Park, California: Sage Publications.

Sutherland, L. R., & Verhoef, M. J. (1994). Why do patients seek a second opinion or alternative medicine? *Journal of Clinical Gastroenterology, 19:*194–197.

Verhoef, M. J., Sutherland, L. R., & Brkich, L. (1990). Use of alternative medicine by patients attending a gastroenterology clinic. *Canadian Medical Association Journal, 142:*121–125.

APPENDIX A

Interview Guide

Grand Tour Question
Could you describe to me your reasons for using herbal supplements?

Potential Probing Questions
Where do/did you get the idea to try or use herbal supplements?

Where do you buy/purchase your herbal supplements?

How do you feel as a result of using herbal supplements?

APPENDIX B

Participant Information

Participant Number _____

1. Date of Birth _____

2. Individual Income (approximately) _____

3. Household Income (approximately) _____

4. Current Occupation (if employed) _____

5. Previous Occupation (if retired) _____

6. Number of Years of Education _____

7. Highest Level of Education Achieved _____

Committee A _____

Committee B _____

Health Research Ethics Administration Board Request for Ethics Review

Note: This form has been designed to be used by researchers in a wide variety of fields. Some questions may not be pertinent for this particular project.

Section A: General information

A1. Title of Project:

What do seniors born in North America, of European descent, living in Edmonton say are the reasons for including herbal supplements in their diet for the maintenance of their health?

A2. Name of Principal Investigator: Brett Hodson

Title(s): _____

Department / Program: _Health Promotion / MSc._ _____

Mailing address for ethics information: _____

_____

Telephone: _____ Fax: _____ E-Mail: _____

Signature: _____ Date: _December 8, 1997_ _____

A3. Name of Co-Investigator: (Required for Students, Residents, Visiting Scholars, etc.)

Name: Dr. Allison McKinnon

Title(s): Assistant Professor / Program Supervisor

Department/Program: Department of Occupational Therapy

Mailing address: _____

_____

Telephone: _____

Signature: _____ Date: _____

A4. Authorizing Signatures: (For U of A staff, must be signed by Department Chair or Associate Dean, Research. For CHA or Caritas staff, must be signed by administrative supervisor of Principal Investigator.)

I support the implementation of this project.

_____   _____
(Signature)   (Date)

_____   _____
(Name: Please print)   (Title)

A5. Co-Investigator(s) / Thesis Committee:

Name   Department / Program   Telephone

_____   _____   _____

_____   _____   _____

_____   _____   _____

_____   _____   _____

_____   _____   _____

_____   _____   _____

A6. Expedited review:

If the study procedures are limited to any of the following, please check the appropriate box. (See guidelines, page 7)

_____ examination of patient or medical or institutional records

_____ secondary analysis of data

_____ use of biological specimens normally discarded

_____ collection of blood and urine specimens

_____ modification of previously approved protocol (specify title and approval date)

_____

_____

A7. Which one of the following best describes the type of investigation proposed? Check more than one if appropriate.

_____ clinical trial

_____ multi-centre trial

_____ pilot study

_____ drug study

_____ technology assessment / development

__X_ qualitative study

_____ epidemiological study

_____ sequel to previously approved project

_____ first application in humans

_____ other (specify) _____

A8. Where will the research be conducted? (Note that administrative approval is required to carry out research in any Capital Health or Caritas facility):

_____ Capital Health Site (specify) _____

_____ Caritas Site (specify) _____

_____ U of A Site (specify) _____

__X__ Other (specify) Participants' homes _____

Funding/Budget

A9. How is the proposal funded?

_____ funding approval (specify source) _____

_____ funding request pending (specify source) _____

__X__ no external funding required _____

A10. Are any of the investigators involved in this study receiving any direct personal renumeration or other personal or family financial benefits (either direct or indirect) for taking part in these investigations? (See guidelines, page 7)

_____ yes   If yes, append a letter detailing these activities to the Chair of the appropriate review committee.

__X__ no _____

Attach a budget summary. Note that the summary must include details of investigator payments and recruitment incentives (if present).

Additional Documentation

A11. If any of the following applies to this study, attach the appropriate letters of approval / support. (See guidelines, page 8)

Health Protection Branch or other Canadian federal agency approval:

__X__ Not applicable

_____ Attached

_____ Pending

Radiation Safety Committee Approval (required for all studies involving radioisotopes and non-routine X-rays):

__X__ Not applicable

_____ Attached

_____ Pending

Electromechanical or Biohazardous Materials Safety Approval:

__X__ Not applicable

_____ Attached

_____ Pending

Consent Template (On Letterhead)

Part 1
Title of Project:

What do seniors born in North America, of European descent, living in Edmonton say are the reasons for including herbal supplements in their diet for the maintenance of their health?

Principal Investigator(s): Brett Hodson

Co-Investigator(s): Dr. Allison McKinnon, University of Alberta

Part 2 (to be completed by the research subject)

Do you understand that you have been asked to be in a research study?	Yes No
Have you read and received a copy of the attached Information Sheet?	Yes No
Do you understand the benefits and risks involved in taking part in this research study?	Yes No
Have you had an opportunity to ask questions and discuss this study?	Yes No
Do you understand that you are free to refuse to participate or withdraw from the study at any time? You do not have to give a reason and it will not affect your care. *(Use wording appropriate to your subject group)*	Yes No
Has the issue of confidentiality been explained to you? Do you understand who will have access to your records?	Yes No
Do you want the investigator(s) to inform your family doctor that you are participating in this research study? If so, please provide your doctor's name:	Yes No

————————————————————— *(N.B. This question is optional).*

This study was explained to me by: ————————————————————

I agree to take part in this study.

———————————————	————	———————————————
Signature of Research Participant	Date	Witness
———————————————		———————————————
Printed Name		Printed Name

I believe that the person signing this form understands what is involved in the study and voluntarily agrees to participate.

———————————————	————
Signature of Investigator or Designee	Date

THE INFORMATION SHEET MUST BE ATTACHED TO THIS CONSENT FORM AND A COPY GIVEN TO THE RESEARCH SUBJECT

Information Sheet (On Letterhead)

Research Title: What do seniors born in North America, of European descent, living in Edmonton say are the reasons for including herbal supplements in their diet for the maintenance of their health?

Investigator: Brett Hodson, BPE   Program Supervisor: Dr. Allison McKinnon, PhD
MSc, Health Promotion Student   Assistant Professor

Purpose

The purpose of this research study is to explore and describe the reasons North American-born seniors, of European descent, living in Edmonton have for using herbal supplements for the maintenance of their health.

Procedure

1. The researcher will ask for you to describe your reasons for using herbal supplements in your diet. The length of the interview will be approximately one to one-and-a-half hours long.

2. The discussion will be tape-recorded. The researcher and the person transcribing the tapes will listen to the tapes.

3. The tapes will be transcribed. The researcher and the thesis supervisor will read the transcript of the tapes.

4. Anything that could be used to identify you, including your name and the names of others, will be erased from the transcript of the tapes.

5. The researcher will contact you if any information is not clear after the tapes have been transcribed.

Participation

There are no known risks to you if you take part in this study. Results of this study may help health professionals and caregivers better understand reasons for herbal supplement use by seniors.

You do not have to be in this study if you do not wish to be. If you decide to be in this study you may drop out at anytime by telling the researcher. You do not have to answer any questions or discuss any subject in the interview, or at any other time, if you do not want to.

Your name will not appear in this study. A code number will be used instead of your name, and will appear on any forms or question sheets. Your name, and the names of others, will be erased from the transcripts of the tapes. As stated by University Policy all tapes, transcripts of the tapes, and notes will be stored in a locked cabinet separate from consent forms and code lists for at least seven (7) years after the research has been completed. Consent forms will be kept in a locked cabinet for at least five (5) years. Data may be used for another study in the future, if the researcher receives approval from the appropriate ethics review committee.

We may publish or present the information and findings of this study in journals or at conferences, but your name or any material that may identify you will not be used. If you have any questions about this study at this or any other time, you can call the researcher or his supervisor at the numbers above.

If you have any concerns about any part of this study, you may call the Capital Health Patients Concerns Office. The researcher and the research supervisor have no affiliation with the Capital Health Patients Concerns Office.

Request for Summary: (optional)
If you wish to receive a summary of the study when it is finished, please complete the next section:

Name: _____

Address: _____

_____

_____

Value Orientations of the Copper Inuit

NANCY A. EDGECOMBE

INTRODUCTION

The provision of nursing care to the aboriginal people of Canada offers its own unique challenges, one of which is working with a client group who are culturally distinct. It involves not only the assessment of the individual client or client group, but also a study of the client culture. Brink (1990) depicts nursing as being primarily concerned with human behavior and points out that "what affects human behaviour eventually affects nursing" (p. 2). Cultural variables shape human behavior and are therefore a legitimate part of nursing knowledge. "Assessing and understanding of cultural variables leads to a better understanding of patient behaviour and the way the patient perceives the illness or health situation" (Tripp-Reimer and Brink, 1984, p. 78). Behaviors reflect values and beliefs, which are culturally grounded.

Although aboriginal people are accepted as being culturally distinct from other groups they are seldom identified as being culturally distinct from one another. Yet, although there may be similarities, there are also differences. It is important for the delivery of nursing care to aboriginal groups to identify these differences. One area in which differences may exist is in their values. The purpose of the study is to identify and describe the value orientations of the Copper Inuit.

VALUES AND VALUE ORIENTATION

Values "are the standards we live by, the goals we hope to achieve. They are basic to our preferences and our decisions and give meaning to all we do" (Werkmeister, 1967, p. 59). Values, as described by Frondizi (1973), have both polarity and hierarchy. Polarity exists because things are considered to have negative or positive aspects, to have negative or positive value. The value of things also varies in importance as illustrated by the preference of one value over another. Preferences can be rank ordered to form a hierarchy of values.

Values are one of the cultural determinants of a person's personality (Brink, 1982). All human beings exist within a physical environment in which they must live. All people share certain life experiences such as birth, aging, and death, and must learn how to survive within their environment as a member of their society. Humans are also social animals and exist in a state of interdependence with other individuals and groups within their own society and culture. Socialization serves to *enculturate* (educate) individual members to the knowledge and expectations of their culture. At the same time each individual will have experiences that are unique to them or to their social group within society. Cultural determinants, therefore, are common to all humans (universal), common to all members of a group (communal), common to a specific social role (role), and specific to the individual (idiosyncratic) (Brink, 1982; Kluckhohn and Mowrer, 1944; Murray and Kluckhohn, 1956).

To live harmoniously within society, an individual must share standards or values that are consistent with the standards or values of other individuals of the group within which the individual lives and works. These shared values are essential.

Social life would be impossible without them; the functioning of the social system could not continue to achieve group goals; individuals could not get what they want and need from other individuals in personal terms, nor could they feel within themselves a requisite measure of order and unified purpose (Kluckhohn, C., 1951, p. 400).

Personal values exist within the broader value orientations of society and variation within orientations does exist.

VALUE ORIENTATIONS

Value orientation refers to the way in which complex principles related to values are rank ordered by individuals within cultural groups. This relates to a premise that societies have the same dominant and alternative cultural orientations, and that individuals or groups may vary in the degree to which they follow the values and norms of the dominant society (Kluckhohn, F., 1951, 1956).

The theory of value orientation is based on three assumptions (Kluckhohn and Strodtbeck, 1961, p. 10):

1. That there is a limited number of common human problems for which all peoples at all times must find solutions.

2. That while there is variability in solutions of all of the problems, they are neither limitless nor random, but are definitely variable within a range of possible solutions.

3. That all solutions are present in all societies at all times but are differentially preferred.

Problems crucial and common to all human groups can be classified into five orientations or groups: Human Nature Orientation, Man-Nature Orientation, Time Orientation, Activity Orientation, and Relational Orientation. Within each orientation there are at least three possible alternatives in any society.

Man-Nature orientation considers a person's relationship with nature as being either (1) Subjugated-to-nature, (2) in Harmony-with-nature, or (3) having Mastery-over-nature. Subjugation-to-nature is a belief that humans are helpless to control or alter the natural order, that there are powers over which they have no control. Harmony-with-nature is a belief that humans are part of a larger whole, which includes nature and supernature, that anything which affects one will affect the other. Mastery-over-nature is a belief that mankind is superior to nature and can control nature through their own will and efforts (Kluckhohn, 1951, 1956; Kluckhohn and Strodtbeck, 1961).

The Relational orientation refers to a person's relationship with other people in their group, which can be either Lineal, Collateral, or Individualistic. In the Lineal Orientation, it is the group goals that are of primary concern to the individual and these goals have continuity over time. Relationships in a Lineal Orientation are based on status relative to one's position within a social hierarchy. Decisions are made by those individuals who possess authority based on their social status. Frequently, age is associated with status. The elders in the society are the decision makers. In the Collateral Orientation, the goals of a laterally extended group, such as the family or community, have primacy for individuals within the group with no continuity over time. Decisions are made through group consensus. In the Individualistic Orientation, the goals of the individual take preference over the goals of the group or of society. Decisions are made by individuals independent of the group.

Time Orientation relates to the temporal focus of human life, which can be either in the Past, the Present, or the Future. Kummel (1966, p. 43) explains the relationship between past, present, and future as being

> essentially one of succession: while a particular time exists as present, there is a time which "not yet" is but which will sometime come into being, as well as a time, already having been, "no longer" exists. Time is therefore never present as a whole but is divided into the elements of a succession: two periods, delimited by the present and continually passing into one another, so that what was previously a future is "now" a present and will soon be a past.

A Past Time Orientation places importance primarily on the maintenance or restoration of traditional activities and beliefs. A Present Orientation places importance on the events and activities of the current moment. Finally, a Future Time Orientation places importance on activities and events that may happen at some later date (Kluckhohn, 1951, 1956; Kluckhohn and Strodtbeck, 1961).

The Activity Orientation relates to a people's method of self-expression through activity. Activities of this kind are classified as Doing, Being, or Being-in-Becoming. Doing activities are those associated with accomplishing some specific function. Being activities are those associated with what the person is, but are not associated with specific functions or personal development. Being-in-becoming activities are associated with what the person is and with personal development and have no specific function associated with them. (Kluckhohn, 1951, 1956; Kluckhohn and Strodtbeck, 1961).

Human Nature Orientation considers the character of innate human nature. This refers to philosophic views about the natural moral status of human beings. The views are that human beings are either innately Good, Evil, or Neutral (mixture of good and evil). A belief that human nature is innately Evil is that people can be born either naturally evil and unchangeable, or born evil but perfectible (Kluckhohn, 1951, p. 378). A belief that human nature is innately Good includes the belief that people are either naturally Good and unalterable, or naturally Good but corruptible (Kluckhohn, 1951, p. 378). A belief that Human Nature is Neutral refers to a belief that humans are a mixture of good and evil, or that they are neither good nor evil but are either invariant or subject to influence (Kluckhohn, 1951, 1956; Kluckhohn and Strodtbeck, 1961).

Kluckhohn (1951) suggested that how a society judges its members is based upon how congruent an individual member's Value Orientation is with the dominant Value Orientation of the society. A person's Value Orientation may differ from the society's dominant Value Orientation just as a person's culture may vary from the dominant culture of that society (as in ethnic groups).

VALUE ORIENTATION RESEARCH

Original Study

Kluckhohn and Strodtbeck (1961) studied five communities in the American southwest: a Mormon, a Zuni, a Navaho, a Spanish American, and a Texan community. All five communities had been the focus of social research for several years both independently and comparatively. A sample from each community was interviewed and asked twenty-two questions related to four of the five Value Orientations: Relational, Time, Activity, or Man-Nature. The preferences for each question were then statistically analyzed to determine within-culture regularity and between-culture difference. The knowledge available from the social science research was used to validate the general results and to provide a more detailed analysis of intracultural variations.

Kluckhohn and Strodtbeck (1961) were able to generate value-orientation profiles for the five communities involved. On analysis "significant within-culture regularities and significant between-culture differences" (p. 138) were identified. The overall Value Orientation profiles are illustrated in Table 1 (Appendix A).

The Spanish-American data demonstrated strong intracultural variation in regard to Relational Orientation. Responses associated with Relational Orientation showed that respondents were "only slightly more individualistic than lineally orientated in their dominant value orientation position" (p. 142). Generally the first-order preference for men was the Individualist alternative and for women the Lineal alternative.

The overall Time Orientation proved to be Present over Past over Future. There was, however, a strong Present over Future over Past in all but the question on ceremonial innovation, where a notable preference for Past orientation affected the overall results. Although the dominant Man-nature orientation was one of Subjugation-to-nature, there was variation as to the second-order choice, Harmony-with-nature being slightly favored to Mastery-over-nature.

The dominant Value Orientation for Activity was clearly Being over Doing. Women, however, generally selected the Being alternative more often than men, who favored the Doing alternative. The only exception to this was in respect to the question on attitude toward men's work habits, where women also favored the Doing alternative.

The degree of variation for the dominant Relational orientation and the variation within the Time orientation suggested a transitional process occurring within the culture. The gender difference in relation to Activity orientation reflects the distinct gender roles within the culture.

Results of the Texan data analysis revealed that Individualistic was the preferred choice in all but one of the Relational questions where Collateral was chosen over Individualistic. Within the Time orientation questions, there was variation between a dominance of Present over Future versus Future over Present. The final outcome was Future over Present over Past. Although the dominant Man-Nature Orientation was clearly Mastery-over-nature there was variation between Subjugation-to-nature and Harmony-with-nature for the second-order alternative. Activity orientation was clearly one of Doing over Being. No variation in Value Orientations between men and women was identified.

Although the overall Mormon Relational Orientation was Individualistic over Collateral over Lineal there was a high degree of variation between Individualistic and Collateral in the individual questions. For Time, the results were similar to the Texan groups with slightly more emphasis on the Past. Interestingly, on the question on ceremonial innovation, approximately half the women and a considerable number of men chose the Future alternative. The Mormon group was consistent in a Mastery-over-nature over Harmony-with-nature over Subjugation-to-nature. A Doing Orientation was favored over Being for Activity Orientation. On the whole, there was no variation between men and women.

The Zuni showed marked variations within all orientation areas. The overall Relational Orientation was Collateral over Lineal over Individualistic. When looking at the individual questions, however, there was no consistent pattern. A Present Time Orientation proved to be only slightly more preferred over Past Orientation. The Man-Nature Orientation was Harmony-with-nature over Mastery-over-nature over Subjugated-to-nature. Men tended to choose Subjugation-to-nature more frequently than women. Although there was variation within the Activity Orientation, it was in relation to the two more indecisive questions in the set, which were related to job choice. This did not affect the overall orientation of Doing over Being. No variation between men and women was identified.

The Navaho response indicated a dominant Collateral orientation. There was variation, however, for the second-order alternative between Lineal and Individualistic, with Lineal being preferred overall. Present Time Orientation was the first order preference. There was, however, variation between Past and Future for the second-order alternative; men predominantly choosing Past and women choosing Future. The overall Man-Nature Orientation was Harmony-with-nature over Mastery-over-nature over Subjugated-by-nature. The men consistently chose the Harmony-with-nature, while the women showed more variation and a tendency towards Mastery-over-nature. The Navaho, as a group, were decisively Doing over Being in their Activity Orientation.

Analysis of data from the social science research was done in an attempt to understand the variations that had been identified. The Spanish-American community was indeed going through a transitional process from a strong lineal social organization based on tradition to a more individualistic organization based on the modern socioeconomic situation. Similarly, there was a decrease in the religious dominance, which had tended to be fatalistic.

The overall Value Orientation profiles of the Mormon and Texan groups varied only in the intensity of preferences. Both were typical rural American communities with links to the rest of rural America and access to the modern conveniences of the time. They did differ somewhat in social organization, which may have accounted for the variations. The Mormon community is centered around a single focus, the church. The Texan community has no similar focal point.

Examination of the Zuni culture identified several factors that may have accounted for the variations found. The Zuni were culturally isolated from all the other groups, especially in regard to language and social and religious organization. It is a complex, yet strongly integrated culture, which has been subject to contraction and the influence of other cultures. In a response to the hostile desert environment and the cultural influence from the Apache, Navaho, Spanish, and Anglos over the years, the Zuni have responded by increasing their cultural isolation in some aspects of their culture while assimilating in other areas. The result has been a society where the clan is the major societal grouping, which has integrated over time. The Zuni showed no distinctive preference in orientation except in the relational orientation where a significant Collateral Orientation was found.

The variations found within the Navaho Value Orientation profile were considered to be the effects of the influence of the American culture, the Navaho being less isolated from the surrounding communities and having more contact with the outside world through education and work. As a result, there is discord between the traditional cultural beliefs and the Anglo-American.

Other Studies on Value Orientations

Since the original study done by Kluckhohn and Strodtbeck (1961), the value orientations of other cultures have been studied using value orientation profiles.

Caudill and Scarr (1962) used an adapted version of the original Kluckhohn and Strodtbeck Value Orientation schedule to ascertain Japanese value orientations in post-World War II Japan. The aim of their study was to identify the Value Orientations of senior school children and their parents, and to compare the changes in Value Orientation between generations and between rural and urban settings. The sample consisted of senior school children and one of their parents. If the student was female her mother was tested and if the student was male the father was tested. The students were selected from either rural or urban environments.

In order to reflect the socio-environment of Japan, the scenarios were adapted to more relevant issues. For example, the community activity of well drilling of the original study was changed to the activity of building a bridge. The study was translated into Japanese and the translation verified by then having it translated back into English.

The results of the study reported the Value Orientation of the sample in the areas of Activity, Relational, and Man-Nature Orientations. The findings, reported in List 1 (Appendix A), indicated that despite the western influence in post-World War II Japan, the traditional values were being communicated to the younger generation.

Lengermann (1971) modified the Kluckhohn and Strodtbeck Value Orientation Questionnaire in order to study the "attitudinal modernity in various working class groups" (p. 151) in Trinidad and Tobago. This modified questionnaire consisted of 20 questions, five for each of the four Value Orientation items (Time, Activity, Man-Nature, and Relational).

In her analysis of the data, Lengermann identified both the rank ordering of preferences, and the patterns of first and second preferences. The overall rank ordering is shown in List 2 (Appendix A). The patterns of first and second preferences allowed the identification of the most frequently chosen orientation, the Dominant Value Orientation (DOV), and the next preferred orientation, the Major Variant (MV).

In the analysis of the data Lengermann (1971) indicated that the sample had adopted modern attitudes "towards practical, everyday situations" (p. 159) but had retained their fundamental "traditional" orientations when confronted with uncommon problems. The sample demonstrated a modern, "core American" Value Orientation of Individualism in dealing with problem solving of everyday problems. However, when faced with less commonplace problems, they were more likely to rely on the group support of Collateral Orientation. Similarly, when dealing with practical matters they tended to be Future Orientated, yet Present Orientated regarding matters of a more abstract nature such as philosophy and socialization of children. In respect to Relational Orientation there was no significant preference and this would support a culture in transition.

Papajohn and Spiegel (1975) used the Value Orientation Questionnaire to identify the Value Orientation of three immigrant families: one Greek, one Italian, and one Puerto Rican, as illustrated in Table 2 (Appendix A). The Value Orientation Questionnaire was used as an assessment tool in evaluating change of values as part of the process of acculturation in immigrant families. The three families studied were at different stages of acculturation. Individuals in each family group were found to be at different stages of acculturation and this was reflected in the diversity of Value Orientation in each group. They also illustrated that when there is no consensus of Value Orientation in a group, conflict will result. This study illustrates that acculturation does affect values and that the rate of change is an individual phenomenon.

Within the dominant middle-class culture, other American subcultures exist. One such subculture is the Appalachian people of the Appalachian Region of northeastern United States. Tripp-Reimer and Friedl (1977) identified only the Dominant Value Orientations and compared them to the core American profile as identified by Kluckhohn and Strodtbeck (1961). The findings, displayed in List 3 (Appendix A), reveal a value system different from the dominant American culture of the middle class.

Bachtold and Eckvall (1978) also used the Value Orientation Questionnaire to identify the Value Orientation profile of a group of Hupa Indians of northwestern California. Their findings listed in List 4 (Appendix A) reflected the Hupa traditional culture.

As part of a health ecology project, Egeland (1978) identified the Value Orientation profiles of five ethnic groups (Bahamian, Haitian, Southern Black, Cuban, and Puerto Rican) in Miami (see Table 3, Appendix A). She created and used a modified version of the original Kluckhohn and Strodtbeck Value Orientation questionnaire. Two of the Relational questions, which dealt with livestock inheritance and water allocation, were omitted. Four health scenarios were added: two relating to the Relational Orientation (Care for the Invalid and a Crippled Child story), one relating to Time (aged parent), and one relating to Man–Nature (relief of pain). Although there were similarities between cultures, the finding supported the theory that the value orientations of different cultural groups are unique. In addition, the validity of the revised Value Orientation schedule was questioned.

DeMay (1982) used an Urban Value Orientation Schedule, developed by Richard Kluckhohn (the son of Clyde and Florence Kluckhohn), in a study of the Value Orientations of health professionals in two different cultures. This was a modified version of the original rural schedule (Kluckhohn and Strodtbeck, 1961). This urban schedule includes a third alternative in the activity alternatives, Being-in-becoming.

DeMay's study compared the value orientations of United States Air Force (USAF) health care professionals and Filipino civilian health care professionals working at Veteran's Administration Hospital (see Table 4, Appendix A). The resulting Value Orientation profiles were significant because neither group represented the core American values identified by Kluckhohn and Strodtbeck (1961). This was especially evident in Time orientation where Present was the first-ranked alternative. Since this study was done 20 years after the original study, this may be the result of a change in core values or it may represent the values of the particular subculture (health professional).

The original Value Orientation Schedule (Kluckhohn and Strodtbeck, 1961) was used by Brink (1984) to determine the Value Orientation profile of a sample of Annang-speaking people of Nigeria (see Table 5, Appendix A). The Annang were going through a time of transition, as illustrated by the range of education level and occupation found in the sample. The overall Annang Value Orientation was consistent with traditional values. However, when sub-groups within the population were examined, the variation associated with the cultural transition is apparent.

Burke and Maloney (1988) included Value Orientation as one of their dependent variables in a study of child bearing and health care (Burke and Maloney, 1988). For this study a Women's Value Orientation Schedule was developed. The Women's Value Orientation Questionnaire consisted of 19 questions "framed in terms of everyday situations ranging from child training to ways of working in the home or for pay" (p. 19). Five of the questions were from the original Kluckhohn and Strodtbeck (1961) schedule. Eight of the questions were edited to update the stories and change the sexist terminology. The scenarios of another six questions were changed to scenarios reflecting maternal and child situations. These new scenarios are notable and were never proven to be consistent with the original questions. The findings identified differences between Maternal and Child Health Nurses and women of three cultural groups: Euro-Canadian, Urban Cree, and Rural Cree (see Table 6, Appendix A). This study provided the first Canadian data on Value Orientations.

Gushuliak (1990) examined the relationship between Leut membership, age of Hutterian women, and Value Orientation in three Hutterian colonies in western Canada. The findings identified a distinct Value Orientation for Hutterian women (see Table 7, Appendix A). The Relational Orientations for all three Leuts was Collateral over Lineal over Individualistic, but not at a significant level. Present orientation for Time was consistent between the groups. There was variation in the second-order preference between Past and Future. The significance of the rank ordering of Time Orientation also varied between Leuts. The Activity orientation of Doing over Being was uniform between the Leuts but at different levels of significance. The Man-Nature Orientation was Subjugated-to-nature over Harmony-with-nature over Mastery-over-nature, but with no level of significance. The similarities in the value orientations between colonies was prominent while the differences were of a minor nature.

Norris (1992) identified the Value Orientation profiles of a group of parents of pre-school children and the relationship of these orientations to attitudes towards participation in their child's care while in hospital. Table 8 (Appendix A) summarizes the value orientation of this group by age and sex. Interestingly, there is within-group variation based on age and sex. The overall Relational Orientation was Collateral over Individualistic over Lineal, which was also the men and the under-35 ranking preference. In comparison, the women and over-35 ranking was Individualistic over Collateral over Lineal. The overall Time Orientation was Present over Future over Past. Men, however, preferred a Future over Present over Past Orientation. The Activity Orientation was Doing over Being except for the men who favored Being over Doing. The Man-Nature orientation was consistently Mastery-over-nature over Subjugated-to-nature over Harmony-with-nature.

This would suggest that in three of the Orientation subsets, Relational, Time, and Activity, men and women may have different value orientations. The results also suggest that Relational Orientations may differ between age groups. However, the sample size of this study is not large enough to be conclusive.

Summary

As the literature demonstrates, Value Orientation profiles are useful tools in cultural assessment. Value Orientation profiles allow us to compare basic values between cultures, individuals, and groups. Individual profiles can be compared to the overall profile of the individual's social group. These comparisons can identify areas where Value Orientations are dissimilar and thereby identify areas of potential conflict.

NATIVE VALUES

Assumptions have been made that what is known about the value systems of other North American groups can be generalized to all native groups including the Inuit (Sealey and McDonald, 1979). However, native groups are not all the same any more than all European groups are the same, despite their similarities. When one examines native cultures, differences are apparent. Their cultures and social organizations are varied. It therefore seems likely that there is also variability in their Value Orientations even though similarities may exist.

Native ethics are considered to place a high value on noninterference, noncompetitiveness, and sharing (Brant, 1990, p. 535). This results in respect for the individual and at the same time an emphasis on the group good and goals. The native perspective of Time is described as being a mixture of Past and Future. The emphasis is on Doing activities "when the time is right—that is, when the whole array of environmental factors converge to ensure success" (p. 536). The motivations for activities are described as being intrinsic with no expectation of extrinsic reward, which would be consistent with a Being Orientation.

Sealey and McDonald (1979) classified value systems as being either generalist or specialist in nature. They depicted Native American cultures as being generalists. The dominant characteristics were Harmony-with-nature, Present and Past Time Orientation, sharing, and noninterference. Even with the assumption that native groups have similar dominant values or ethical themes, little is known of the rank ordering of Value Orientations within and between native groups.

The original work on Value Orientation by Kluckhohn and Strodtbeck (1961) demonstrated that while there were similarities as to how the Navaho and Zuni differed from dominant American Value Orientation, there were also differences between the two groups. This would indicate that comparable differences may exist among the various native groups.

IMPLICATIONS FOR HEALTH SERVICES

Health practices and beliefs are associated with cultural values as are the choices made about accessing health care. Conflicting Value Orientations within or between groups can result in discord between the groups (Papajohn and Spiegel, 1975; Swanson and Hurley, 1983; Egeland, 1978). The Value Orientations of the health service providers are reflected in the health programs provided. Health care providers tend to possess the Value Orientation of the dominant culture of a society (Swanson and Hurley, 1983) and may therefore conflict with alternative cultures. Such value conflicts result in barriers between the client and the health services (Tripp-Reimer and Friedl, 1977; Egeland

1978). These barriers can create misunderstandings, misutilization of services, poor attendance, and noncompliance with regimens.

INUIT HEALTH CARE

Primary health care of the Inuit is provided by nurses who are predominantly Non-Inuit. In addition, Inuit requiring hospitalization or specialized health care are transported south to urban centers. Health care and health promotion programs are based on the Value Orientation of those planning them. They are often programs developed for urban centers in Southern Canada, which have been carried over into the Northwest territories. The success of such programs is limited and attendance is poor. The communities take little if any ownership of the programs. As nurses leave, the programs cease. Patients transported to southern centers are exposed to a system and personnel with little if any knowledge of their culture or values, which results in further conflict.

Information on Inuit values could be used by nurses in the north to plan health programs more appropriate to the population they serve. It would also be useful for nurses in the referral centers of southern Canada to plan care with an understanding of the cultural values meaningful to the patient. Knowledge of Value Orientation profiles would also allow for the identification of potential areas of conflict between the values of individual nurses and their clients.

PURPOSE OF THE STUDY

The purpose of this study is to identify and describe the Value Orientation profile of the Copper Inuit living in Coppermine, NWT (Northwest Territories).

DEFINITION OF TERMS

Value orientation: The rank-ordered value preferences that are the bases for problem-solving decisions in everyday life. Value orientations will be measured by the Kluckhohn and Strodtbeck Value Orientation Questionnaire.

THE RESEARCH DESIGN

A descriptive field study, in conjunction with the Kluckhohn and Strotdbeck Value Orientation Questionnaire, will be used to determine the Value Orientations of a stratified sample of Copper Inuit. The study will be conducted in the hamlet of Coppermine in the Kitikmeot Region of the Northwest Territories.

THE COPPER INUIT

The Copper Inuit are a culturally distinct subgroup within the Inuit peoples. Like other Inuit peoples, they existed in a dichotomous relationship with the land and sea, the summer and the winter. The resources available to them and their social environment are unique. Consequently they are also unique.

Geography

The traditional territory of the Copper Eskimo as outlined by Damas (1984, p. 397) was as follows:

> The normal western boundary of the Copper Eskimo country on the mainland of Canada seems to have been Wise Point (Stefansson 1913:167). In the northwest the south coast of Banks Island was visited in the region from DeSalis Bay to Nelson Head. In the south the Copper Eskimo knew of Great Bear Lake (Stefansson 1919:260) and also visited Beechey Lake on the Back River (Rasmussen 1932:119) and Contwoyto Lake (Damas 1962–1963). In the east, Perry River is regarded as having been the boundary between Copper Eskimo and Netsilik countries (Damas 1968). Much of Victoria Island was hunted over but usually the area south of a line drawn from Walker Bay to Denmark Bay is considered to be their region of travel and occupation.

Jenness (1922, p. 14) described the mainland coast as being

> low, sloping back in undulated ridges to an interior plateau. The ridges run usually east west at no great distance from each other, and are connected by numerous short transverse ridges that enclose a network of lakes and ponds of every size and shape. The coast becomes more rocky east of the Coppermine river, and granite makes its first appearance.

The numerous islands of Coronation Gulf are described as having high cliffs along their east and south shores. The south coast of Victoria Island was described as having high cliffs of dolomite ranging from 40 to 80 feet in height.

The area of the Copper Inuit is above the Arctic Circle. Winters are long and extend well into spring and start in early fall. Summer is limited to July and August and snow may occur even then. During the winter months the sun appears only low on the horizon for short periods and fails to rise at all for several weeks. In contrast, in the summer months it is daylight 24 hours a day and for periods the sun never sets. The result is a distinct winter–summer dichotomy affecting not only the Inuit but also the resources available to them.

Snow remains on the ground well into summer and the permafrost never leaves the land. This limits the variety and quantity of vegetation able to survive this environment. The southern regions of the Copper Inuit lands did extend into the tree line and here "in the valleys of the Tree and Coppermine rivers . . . occasional beds of willow that grow to a height of five or six feet" (Jenness, 1922, p. 14). For the most part, however, vegetation was limited to heather, moss, grass, and tiny flowering plants (Jenness, 1922). Several edible varieties of plant life existed such as crowberries, cloudberries, bearberries, and sorrel, in limited amounts, but the Copper Inuit had not incorporated them into their diet as had some other Eskimo groups (Jenness, 1922, p. 97).

The restrictions on plant life influence the disposition of wildlife in the area. During the summer when there were plants for grazing, caribou migrated north into the area and remained until fall when they migrated south. The caribou remained constantly on the move as they depleted local growth. Smaller grazing animals such as lemmings and Arctic hare also thrived. This small game allowed small carnivores such as fox and wolf to survive. Polar bear and musk-ox could be found in only some areas of the Copper Inuit region with musk-ox in the area of Bathurst Inlet, and polar bear in the area beyond Kent peninsula and near Cape Baring in the summer. The area is the summer nesting ground for a variety of birds such as falcons, snow buntings, hawks, snowy owl, sandpipers, plovers, gulls, terns, ducks, and loons (Udvardy, 1977). A few birds, such as the ptarmigan, stay in the area year round.

In the winter months "the straits and gulfs of the Copper Inuit regions are covered by a continuous sheet of ice from October or November until sometime in July" (Damas, 1984, p. 398), preventing free and easy access to marine life. Seals remained throughout the winter, maintaining holes for breathing. In the spring, they converged at the flow edge where they would lie at the edge of the ice, basking in the sun.

THE ETHNOGRAPHIC PRESENT

Culture Contact

The first documented contact with the Copper Inuit was in 1771 by Samuel Hearne who, while travelling overland with a party of Chipewyan Indians, came upon two camps of Inuit near the mouth of the Coppermine River. Captain Franklin also found evidence of Eskimos in the area when he visited in 1821. There were other brief encounters: Richardson, 1848; McClure, 1851; Collinson, 1850–51; Hanbury, 1902; Klengenburg, 1905–06; and Mogg, 1907. However, the first significant contact with the Inuit of this region was by Stefansson in 1910. Stefansson was followed by Jenness in 1922 and Rasmussen in 1923. By 1920 both the Anglican and Roman Catholic churches, the Royal Canadian Mounted Police (RCMP), and the Hudson Bay Company (HBC) were present in the area. From this time onward, European involvement continued to increase (Jenness, 1922; Damas, 1984; Buliard, 1953).

Culture

The Language of the Copper Inuit was a regional dialect, Innuniagtun. Jenness (1922) described it as being substantially different from other Inuit languages, but varying only in intonation between the people within the Copper Inuit region. Like other Inuit languages, Innuniagtun had no written form until developed by church groups. The written form of Innuniagtun is in Roman orthography. This is a phonetic representation of the language.

The Copper Inuit trace their ancestry through both the maternal and paternal lines. The basic social unit was the family, consisting of a man and woman and their descendants. In the average family four or five children were born, three of which may have survived. Unwanted children were either adopted by another family or alternatively killed by suffocation or abandonment. Children adopted into the family held full membership. When a twin birth occurred, one infant was killed because it was not possible to provide for both infants.

In kinship terms there was no distinction between parallel or cross cousins. Kinship terms for siblings were determined by the age and gender of the individual in relation to oneself. A man would address his older brother as *angayua* and his older sister as *alekka;* similarly, a woman would call her older sister *angayua* and her older brother *alekka.* Kinship terms related to sibling's offspring were based on relationship rather then gender, with *kangiganga* for brother's child and *oyorua* for sister's child. Similarly, maternal and paternal aunts and uncles have different kinship terms (Jenness, 1922).

Upon marriage, children formed a new and distinct family of their own, living separately from other family members. Although there did not seem to be any formal arranging of marriages, if the bridegroom was going to move away with his new bride, a small payment was made to the girl's parents. If the couple remained in the area, they simply moved into their own home. Marriage by capture was common, but usually involved women who had already been married. During the initial period of the marriage, it was common for the marriage to be dissolved by either party. Once children had been born, marriages were relatively stable. Polygamy occurred on occasion but was not the norm. Under special circumstances wife sharing or exchanging did occur. Such exchanges served to create a lasting bond between a visitor and the group he was visiting. Similar bonds were also formed by becoming a "dancing associate" or "flipper-associate" with someone in a group. In case of divorce, a woman would return to her kinsfolk (Jenness, 1922).

Both men and women had complementary roles necessary for survival. Men did most of the hunting, building of shelters (igloos in winter and tents in summer), and made tools and weapons. During migrations, men were responsible for the preparation and operation of the dogs and sled. Women were responsible for all cooking, sewing, dressing of skins, and maintenance of the shelter once it was built. This included the gathering of fuel and the maintaining of seal lamps. Everyone participated in fishing both with rod and line; however, only men used spears for fishing in the weirs.

Property was distinguished as either personal, family, or communal. Personal property consisted of anything used by the individual in daily life, such as tools (weapons for a man or lamps and sewing kit for a woman). Such personal property belonged to the individual and would go with them if they left the family in divorce or marriage. It was not unusual for friends and relatives to borrow from each other. When an owner died, a portion of that person's personal property was laid on the owner's grave. The remaining articles were distributed among the kinsfolk based on group discussion with no priority to any one individual.

All food and skins acquired by family members was considered to be family property although some must be shared with neighbors, the amount depending on the abundance of food in the community at that time. Land was considered the property of the community, which used it as hunting and fishing grounds. Visitors were restricted from using local natural resources unless they established a bond with the community.

Leadership was flexible based on the characteristic of the individual who earned respect from other community members. "A man acquires influence by his force of character, his energy and success in hunting, or his skill in magic. As long as these last him age but increases his influence, but when they fail his prestige and authority vanish" (Jenness, 1922, p. 93). There was no organized council to oversee the conduct of community members. Minor disputes such as theft or abduction were settled between the individuals involved through compensation or vengeance. As a result, murder in response to a dispute was common.

The Copper Inuit spiritual system was animistic. Birds, animals, and even land forms were considered to have supernatural power. Spirits of the dead may also affect the living. Water or oil was poured into the mouth of killed animals to quench their thirst. Oil was rubbed into the skins of killed birds. Offerings were also left beside the larger animals, such as polar bears, when they were killed. The Copper Inuit made clear distinctions between animals of the land and of the sea, and the products of the two were kept and used separately. Caribou, a land food, could not be cooked or their skins sewn while living on sea ice. At no time were caribou and seal meat to be cooked in the same pot. Similarly, seal skin was not to be tanned or sewn while fishing was taking place at a fresh water site. Failure to follow the rules related to this land–sea dichotomy would cause storms, famine, or other misfortune.

Shaman were Inuit who acted as "mediators and intercessors between living Eskimos and the supernatural world of shades and spirits" (Jenness, 1922, p. 191). The shaman was a person able to control certain spirits of either certain animals or shades of the deceased. A person became a shaman in one of two ways. Either a spirit would make itself available to the person or the person could purchase knowledge about how to approach a spirit from an existing shaman. Once contact had been made, the spirit would ask the person to perform a deed, such as kill a specific animal and eat a certain part of that animal. If the person did as asked, the spirit would promise to serve that person and to bestow magical powers on them.

Shamans had the power to change their forms and take on the form of an animal. The chief function of the shaman was to hold séances to learn about some future event, such as success at hunting, or to determine the cause of illness or misfortune in order to take corrective action. Illnesses were attributed to bewitchment by spirits with whom the shaman could intercede. However, some shaman used their power for their own gain. They were often feared because their connection to the spirit world allowed them to influence spirits to do harm as well as good.

The Copper Inuit had minimal contact with other native groups because of geographic distance and natural barriers. They did trade extensively among themselves. Access to many resources such as copper, polar bear, wood, and musk-ox were localized. This resulted in a trade economy, primarily in the large camps found along the coast while waiting for the sea ice to form. Although the Copper Inuit did not have direct contact with whites until the 1900s, their economy was indirectly affected by polar exploration. The "Investigator," a ship sent out in search of the lost Franklin expedition of 1845, was abandoned by its crew in the region after being ice locked for two years (Hickey, 1984, p. 17). This crew left behind a large cache of supplies.

The Copper Inuit near Berkley Point, Victoria Island found the ship and its valuable cache and over the next 30 years salvaged the site (Hickey, 1984; pp. 18–19, 24). Hickey (1984) showed that this influx of a large quantity of valuable and exotic goods may have affected the economic balance of the Copper Inuit culture; the result being a de-emphasis on the extended family and an emphasis on the individual.

As the western goods were only accessible to those Inuit frequenting Banks Island and the environment, there would not be support for a large number of Inuit. The only way for most Copper Inuit to obtain the other goods was to trade for them. The value of these items was far greater than the value of most goods traded. Inuit without access responded in one of two ways: to obtain these valued goods, a family would have to trade proactively for future goods (go into debt), or enter into some kind of partnership with the other party. Either response would likely lead to a shift to a more individualistic existence.

Hickey (1984, p. 25) contends that to maintain the egalitarian nature of their society, the Copper Inuit responded in two ways;

> First, by entering into either closer kin relationships (real or fictive) or into formal exchange partnerships which allowed 'debts' to be deferred, second, the 'debtor' could extend similar relationships out to others in order to obtain such materials as native copper, soapstone, driftwood and wood from the tree-line at the southern margins of their territories (both of which, it appears, were preferred to the Investigator's hardwood), and—for the caribou-poor Bankslanders—an annual supply of vitally important caribou skins for clothing and other uses.

A land-based specialization occurred, based on geographic location, to restrict access to the valuable land-based resources that were used in trade (Hickey, 1984, pp. 26–27). As sea resources were not regional and were accessible to all, there was little change in the winter social groupings. The land–sea dichotomy did change, however, with groups leaving the sea ice earlier in the spring to work the land for trade resources (Hickey, 1984, p. 27). The result was the decline of basking seal hunting (Hickey, 1984, p. 27) and spring caribou hunting (Jenness, 1922, p. 123, cited in Damas, 1984, p. 398).

Modern Copper Inuit

The Copper Inuit territories fall within the Kitikmeot Region of the Northwest Territories and will fall for the most part within the proposed Nunavut Territory. Like other areas of the Canadian Arctic, they have been greatly influenced by the development that took place as a result of the defense installations following World War II. During 1950, the Federal government constructed schools and nursing stations at some locations, and movement into permanent settlement gradually occurred. Today the Copper Inuit reside primarily in the communities of Coppermine, Cambridge Bay, Holman Island, Bay Chimo, and Bathurst Inlet.

Although the elderly may be unilingual in Innuniagtun, most people are at least verbally bilingual in both English and Innuniagtun. The school system may be conducted in Innuniagtun in the primary grades with a gradual transition to English. Newspapers and some other publications are available in both languages and translation service exists to translate material such as government documents into both languages. All communities have local radio, which is predominantly in Innuniagtun. Until 1992, programming in Inuit Languages was available through Canadian Broadcast Corporation North (CBC North) several hours a day, produced by Inuit Broadcast Corporation (IBC). In January of 1992, Television Northern Canada (TVNC) began broadcasting. This network produces 11 hours a day of native broadcasting. Most programs on this network are about regions in the Northwest Territories, and many are in one of the seven native languages of the Northwest Territories including Innuniagtun.

Economy of the Copper Inuit has undergone major changes. Hunting and fishing still provide the main supply of protein for the population. Since the decline of the fur trade in the 1970s, hunting has not been a significant source of income. The main employers in the area are the various agencies of the territorial government, and service industries. As a result, there is a high level of unemployment and, even with education, limited potential in the area.

The Copper Inuit, like other Inuit groups, have quickly adjusted to modern technology while at the same time retaining their own culture. Igloos and skin tents have been replaced by two- and three-bedroom homes; dog teams have been replaced by skidoos; CB radios provide communication for hunters and families while out on the land, and children are familiar with computers. At the same time, caribou clothing is still preferred on winter hunting trips and igloos are used on hunting trips. Inuit traditional skills are preserved through the Inuit Traditional games. Events in these games include seal skinning and duck plucking, and athletic events such as high kicking, bench reach, and walrus pull. These events demonstrated the skills necessary for the traditional lifestyle. During the summer months many families leave the communities to live in camps along the Arctic coasts. In addition Inuit traditional entertainment, such as drum dancing and singing, are part of many community social occasions.

The Copper Inuit have adopted Christian religions that were introduced by the missionaries in the early 1900s. Today all communities have at least one church and in the larger communities several denominations may be represented. With the adoption of Christianity, shamanism seemed to have disappeared.

With the establishment of permanent communities a more structured political system has also evolved. Each settlement has its own elected local government consisting of a mayor and council. Ridings within the region elect members to the Legislative Assembly of the Northwest Territories (NWT) and the area is within one of the two federal ridings of the NWT. The Kitikmeot Region Inuit Association is an affiliate of the Inuit Tapirisat of Canada. This organization represents the interests of the Inuit on various issues concerning the development of the north and the preservation of the Inuit Culture on a national level (Devine, 1982).

Coppermine

Coppermine is a community of 888 people (Statistics Canada, 1986) of which 98% are Inuit (Bureau of Statistics, Government of the Northwest Territories, 1983a). Of these between 50% and 60% are over the age of 18 years (Bureau of Statistics, Government of the Northwest Territories, 1983b). It is situated on Coronation Gulf, immediately west of the mouth of the Coppermine River on the mainland Arctic Coast, latitude 67° 50′ N and longitude 115° 06′ W. It is 563 air km north of Yellowknife and 1603 air km north of Edmonton (Devine, 1982, p. 108).

The main sources of income are local government services, local merchants, and activities such as hunting, fishing, and carving. The community has two stores, the Coppermine Eskimo Co-operative Ltd., and the Northern Store (formerly the Hudson Bay Company). Consumer prices are approximately 50% to 59% higher than in Edmonton. Water is available from the Coppermine River and is delivered by both a utilidor (pipeline) or by water trucks to holding tanks in the homes. Sewage is collected in sewage pump-out tanks and then deposited in a disposal area 2.2 km from the community. The community receives scheduled air service on a regular basis, and in the fall nonperishable materials are transported to the community by barge from the railhead at Hay River, NWT. The community has a four-nurse Health Center, a three-man Royal

Canadian Mounted Police (RCMP) detachment, and a school for grades K through 9. For recreation there is a community hall, playground, curling rink arena, and summer swimming pool (Devine, 1982).

Target Population

The target population will be all adults over the age of 18, of Coppermine NWT. Criteria for inclusion in the study will be as follows:

a. Both parents being Inuit and at least one being from the Coppermine area
b. Currently residing in the Kitikmeot region

Subjects may elect not to participate when asked.

Sample Selection Procedure

The target population will be identified by the use of a settlement list obtained from the Hamlet office in Coppermine. Names on the list will be divided initially into males and females. The sample will be further divided into two age groups: over 40 and under 40. From a total sample of 60 people, the division would be as follows: 30 males (15 over 40, 15 under 40) and 30 females (15 over 40, 15 under 40). The names on the lists will then be numbered and subjects chosen by use of a random number table. Following Cohen (1988, p. 55), setting alpha at 0.05 and using t-tests, a large affect (0.80) will be required to achieve a power of 0.85. The lower the affect achieved, the lower the power.

As with all studies, attrition is to be expected. In this study attrition can occur in two ways: subjects can drop out prior to the completion of the questionnaire, or subjects may ask to be withdrawn from the study once the questionnaire is completed. Whatever the reason for withdrawal, another subject will be chosen in the same manner as the original.

Research Instrument

The research instrument to be used in this study is the Kluckhohn and Strodtbeck (1961) Value Orientation Questionnaire. It consists of 22 items with four subscales: man–nature, time, activity, and relational. Relational Orientation is evaluated by 7 items, with man–nature, activity, and time orientation each having 5 items. Within the items, relational, time, and man–nature each have three alternative choices, and activity has two alternative choices.

For the purpose of this study, the Value Orientation Questionnaire has been modified in two ways. The language of the questionnaire was sexist by modern standards, and gender terms have been changed to make the questionnaire gender neutral. Second, the questionnaire was designed for rural agricultural populations. This tool has been modified for use in urban settings (Egeland, 1978; DeMay, 1982) with varying success. Such modifications were done to provide culturally relevant value stories. However, it has never been established that such changes are necessary. It is the philosophic meaning of the alternative solutions representing the variant values (Egeland, 1978) that is the basis for the rank-ordering of value orientations. It then may be possible for individuals to respond to the problems presented in the original questionnaire even if the situations differ from their own experience. Therefore, the stories of the original questionnaire will be asked in conjunction with modified questions.

In the modified questions, terms of reference relating to agricultural activities will be modified to be relevant to the Copper Inuit fishing traditions (questions 4, 7, 10, 16, 17, and 18). In addition, questions related to water supply will be asked in their original form and in a modified form to reflect northern water supplies (questions 2 and 20). The questionnaire will therefore consist of a total of 30 questions (see Appendix B).

DATA COLLECTION PROCEDURES

Data will be collected by the interview method. Questions will be asked either by the researcher or the interpreter. The interpreter will receive instruction regarding the purpose of the questionnaire and the necessity of asking the questions exactly as written without further explanation. All interviews will be tape recorded. Transcripts will be made of the interviews conducted in English. Recordings from interviews conducted in Innuniagtun will be reviewed with the interpreter for relevant information and field notes will be made of this information. The field notes and transcripts will be used to analyze variations within questions for each subset.

A field journal will be kept to document the research. The field journal will consist of three types of entries: a daily agenda or appointment calendar, observational notes, and recall notes. The daily agenda will consist of a record of the daily activities of the researcher and will be cross indexed with the observational and recall notes. Observational notes will consist of notes taken by the researcher during community activities such as public meetings and community functions. These notes will include a description of these events, social interactions, and behaviors. Recall notes will consist of recollections made at a later date by the researcher.

On a monthly basis, the researcher will write a progress report to members of her thesis committee informing them of observations and the progress of data collection. This correspondence will include a summary of the observations recorded in the field notes and of the results of the individual interviews. Concerns and questions arising from the data collection will also be included in these letters.

Reliability and Validity

The Value Orientation Profile (Kluckhohn and Strodtbeck, 1961) has been shown to have construct validity through previous usage in a variety of cultures (Kluckhohn and Strodtbeck, 1961). Content validity of the tool has also been established from the initial work done by Kluckhohn and Strodtbeck (1961) when the tool was reviewed with experts in the field of anthropology, sociology, and statistics. Concurrent validity was established from the initial work done by Kluckhohn and Strodtbeck (1961) comparing their findings with the anthropological research done with the populations at the same time (work done by R. Kluckhohn, C. Kluckhohn, J. Roberts, F. Kluckhohn, F. Strodtbeck, and K. Rommey), which supported their findings. This qualitative data illustrated that the behavior of community members reflected the Value Orientations of the culture and where possible explain variations.

Modifications made to the tool for this study will be evaluated through several judge panels to assess content validity. First, the revised questionnaire will be circulated to persons familiar with value orientation research and who have used the Value Orientation Questionnaire. They will be asked to judge whether the changes are appropriate and consistent with the intent of the question. Second, prior to translation, the revised questionnaire will be shared with a group of Inuit to determine if the changes are appropriate and to assess the questionnaire for any problems related to translatability. Third, following translation, several bilingual Copper Inuit will be asked to evaluate the translation for content and consistency with the original document. Finally, once in the community of Coppermine, a final check of the translation of the document will be done, with individuals not within the sample, and final changes made.

Reliability of the tool is more difficult to establish. To date, no test retest of the tool has been successfully accomplished. One problem may be that values themselves may change over time. DeMay (1982, p. 76) discusses this possibility from the findings of a Filipino sample who had adapted "American" values. Gushuliak's (1990) attempt to do a test retest was unsuccessful due to small sample size and attrition.

The equivalence reliability of the Value Orientation Profile has been demonstrated in previous studies. This is based on the alternative forms of questions offered for each orientation group.

The analysis of the data looks at consistency of preference of the individual within each value orientation subset. The consistency of the original tool has been demonstrated in the original study (Kluckhohn and Strodtbeck, 1961). The reliability of the modified questions will be determined by examining their consistency with the original questions.

Data Analysis

Data analysis of the questionnaire will be done as outlined by Kluckhohn and Strodtbeck (1961) in the original study. This method of analysis has also been used by Egeland (1978), DeMay (1982), Gushuliak (1990), and Brink (1984). This analysis involves three stages: (1) Total Item Patterning, (2) Intra Item Patterning, and (3) Total Orientation Patterning.

Total Item Patterning looks at each value orientation subset (e.g., time), and compares the expected frequency to the observed frequency of the alternatives. The expected frequency is that each alternative (past, present, and future) would occur with equal regularity. The Kendall S statistic will be used to compare the expected with the observed.

Intra Item Patterning looks at the consistency of the rank ordering of responses for each question of the subsets. The expected preferences of rank ordering will be compared with the observed rank ordering for each question. A consistent preference for one value over another within the subset will be expected. This will be tested through binomial analysis.

Total Orientation Patterning looks at the consistency of the rank-ordered responses of each value orientation subset (e.g., time). It compares the expected rank ordering of the subset with the observed rank ordering of the subset. A t-test will be used to compare the expected and observed mean frequencies. In this manner, the significance of patterns can be determined.

The field journal will be used to compare observed behaviors with ascribed values. Both individual items as well as the overall patterning will be analyzed in light of the observations made in the field journal.

Ethical Considerations

The human rights of individuals will be protected in several ways. In accordance with the policy of the University of Alberta Faculty of Graduate Studies, this proposal will require approval of the ethics committee of the Faculty of Nursing. Following ethical clearance, an application for license to conduct research in the Northwest Territories will be submitted to the Science Institute of the Northwest Territories (see Appendix C).

Permission to conduct the research will be requested from the hamlet council of Coppermine, NWT (Appendix C). The Hamlet will be requested to provide access to the settlement list and to allow the researcher to take observational notes of activities in Coppermine. The council will be given a written summary of the proposal, a copy of the questionnaire, and all information about consents. Individual committees and agencies will be approached for permission to attend meetings and make observations. The purpose of the study will be explained to them and if requested the general written summary of the proposal of the consent form will be given to them (see Appendix F). In addition, the Kitikmeot Regional Health Board will be given a written summary of the proposal with a request for a written statement of support of the study.

Subject participation will be voluntary and the subjects will be free to withdraw at any time. An informed consent in both English and Innuniagtun will be obtained from each subject (see Appendix F). This consent will briefly describe the study and the expectations of the subject. In addition, the researcher will provide a verbal explanation of the study (see Appendix F) as well as an opportunity for questions at the time of obtaining the consent.

REFERENCES

Bachtold, L. M., & Eckvall, K. L. (1978). Current value orientation of American Indians in northern California: The Hupa. *Journal of Cross Cultural Psychology, 9*(3):367–375.

Brant, C. (1990). Native ethics and rules of behaviour. *Canadian Journal of Psychiatry. 35*, 534–539.

Brink P. J. (1982) Cultural assessment. In B. Jennings (ed.), *Woman's Health: Ambulatory Care* (pp. 69–82). New York: Grune and Stratton.

Brink, P. J. (1984). Value orientations as an assessment tool in cultural diversity. *Nursing Research, 33*(4),198–203.

Brink, P. J. (Ed.) (1990). *Transcultural nursing: A book of readings*. Prospect Heights, IL: Perception Press.

Bureau of Statistics, Government of the Northwest Territories. (1983). *Population 15 years and over: By mother tongue, home language, official language, place of birth, ethnic group, educational level and sex*. Yellowknife, NWT: Government of Northwest Territories.

Bureau of Statistics, Government of the Northwest Territories. (1983). *Population families and children dwelling and households*. Yellowknife, NWT: Government of Northwest Territories.

Burke, S. O., & Maloney, R. (1986). The women's value orientation questionnaire: An instrument revision study. *Nursing Papers, 18*(1),33–44.

Caudill, W., & Scarr, H. A. (1962) Japanese value orientation and cultural change. *Ethnology, 1*, 53–91.

Cohen, J. (1988). *Statistical power analysis for the behavioural sciences* (2nd ed.), Hillside, NJ: Lawrence Erlbaum Associates.

Damas, D. (1984). Copper Eskimo. In C. Sturtevant (ed.), *Handbook of North American Indians* (vol. 5, pp. 397–414). Washington, DC: Smithsonian Institution.

DeMay, D. A. (1982). *Health care professional value orientation: A comparative study.* Unpublished master's thesis, University of California, Los Angeles.

Devine, M. (1982). *NWT data book: 1982–1983.* Yellowknife, NWT: Outcrop Ltd..

Egeland, J. (1978). Ethnic value orientation analysis. In *Miami health ecology project report.* Miami, FL: University of Miami, School of Medicine.

Frondizi, R. (1963). *What is a value?* LaSalle, Illinois: Open Court Publishing Co.

Gushuliak, T. (1990). *Value orientations of Hutterian women.* Unpublished master's thesis, University of Alberta, Edmonton, AB.

Hammersley, M., & Atkinson, P. (1983). *Ethnography: Principles and practice.* New York: Tavistock Publications.

Hickey, C. (1984). An examination of processes of cultural change among nineteenth century Copper Inuit. *Etudes Inuit, 8*(1),13–35.

Jenness, D. (1922). *Report of the Canadian Arctic Expedition 1913–1918* (Vol XII). Ottawa, ON: F. A. Acland.

Kluckhohn, C. (1951). Values and value orientations in the theory of action. In T. Parsons (ed.), *Toward a general theory of action.* Cambridge: Harvard University Press.

Kluckhohn, C., & Murray H. A. (1956). Personality formation: The determinants. In C. Kluckhohn & H. A. Murray (eds.), *Personality in nature, society and culture.* New York: Alfred A. Knopf.

Kluckhohn, F. (1951). Dominant and substitute profiles of cultural orientation: Their significance for the analysis of social stratification. *Social Forces, 28*(4):376–394.

Kluckhohn, F. (1953). Dominant and variant value orientations. In C. Kluckhohn & H. A. Murray (eds.), *Personality in nature, society and culture* (pp. 342–357). New York: Alfred A. Knopf.

Kluckhohn, F. R., & Strodtbeck, F. L. (1961). *Variations in value orientations.* New York: Row Peterson and Co..

Kummel, F. (1966). Time as succession and the problem of duration. In J. T. Fraser (ed.), *The voices of time,* (pp. 31–55). New York: George Braziller Inc.

Lengermann, P. M. (1971). Working-class values in Trinidad and Tobago. *Social and Economic Studies, 20*(2):151–163.

Murray, H. A., & Kluckhohn, C. (1956). Outline of a conceptualisation of personality. In C. Kluckhohn & M. A. Murray (eds.), *Personality in nature, society and culture,* (pp. 342–357). New York: Alfred A. Knopf.

Norris, C. M., (1992). *The relationship between parental value orientations and parental participation in hospital care.* Unpublished master's thesis, University of Alberta, Edmonton, AB.

Papajohn, J., & Spiegel, J. (1971). The relationship of culture value orientation change and Rorschach indices of psychological development. *Journal of Cross-Cultural Psychology, 2*(3): 257–272.

Papajohn, J., & Spiegel, J. (1975). *Transactions in families.* London: Jossey-Bass Publishers.

Rasmussen, K. (1932). *Intellectual culture of the Copper Eskimo. Report of the fifth Thule expedition 1921–24* (vol. 9). Copenhagen.

Sealey, D. B., & McDonald, N. (1979). *The health care professional in a native community: A cross-cultural study guide.* Faculty of Education, University of Manitoba.

Statistics Canada. (1987). *Population and dwelling counts—provinces and territories. Northwest Territories.* Ottawa, ON: Minister of Supply and Services Canada.

Stefansson, V. (1913). *My life with the Eskimo.* New York: Macmillian.

Stefansson, V. (1919). The Stefansson–Anderson arctic expedition: Preliminary ethnological report. *Anthropological papers of the American Museum of Natural History,* vol. 14. New York: American Museum of Natural History.

Swanson, A. R., & Hurley, P. M. (1983). Family systems: Values and value conflicts, *Journal of Psychosocial Nursing and Mental Health Services, 21*(7):24–30.

Tripp-Reimer, T., & Friedl, C. (1977). Appalachians: A neglected minority. *Nursing Clinics of North America, 12*(1):41–54.

Tripp-Reimer, T., & Brink, P. J. (1984). Cultural assessment: Content and process. *Nursing Outlook, 32*(2):78–82.

Udvardy, M. (1977). *The Audubon society field guide to North American birds, western region.* New York: Alfred A. Knopf.

Werkmeister, W. H. (1967). *Man and his values.* Lincoln, NB: University of Nebraska Press.

APPENDIX A: TABLES AND LISTS

TABLE 1	Value Orientations American Southwest			
	Relational	*Time*	*Activity*	*Man–Nature*
MORMON	Indy>Col>Lin	Fut≥Pres>Past	Doing>Being	Mast≥Har>Sub
TEXAN	Ind>Col>Lin	Fut≥Pres>Past	Doing>Being	Mast>Har≥Sub
ZUNI	Col>Lin≥Ind	Pres≥Past>Fut	Doing≥Being	Har≥Sub>Mast
NAVAJO	Col>Lin≥Ind	Pres>Past≥Fut	Doing>Being	Har≥Mast≥Sub
SPANISH AMERICAN	Ind≥Lin≥Col	Pres>Fut>Past	Being>Doing	Sub>Mast>Har

Abbreviations: Past = Past, Fut = Future, Pres = Present, Being = Being, Doing = Doing, Lin = Lineal, Col = Collateral, Ind = individualistic, Har = Harmony-with-nature, Mast = Mastery-over-nature, Sub = Subjugated-to-nature
Key = no preference, ≥ non significant preference, > significant preference

TABLE 2	Greek, Italian, Puerto Rican Value Orientation Profile			
	Relational	*Time*	*Activity*	*Man–Nature*
GREEK	Lin>Ind>Col	Pres>Past>Fut	Be>Do>BIB	Sub>Har>Mast
ITALIAN	Col>Lin>Ind	Pres>Past>Fut	Be>BIB>Do	Sub>Har>Mast
PUERTO RICAN	Col>Lin>Ind	Pres>Fut>Past	Be>Do>BIB	Sub>Har>Mast

Abbreviations: Past = Past, Fut = Future, Pres = Present, Be = Being, Do = Doing, BIB = Being-in-becoming, Lin = Lineal, Col = Collateral, Ind = Individualistic, Har = Harmony-with-nature, Mast = Mastery-over-nature, Sub = Subjugated-to-nature
Key = no preference, > preference

TABLE 3	Value Orientation Profiles: Southern Blacks, Bahamian, Cuban, Haitian, and Puerto Rican			
	Relational	*Time*	*Activity*	*Man–Nature*
SOUTHERN BLACKS	Lin≥Col≥Ind	Pres≥Fut≥Past	Being≥Doing	Sub≥Mast>Har
BAHAMIAN	Ind>Lin>Col	Pres≥Past≥Fut	Doing≥Being	Sub≥Mast≥Har
CUBAN	Ind≥Col≥Lin	Pres≥Past≥Fut	Doing≥Being	Mast≥Sub≥Har
HAITIAN	Lin>Ind≥Col	Pres>Past≥Fut	Doing>Being	Sub>Mast>Har
PUERTO RICAN	Ind>Col≥Lin	Pres≥Fut≥Past	Doing≥Being	Har≥Sub≥Mast

Abbreviations: Past = Past, Fut = Future, Pres = Present, Being = Being, Doing = Doing, Lin = Lineal, Col = Collateral,
Ind = Individualistic, Har = Harmony-with-nature, Mast = Mastery-over-nature, Sub = Subjugated-to-nature
Key = no preference, ≥ non significant preference, > significant preference

TABLE 4	USAF and Filipino Health Personnel Value Orientation Profiles			
	Relational	*Time*	*Activity*	*Man–Nature*
USAF HEALTH PERSONNEL	Ind>Col>Lin	Pres≥Fut>Past	BIB≥Do≥Be	Mast>Har≥Sub
FILIPINO HEALTH PERSONNEL	Ind≥Col≥Lin	Pres=Fut>Past	Do≥BIB>Be	Mast≥Har≥Sub

Abbreviations: Past = Past, Fut = Future, Pres = Present, Being = Being, BIB = Being-in-becoming, Doing = Doing, Lin = Lineal,
Col = Collateral, Ind = Individualistic, Har = Harmony-with-nature, Mast = Mastery-over-nature, Sub = Subjugated-to-nature
Key = no preference, ≥ non significant preference, > significant preference

TABLE 5	Annang Value Orientation Profiles			
	Relational	*Time*	*Activity*	*Man–Nature*
ANNANG	Col>Ind>Lin	Pres>Fut>Past	Being>Doing	Sub>Mast>Har
MALES & FEMALES	Col>Ind>Lat	Pres>Fut>Past	Being>Doing	Har>Sub>Mast Mast>Sub>Har
TRADITION HEALERS	Ind>Col>Lin	Pres>Fut>Past	Being>Doing	Har>Sub>Mast
NURSES	Lin>Col>Ind	Fut>Pres>Past	Doing>Being	Mast>Sub=Har
EDUCATED MALES	Lin=Col=Ind	Pres>Fut>Past	Being>Doing	Sub=Mast=Har
EDUCATED FEMALES	Lin=Col-Ind	Pres=Fut=Past	Being=Doing	Mast>Har>Sub

Abbreviations: Past = Past, Fut = Future, Pres = Present, Being = Being, Doing = Doing, Lin = Lineal, Col = Collateral, Ind =
Individualistic, Har = Harmony-with-nature, Mast = Mastery-over-nature, Sub = Subjugated-to-nature
Key = no preference, ≥ non significant preference, > significant preference

| TABLE 6 | Value Orientation Canadian Women | | | |

	Relational	Time	Activity	Man–Nature
NURSES	Ind>Col>Lin	Pres>Fut>Past	Doing>Being	Sub>Har>Mast
EURO CANADIAN	Ind>Col>Lin	Pres>Fut>Past	Doing>Being	Har>Sub>Mast
RURAL CREE	Col>Ind>Lin	Pres>Past>Fut	Doing>Being	Har>Sub>Mast
URBAN CREE	Col>Lin>Ind	Pres>Past>Fut	Doing>Being	Har>Sub>Mast

Abbreviations: Past = Past, Fut = Future, Pres = Present, Being = Being, Doing = Doing, Lin = Lineal, Col = Collateral,
   Ind = Individualistic, Har = Harmony-with-nature, Mast = Mastery-over-nature, Sub = Subjugated-to-nature
Key = no preference, > preference

| TABLE 7 | Hutterian Women Value Orientation Profile | | | |

	Relational	Time	Activity	Man–Nature
DARIUS-LEUT COLONY	Col≥Lin≥Ind	Pres=Past≥Fut	Doing≥Being	Sub≥Har≥Mast
LEHRELEUT COLONY	Col≥Lin≥Ind	Pres≥Fut>Past	Doing>Being	Sub≥Har≥Mast
SCHMIEDE-LEUT COLONY	Col≥Lin≥Ind	Pres>Past=Fut	Doing≥Being	Sub≥Har≥Mast

Abbreviations: Past = Past, Fut = Future, Pres = Present, Being = Being, Doing = Doing, Lin = Lineal, Col = Collateral,
   Ind = Individualistic, Har = Harmony-with-nature, Mast = Mastery-over-nature, Sub = Subjugated-to-nature
Key = no preference, ≥ non significant preference, > significant preference

| TABLE 8 | Value Orientation Parents of Preschool Children | | | |

	Relational	Time	Activity	Man–Nature
OVERALL	Col≥Ind>Lin	Pres>Fut>Past	Doing≥Being	Mast>Sub>Har
FEMALES	Ind≥Col>Lin	Pres>Fut>Past	Doing>Being	Mast>Sub≥Har
MALES	Col≥Ind≥Lin	Fut≥Pres>Past	Being≥Doing	Mast>Sub≥Har
UNDER 35	Col>Ind>Lin	Pres>Fut>Past	Doing>Being	Mast>Sub>Har
OVER 35	Ind≥Col>Lin	Pres>Fut>Past	Doing≥Being	Mast≥Sub≥Har

Abbreviations: Past = Past, Fut = Future, Pres = Present, Being = Being, Doing = Doing, Lin = Lineal, Col = Collateral,
   Ind = Individualistic, Har = Harmony-with-nature, Mast = Mastery-over-nature, Sub = Subjugated-to-nature
Key = no preference, ≥ non significant preference, > significant preference

LIST 1	Japanese Value Orientation Profile

RELATIONAL	Col > Lin > Ind
TIME	Fut > Pres > Past
MAN–NATURE	Mast > Har > Sub

Abbreviations: Past = Past, Fut = Future, Pres = Present, Lin = Lineal, Col = Collateral, Ind = Individualistic, Har = Harmony-with-nature, Mast = Mastery-over-nature, Sub = Subjugated-to-nature
Key = no preference, > preference

LIST 2	Trinidadian Value Orientation Profile

RELATIONAL	Ind > Col ≥ Lin
TIME	Pres ≥ Fut > Past
ACTIVITY	Doing > Being
MAN–NATURE	Har ≥ Sub ≥ Mast

Abbreviations: Past = Past, Fut = Future, Pres = Present, Being = Being, Doing = Doing, Lin = Lineal, Col = Collateral, Ind = Individualistic, Har = Harmony-with-nature, Mast = Mastery-over-nature, Sub = Subjugated-to-nature
Key = no preference, ≥ non significant preference, > significant preference

LIST 3	Appalachian Dominant Value Orientation

RELATIONAL	Lineal
TIME	Present
ACTIVITY	Being
MAN–NATURE	Subjugation

LIST 4	Hupa Value Orientation Profile

RELATIONAL	Ind > Col > Lin
TIME	Pres > Fut
ACTIVITY	Doing > Being
MAN–NATURE	Mast = Sub > Har

Abbreviations: Fut = Future, Pres = Present, Being = Being, Doing = Doing, Lin = Lineal, Col = Collateral, Ind = Individualistic, Har = Harmony-with-nature, Mast = Mastery-over-nature, Sub = Subjugated-to-nature
Key = no preference, > significant preference

APPENDIX B: VALUE ORIENTATION QUESTIONNAIRE

1. Job Choice (Activity: item A1 & A2)

A person needed a job and had a chance to work for two people. The two bosses were different. Listen to what they were like and say which you think would be the best one to work for.

A (Doing)

One boss was a fair enough person, who gave somewhat higher pay than most people, but was the kind of boss who insisted that people work hard, stick on the job. This boss did not like it at all when a worker sometimes just knocked off work for a while to go on a trip or to have a day or so of fun, and thought it was right not to take such a worker back on the job.

B (Being)

The other boss paid just average wages but was not so firm. This boss understood that a worker would sometimes just not turn up—would be off on a trip or having a little fun for a day or two. When employees did this boss would take them back without saying too much

> Part 1: Which of these bosses do you believe that it would be better to work for in most cases?
> Which of these bosses would most other Inuit think it better to work for?
> Part 2: Which kind of boss do you believe that it is better to be in most cases?
> Which kind of boss would most other Inuit believe that it is better to be in most cases?

2. Well Arrangements (Relational: Item R1)

When a community has to make arrangements for water, such as drill a well, there are three different ways they can decide to arrange things like location, and who is going to do the work.

A (Lin)

There are some communities where it is mainly the older or recognized leaders of the important families who decide the plans. Everyone usually accepts what they say without much discussion since they are the ones who are used to deciding such things and are the ones who have had the most experience.

B (Coll)

There are some communities where most people in the group have a part in making the plans. Lots of different people talk, but nothing is done until almost everyone comes to agree as to what is best to be done.

C (Ind)

There are some communities where all the people hold to their own opinion, and they decide the matter by vote. They do what the largest number want even though there are still a very great many people who disagree and object to the action.

Which way do you think is usually best in such cases?

Which of the other two ways do you think is better?

Which way of all three ways do you think most other persons in Coppermine would usually think is best?

3. Child Training (Time: item T1)

Some people were talking about the way children should be brought up. Here are some different ideas.

A (Past)

Some people say that children should always be taught well the traditions of the past (the ways of the old people). They believe the old ways are best, and that it is when children do not follow them too much that things go wrong.

B (Pres)

Some people say that children should be taught some of the old traditions (ways of the old people), but it is wrong to insist that they stick to these ways. These people believe that it is necessary for children always to learn about and take on whatever of the new ways will best help them get along in the world of today.

C (Fut)

Some people do not believe children should be taught much about past traditions (the ways of the old people) at all except as an interesting story of what has gone before. These people believe that the world goes along best when children are taught the things that will make them want to find out for themselves new ways of doing things to replace the old.

Which of these people had the best idea about how children should be taught?

Which of the other two people had the better idea?

Considering again all three ideas, which would most other persons in Coppermine say had the better idea?

4. Livestock Dying (Man–nature: Item MN1)

One time a person had a lot of livestock. Most of them died off in different ways. People talked about this and said different things.

A (Subj)

Some people said you just can't blame a person when things like this happen. There are so many things that can and do happen, and a person can do almost nothing to prevent such losses when they come. We all have to learn to take the bad with the good.

B (Over)

Some people said that it was probably the person's own fault that they lost so many. That the person probably didn't use their head to prevent the losses. They said that, it is usually the case that people who keep up on new ways of doing things, and really set themselves to it, almost always find a way to keep out of such trouble.

C (With)

Some people said that it was probably because this person had not lived their life right—had not done things in the right way to keep harmony between themselves and the forces of nature (i.e., the ways of nature like rain, wind, snow, etc.).

Which way of getting the help do you think would usually be best?

Which way of getting the help do you think is next best?

Which way do you think you yourself would really follow?

Which way do you think most other people in Coppermine would think best?

5. Expectations about Change (Time: item T2)

A. 20–40 AGE GROUP Three young people were talking about what they thought their families would have one day compared with their fathers and mothers. They each said different things.

C (Fut)

The first said: I expect my family to be better off in the future than the family of my father and mother or relatives if we work hard and plan right. Things in this country usually get better for people who really try.

B (Pres)

The second one said: I don't know whether my family will be better off, the same, or worse off than the family of my father and mother or relatives. Things always go up and down even if people do work hard. So one can never really tell how things will be.

A (Past)

The third one said: I expect my family to be about the same as the family of my father and mother or relatives. The best way is to work hard and plan ways to keep things as they have been in the past.

Which of these people do you think had the best idea?

Which of the other two persons had the better idea?

Which of these three people would most other Inuit your age think had the best idea?

B. 40 PLUS AGE GROUP Three older people were talking about what they thought their children would have when they were grown. Here is what each one said.

A (Fut)
One said: I really expect my children to have more than I have had if they work hard and plan right. There are always good chances for people who try.

B (Pres)
The second one said: I don't know whether my children will be better off, worse off, or just the same. Things always go up and down even if one works hard, so we can't really tell.

A (Past)
The third one said: I expect my children to have just about the same as I have had or bring things back as they once were. It is their job to work hard and find ways to keep things going as they have been in the past.

Which of these people do you think had the best idea?

Which of the other two persons had the better idea?

Which of these three people would most other Inuit your age think had the best idea?

6. Facing Conditions (Man-nature: item MN2)

There are different ways of thinking about how God (the gods) is (are) related to people and to other natural conditions which make the animals live or die. Here are three possible ways.

C (With)
God (the gods) and people all work together all the time; whether the conditions which make the crops and animals grow are good or bad depends upon whether people themselves do all the proper things to keep themselves in harmony with their God (gods) and with the forces of nature.

B (Over)
God (the gods) does (do) not directly use power to control all the conditions which affect growth of crops or animals. It is up to the people themselves to figure out the ways conditions change and to try hard to find the ways of controlling them.

A (Subj)
Just how God (the gods) will use power over all the conditions which affect the growth of crops and animals cannot be known by people. But it is useless for people to think they can change conditions very much for very long. The best way is to take conditions as they come and do as well as one can.

Which of these ways of looking at things do you think is best?

Which of the other two do you think is better?

Which of the three ways of looking at things would most other people in Coppermine think is best?

7. Help in Misfortune (Relational: item R2)

A person had a crop failure, or, let us say, had lost most of their sheep or cattle. The family had to have help from someone if they were going to get through the winter. There are different ways of getting help. Which of these ways would be best?

B (Coll)
Would it be best if people depended mostly on their brothers and sisters or other relatives all to help them out as much as they could?

C (Ind)
Would it be best for people to try to raise the money on their own outside the community (own people) from people who are neither relatives nor employers?

A (Lin)
Would it be best for people to go to a boss or to an older important relative who is used to managing things in the group, and ask them to help out until things get better?

Which way of getting the help do you think would actually be the best?

Which way of getting the help do you think is next best?

Which way do you think you yourself would really follow?

Which way do you think most other people in Coppermine would think best?

8. Family Work Relations (Relational: item R3)

I'm going to tell you about three different ways families can arrange work. These families are related and they live together.

C (Ind)
In some groups (or communities) it is usually expected that each of the separate families (by which we mean just husband, wife, and children) will look after its own business separate from all others and not be responsible for others.

B (Coll)
In some groups (or communities) it is usually expected that the close relatives in the families will work together and talk over among themselves the way to take care of whatever problems come up. When a boss is needed they usually choose (get) one person, not necessarily the oldest able person, to manage things.

A (Lin)
In some groups (or communities) it is usually expected that the families which are closely related to each other will work together and have the oldest able person be responsible for and take charge of most important things.

Which of these ways do you think is usually best in most cases?

Which of the other two ways do you think is better?

Which of all the ways do you think most other persons in Coppermine would think is usually best?

9. Choice of Delegate (Relational: item R4)

A group like yours (community like yours) is to send a delegate—a representative—to a meeting away from here (this can be any sort of meeting). How will the delegate be chosen.

B (Coll)

It is best that a meeting be called and everyone discuss things until almost everyone agrees so that when a vote is taken almost all people would agree on the same person?

A (Lin)

It is best that the older, important, leaders take the main responsibility for deciding who should represent the people since they are the ones who have had the long experience in such matters?

C (Ind)

Is it best that a meeting be called, names be put up, a vote be taken, then send the person who gets the majority of votes even if there are many people who still are against this person?

Which of these ways of choosing is usually best in cases like this?

Which of the other two ways is usually better?

Which would most other persons in Coppermine say is usually best?

10. Use of Fields (Man-nature: item MN3)

There were three people who had fields with crops (were farmers). The three people had quite different ways of setting and taking care of crops.

C (With)

One person put in the crops, worked hard, and also set out to living right and proper ways. This person felt that it is the way a person works and tries to keep oneself in harmony with the forces of nature that has the most effect on conditions and the way crops turn out.

A (Subj)

One person put in the crops. Afterwards this person worked on them sufficiently but did not do more than was necessary to keep them going along. This person felt that it mainly depended on weather conditions how they would turn out, and that nothing extra that people do could change things much.

B (Over)

One person put in the crops and then worked on them a lot of time and made use of all the new ideas they could find out about. This person felt that by doing this it would in most years prevent many of the effects of bad conditions.

> Which of these ways do you believe is usually best?
>
> Which of the other two ways do you believe is better?
>
> Which of the three ways would most other persons in Coppermine think is best?

11. Philosophy of Life (Time: item T3)

People often have very different ideas about what has gone before and what we can expect in life. Here are three ways of thinking about these things.

B (Pres)

Some people believe it best to give most attention to what is happening now in the present. They say that the past has gone and the future is much too uncertain to count on. Things do change, but it is sometimes for the better and sometimes for the worse, so in the long run it is about the same. These people believe the best way to live is to keep those of the old ways that one can—or that one likes—but to be ready to accept the new ways which will help to make life easier and better as we live from year to year.

A (Past)

Some people think that the ways of the past (ways of the old people or traditional ways) were the most right and the best, and as changes come things get worse. These people think the best way to live is to work hard to keep up the old ways and try to bring them back when they are lost.

C (Fut)

Some people believe that it is almost always the ways of the future—the ways which are still to come—which will be the best, and they say that even though there are sometimes small setbacks, change brings improvements in the long run. These people think the best way to live is to look a long time ahead, work hard, and give up many things now so that the future will be better.

> Which of these ways of looking at life do you think is best?
>
> Which of the other two ways do you think is better?
>
> Which of the three ways of looking at life do you think most other persons in Coppermine would think is best?

12. Wage Work (Relational: item R5)

There are three ways in which people who do not themselves hire others may work.

C (Ind)

One way is working on one's own as an individual. In this case a person is pretty much one's own boss. These people decide most things themselves, and how they get along is their own business. These people only have to take care of themselves and don't expect others to look out for them.

B (Coll)

One way is working in a group of people where all the people work together without there being one main boss. Every person has something to say in the decisions that are made, and all the people can count on each other.

A (Lin)

One way is working for an owner, a big boss, or a person who has been running things for a long time (a patron). In this case, the people do not take part in deciding how the business will be run, but they know they can depend on the boss to help them out in many ways.

> Which of these ways is usually best for a person who does not hire others?
>
> Which of the other two ways is better for a person who does not hire others?
>
> Which of the three ways do you think most other people in Coppermine would think is best?

13. Belief in Control (Man-nature: item MN4)

Three people from different areas were talking about the things that control the weather and other conditions. Here is what they each said.

A (Subj)

One person said: My people have never controlled the rain, wind, and other natural conditions and probably never will. There have always been good years and bad years. That is the way it is, and if you are wise you will take it as it comes and do the best you can.

B (Over)

The second person said: My people believe that it is a person's job to find ways to overcome weather and other conditions just as they have overcome so many other things. They believe they will one day succeed in doing this and may even overcome drought and floods.

C (With)

The third person said: My people help conditions and keep things going by working to keep in close touch with all the forces which make the rain, the snow, and other conditions. It is when we do the right things—live in the proper way—and keep all that we have—the land, the animals, and the water—in good condition, that all goes along well.

> Which of these people do you think had the best idea?
>
> Which of the other two people do you think had the better idea?
>
> Which of the three people do you think most other persons in Coppermine would think had the best idea?

14. Ceremonial Innovation (Time: item T4)

Some people in a community like your own saw that the religious ceremonies (the church services) were changing from what they used to be.

C (Fut)

Some people were really pleased because of the changes in religious ceremonies. They felt that new ways are usually better than old ones, and they like to keep everything—even ceremonies—moving ahead.

A (Past)

Some people were unhappy because of the change. They felt that religious ceremonies should be kept exactly—in every way—as they had been in the past.

B (Pres)

Some people felt that the old ways for religious ceremonies were best but you just can't hang on to them. It makes life easier just to accept some changes as they come along.

Which of these three said most nearly what you would believe is right?

Which of the other two do you think is more right?

Which of the three would most other Inuit say was most right?

15. Ways of Living (Activity: item A1)

There were two people talking about how they liked to live. They had different ideas.

A (Doing)

One said: What I care about most is accomplishing things—getting things done just as well or better than other people do them. I like to see results and think they are worth working for.

B (Being)

The other said: What I care about is to be left alone to think and act in the ways that best suit the way I really am. If I don't always get much done, but can enjoy life as I go along, that is the best way.

Which of these two persons do you think has the better way of thinking?

Which of the two do you think you are more like?

Which of you think most other Inuit would say had the better way of living?

16. Livestock Inheritance (Relational: item R6)

Some sons and daughters have been left some livestock (sheep or cattle) by a father or mother who had died. All these sons and daughters are grown up, and live near each other. There are three different ways they can run the livestock.

A (Lin)

In some groups of people it is usually expected that the oldest able person will take charge of, or manage, all the livestock held by themselves and the other sons and daughters.

C (Ind)

In some groups of people it is usually expected that each of the sons and daughters will prefer to take his or her own share of the stock and run his or her own share of the stock and run his or her own business completely separate from all the others.

D (Coll)

In some groups of people it is usually expected that all the sons and daughters will keep all their cattle and sheep together and work together and decide among themselves who is best able to take charge of things, not necessarily the oldest, when a boss is needed.

Which way do you think is usually best in most cases?

Which of the other two ways do you think is better?

Which of all three ways do you think most other persons in Coppermine would think is usually best?

17. Land Inheritance (Relational: item R7)

Now I want to ask a similar question concerning farm and grazing land instead of live-stock. Some sons and daughters have been left some farm and grazing land by a father or mother who has died. All these sons and daughters are grown and live near each other. There are three ways they can handle the property.

A (Lin)

In some groups of people it is usually expected that the oldest able person will take charge of or manage the land for themselves and all the other sons and daughters, even if they all share it.

C (Ind)

In some groups of people it is usually expected that each son and daughter will take his or her own share of the land and do with it what he or she wants—separate from all the others.

B (Coll)

In some groups of people it is usually expected that all the sons and daughters will make use of the land together. When a boss is needed, they all get together and agree to choose someone of the group, not necessarily the oldest, to take charge of things.

Which of these ways do you think is usually best in most cases?

Which of the other two ways do you think is better?

Which of all three ways do you think most other persons in Coppermine would think is usually best?

18. Care of Fields (Activity: item A4)

There were two people, both of them farmers. They lived differently.

B (Being)

One person kept the fields all right but didn't work on them more than they had to. This person wanted to have extra time to visit with friends, go on trips, and enjoy life. This was the way they liked best.

A (Doing)

One person liked to work with their fields and was always putting in extra time keeping them free of weeds and in fine condition. Because this person did this extra work, they did not have much time left to be with friends, to go on trips, or to enjoy themselves in other ways. But this was the way this person really liked best.

Which kind of person do you believe it is better to be?

Which kind of person are you really like?

Which kind of person would most other Inuit think it better to be?

19. Length of Life (Man-nature: item MN5)

Three people were talking about whether people themselves can do anything to make the lives of men and women longer. Here is what each said.

B (Over)

One said: It is already true that people like doctors and others are finding the way to add many years to the lives of most people by discovering (finding) new medicines by studying foods, and doing other such things such as vaccinations. If people will pay attention to all these new things they will almost always live longer.

A (Subj)

The second one said: I really do not believe that there is much human beings themselves can do to make the lives of men and women longer. It is my belief that every person has a set time to live, and when that time comes it just comes.

C (With)

The third one said: I believe that there is a plan to life which works to keep all living things moving together, and if a person will learn to live their whole life in accord with that plan, this person will live longer than other people.

Which of these said most nearly what you would think is right?

Which of the other two ways is most right?

Which of the three would most other persons in Coppermine say was most right?

20. Water Allocation (Time: item T5)

The government is going to help a community like yours to get more water by redrilling and cleaning out a community. The government officials suggest that the community should have a plan for dividing the extra water, but don't say what kind of plan. Since the amount of extra water that may come in is not known, people feel differently about planning.

A (Past)
Some say that whatever water comes in should be divided just about like water in the past was always divided.

C (Fut)
Others want to work out a really good plan ahead of time for dividing whatever water comes in.

B (Pres)
Still others want to just wait until the water comes in before deciding on how it will be divided.

Which of these ways do you think is usually best in cases like this?

Which of the other two ways do you think is better?

Which of the three ways do you think most other persons in Coppermine would think best?

21. Work (Home) (Activity: item A5)

There were two people talking about the way they liked to live.

B (Being)
One said that they were willing to work as hard as the average, but that they didn't like to spend a lot of time doing the kind of extra things outside like cleaning up around the yard. Instead they liked to have time free to enjoy visiting with people—to go on trips—or to just talk with whoever was around.

A (Doing)
The other person said they liked best of all to find extra things to work on around the house which would interest her or him. They said they were happiest when kept busy and were getting lots done.

Which of these ways do you think it is usually better for people to live?

Which person are you really more like?

Which way of life would most other Inuit think is best?

22. Nonworking Time (Activity A6)

Two people spend their time in different ways when they have no work to do. (This means when they are actually on the job.)

A (Doing)
One person spends most of this time learning or trying out things which will help them in their work.

B (Being)

One person spends most of their time talking, telling stories, singing, and so on with friends.

Which of these people has the better way of living?

Which of these people do you think you are more like?

Which of these people would most other Inuit think had the better way of living?

23. Water Arrangements (Relational: item R8)

When a community has to make arrangements for water, such as picking a water lake and building a road to it, there are three different ways they can decide to arrange things like location, and who is going to do the work.

A (Lin)

There are some communities where it is mainly the older or recognized leaders of the important families who decide the plans. Everyone usually accepts what they say without much discussion since they are the ones who are used to deciding such things and are the ones who have had the most experience.

B (Coll)

There are some communities where most people in the group have a part in making the plans. Lots of different people talk, but nothing is done until almost everyone comes to agree as to what is best to be done.

C (Ind)

There are some communities where everyone holds to his own opinion, and they decide the matter by vote. They do what the largest number want even though there are still a very great many people who disagree and object to the action.

Which way do you think is usually best in such cases?

Which of the other two ways do you think is better?

Which way of all three ways do you think most other persons in Coppermine would usually think is best?

24. Dogs Dying (Man-nature: item MN6)

One time a person had a lot of dogs. Most of them died off in different ways. People talked about this and said different things.

A (Subj)

Some people said you just can't blame a person when things like this happen. There are so many things that can and do happen, and a person can do almost nothing to prevent such loses when they come. We all have to learn to take the bad with the good.

B (Over)

Some people said that it was probably the person's own fault that they lost so many. That the person probably didn't use their head to prevent the losses. They said that, it is usually the case that people who keep up on new ways of doing things, and really set themselves to it, almost always find a way to keep out of such trouble.

C (With)

Some people said that it was probably because the person had not lived his life right— had not done things in the right way to keep harmony between themselves and the forces of nature (i.e., the ways of nature like rain, wind, snow, etc.).

25. Help in Misfortune (Relational: item R9)

A person had bad luck fishing. The family had to have help from someone if they were going to get through the winter. There are different ways of getting help. Which of these ways would be best?

B (Coll)

Would it be best if the person depended mostly on their brothers and sisters or other relatives to help out as much as each one could?

C (Ind)

Would it be best for the person to try to raise the money on their own outside the community (own people) from people who are neither relatives nor employers?

A (Lin)

Would it be best for the person to go to a boss or to an older important relative who is used to managing things in the group, and ask them to help out until things get better?

Which way of getting the help do you think would actually be the best?

Which way of getting the help do you think is next best?

Which way do you think you yourself would really follow?

Which way do you think most other people in Coppermine would think best?

26. Use of Fish Nets (Man-nature: item MN7)

There were three people who had fishing nets. The three people had quite different ways of setting and taking care of nets.

C (With)

One person put in the nets, worked hard, and also set out to living right and proper ways. This person felt that it is the way a person works and tries to keep himself in harmony with the forces of nature that has the most effect on conditions and the way nets work.

A (Subj)

One person put in the nets. Afterwards this person worked on them sufficiently but did not do more than was necessary to keep them going along. This person felt that it mainly depended on weather conditions how they would turn out, and that nothing extra that people do could change things much.

B (Over)

One person put in the nets and then worked on them a lot of time and made use of all the new scientific ideas they could find out about. This person felt that by doing this it would in most years prevent many of the effects of bad conditions.

Which of these ways do you believe is usually best?

Which of the other two ways do you believe is better?

Which of the three ways would most other persons in Coppermine think is best?

27. Animal Inheritance (Relational: item R10)

Some sons and daughters have been left some dogs by a father or mother who had died. All these sons and daughters are grown up, and live near each other. There are three different ways they can use the dogs.

A (Lin)

In some groups of people it is usually expected that the oldest able person will take charge of, or manage, all the dogs for all the others.

C (Ind)

In some groups of people it is usually expected that each of the sons and daughters will prefer to take his or her own share of the dogs and run his or her own share of the dogs completely separate from all the others.

D (Coll)

In some groups of people it is usually expected that all the sons and daughters will keep all their dogs together and work together and decide among themselves who is best able to take charge of things, not necessarily the oldest, when a boss is needed.

Which way do you think is usually best in most cases?

Which of the other two ways do you think is better?

Which of all three ways do you think most other persons in Coppermine would think is usually best?

28. Property Inheritance (Relational: item R11)

Now I want to ask a similar question concerning property instead of animals. Some sons and daughters have been left some property (summer camp and cabin) by a father or mother who has died. All these sons and daughters are grown and live near each other. There are three ways they can handle the property.

A (Lin)

In some groups of people it is usually expected that the oldest able person will take charge of or manage the camp for himself or herself and all the other sons and daughters, even if they all share it.

C (Ind)

In some groups of people it is usually expected that each son and daughter will take his or her own share of the camp and do with it what he or she wants—separate from all the others.

B (Coll)

In some groups of people it is usually expected that all the sons and daughters will make use of the camp together. When a boss is needed, they all get together and agree to choose someone of the group, not necessarily the oldest, to take charge of things.

Which of these ways do you think is usually best in most cases?

Which of the other two ways do you think is better?

Which of all three ways do you think most other persons in Coppermine would think is usually best?

29. Care of Nets (Activity: item A6)

There were two people, both of whom fished (had nets). They lived differently.

B (Being)

One person kept the nets working all right but didn't work on them more than they had to. This person wanted to have extra time to visit with friends, go on trips, and enjoy life. This was the way they liked best.

A (Doing)

One person liked to work with their nets and was always putting in extra time keeping them clean of debris and in fine condition. Because this person did this extra work, they did not have much time left to be with friends, to go on trips, or to enjoy oneself in other ways. But this was the way this person really liked best.

Which kind of person do you believe it is better to be?

Which kind of person are you really like?

Which kind of person would most other Inuit think it better to be?

30. Water Allocation (Time: item T6)

The government is going to help a community like yours to get more water by providing more water and sewage trucks. The government officials suggest that the community should have a plan for dividing the extra water, but don't say what kind of plan. Since the amount of extra water that may come in is not known, people feel differently about planning.

A (Past)

Some say that whatever water comes in should be divided just about like water in the past was always divided.

C (Fut)

Others want to work out a really good plan ahead of time for dividing whatever water comes in.

B (Pres)

Still others want to just wait until the water comes in before deciding on how it will be divided.

> Which of these ways do you think is usually best in cases like this?

> Which of the other two ways do you think is better?

> Which of the three ways do you think most other persons in Coppermine would think best?

APPENDIX C: LETTER TO COPPERMINE HAMLET COUNCIL

Nancy A Edgecombe
Cambridge Bay, NWT

Hamlet Council
Coppermine, NWT

Dear Council:

My name is Nancy Edgecombe. I am a Master's student at the University of Alberta in the faculty of Nursing. Last year I wrote to you about the possibility of doing research in your community. I would like permission to visit your community for a period of six months to learn about the values of the Copper Inuit people. This six month period would start in the spring of 1993, either in March or April.

I would like your permission to attend community activities and to make notes of my observations at community functions. In order to do my research I will need your permission to use your settlement list. This list will be used to select people at random to be in my study. The people selected will be asked if they would be in my study and will be free not to be involved. Those individuals approached who agree to be in the study will be interviewed and asked a series of questions about some stories I will tell them.

These interviews may be tape recorded if the person agrees. Who talks to me and what they tell me will be kept private. No one's name will appear on my questionnaires or in anything I write about this study. I will be using the answers to the questionnaires and my notes to write a description of the values of the Copper Inuit. Once I have completed my degree the tapes and questionnaires from the study will be destroyed.

I do not know of any risks for being in this study. I plan to give a copy of my study to the Hamlet of Coppermine and the Kitikmeot Health Board when my degree is finished. I expect nurses and doctors to use my study to help them understand the Inuit better. If they understand the Inuit better they will be more sensitive to the Inuit perspective.

Enclosed are: a description of my study, a copy of the questionnaire and a copy of the consent form which will be used. If you have any questions about this study you can contact me or my thesis supervisor, Dr. P. Brink at (phone number supplied). I look forward to your reply. Thank you.

Nancy A. Edgecombe

APPENDIX D: INFORMED CONSENT FOR SUBJECTS

Title of Research—A Value Orientation Profile of the Copper Inuit

Principle Researcher: Nancy A. Edgecombe
Master of Nursing Candidate
Faculty of Nursing
University of Alberta
phone:

Thesis Supervisor: Dr. P. Brink
Associate Dean of Research
Faculty of Nursing
University of Alberta
phone:

My Name is Nancy Edgecombe. I am a Master's student at the University of Alberta. I will be in Coppermine the next few months. I have come to learn about the values of the Copper Inuit people. To do this I would like to tell you some short stories and ask you questions about these stories. I will write down your answers. I would also like to tape our interview so I can listen to your answers again later. This will take about 45 minutes.

If you do not want to talk to me, it is all right. If you do not want me to tape our talk I will not tape it. If you decide to talk to me and later change your mind, just tell me and we will stop talking. If you do not want to answer any of the questions just tell me and we will skip that question. I will not tell anybody that you have talked to me. Your name will not be placed on the questionnaire, and your name will not be mentioned when I write about the study.

I do not know of any risks to you for being in this study. I will be using your answers to the questions and my notes to write a description of the values of the Copper Inuit. Once I have finished my study I will destroy the tapes and the questionnaires.

I plan to give a copy of my study to the Hamlet of Coppermine and the Kitikmeot Health Board when my degree is finished. I expect nurses and doctors to use my study to help them understand the Inuit better. If they understand the Inuit better they will be more sensitive to the Inuit perspective. If you have any questions about me or what we have talked about, you can call me (phone number) or my thesis supervisor Dr. P. Brink.

Consent

The study has been explained to me by Nancy Edgecombe, and she has given me a copy of her explanation. All my questions about the study have been answered. I agree to be in her study.

_____	_____	_____	_____
Informant	Date	Researcher	Date

Living in a Nursing Home with Multiple Sclerosis

CONNIE WINTHER

Nursing homes are institutions for the aged with services and attitudes in place for managing elderly people. There does exist, however, a minority of persons living in nursing homes who are not elderly. In Alberta, 9% of the residents in nursing homes are under the age of 65, and are called the young handicapped (Smith, Schalm, Shaw, Wellock, and Lyle, 1991). Of this young handicapped population, persons with multiple sclerosis (M.S.) make up the largest category. People with M.S. living in nursing homes also have the highest care needs of all the residents, and have the longest length of stay of all residents.

Despite the high care needs of the group, and the large number of persons with M.S. living in long-term care, no investigations to date have taken place to explore their experience of living in a nursing home. Whether or not the experiences of living with M.S. are changed by living in a nursing home are not known. Whether or not the experience of living in a nursing home is the same for an elderly person as for a young handicapped person is not known. Exploration and description of the experiences of people with M.S. living in nursing homes is therefore needed in order to plan programs and meet the needs of this population.

I. LIVING IN A NURSING HOME WITH MULTIPLE SCLEROSIS

Nursing Homes

A nursing home is an institution in which care is provided for persons who are no longer able to manage for themselves due to physical, cognitive, or emotional disability (Pitters, 1995). The typical nursing home resident is female, over 85 years of age, and has high physical care needs (Jacelon, 1995). Typical labels for the residents of a nursing home include "incontinent," "senile," and "feeder," referring to both the physical and cognitive disabilities present within the nursing home population (Jacelon, 1995). In Alberta, 12,832 people were reported to reside in nursing homes in 1992 (Smith et al., 1991). The typical nursing home resident in Alberta is also female, but with a slightly lower average age of 81.

After a 6-month participant observation study of 35 subjects living in a nursing home, Nystrom and Segesten (1996) related the structure and function of a nursing home to the construct of the family. Both the nursing home and the family provide physical care for the weaker individual through the supply of food, shelter, and a comfortable, safe, and protected environment. The registered nurse in the nursing home is likened to the mother of the family with her skilled, experienced, affectionate, and organizing manner. The physician can be seen as the father figure, with his authority and importance despite his frequent absence from the setting. The children, or residents of the nursing home, are the weaker members, with all attention and care being directed toward them. Similarly, Pearson, Hocking, Mott, and Riggs (1993), have stated that only when the nursing home is most like a home, as opposed to a medical institution, can the best quality of life be achieved.

Life in a Nursing Home

Life for the elderly in a nursing home has been the subject of a large number of studies. Few investigations have outlined a positive experience within this environment. Most studies have continued to find that life in a nursing home exists within the confines of the total institution, as described by Erving Goffman in 1961. Living in an institution, people are segregated from the rest of society, their personal identity is stripped away, and treatment is delivered to the group rather than to the individual.

In the nursing home environment, the loss of personal identity begins even before admission to the institution. The decision-making process to admit someone to a nursing home may not even involve that person, as evident in the dialogue of two nursing home residents:

> "I don't want to end up there I said, I'd rather end up on my own."
> "I'm gonna get out of this place one way or another. I called an attorney friend of mine and I'm gonna put the pressure on him to turn us loose. They just put us here, I didn't even know about it." (Running, 1997: 121)

Once in the nursing home, personal identity is deprived by the loss of personal possessions and loss of treatment according to personal needs.

Attempts have been made to make the institution more homelike, and less of a medical institution, and to allow for consideration of individual needs. Clark and Bowling (1990) performed an investigation comparing the everyday life experience of elderly persons in three different types of institutional care: a traditional ward-type nursing home; a small, intimate nursing home; and a geriatric ward in a hospital. Nonparticipant observation was used to document the interactions and moods of the persons living in the three different settings. In all settings, batch treatment was observed, with little regard for individuality. Kayser-Jones (1981) used participant observation to compare nursing home life in Scotland and the United States, and found batch treatment occurred in both countries, although more often in America.

Being treated as part of the total institution strips away the personal identity of individual residents, and depersonalizes the experience of life (Gubrium, 1993). Providing care without any concern for individual differences, and not providing care upon request by an individual, are considered depersonalizing practices. Part of depersonalizing care involves dehumanizing the recipient of the care, which allows for the acceptance of somewhat other unacceptable behaviors. In Clark and Bowling's (1990) nonparticipant observation, only in the small nursing home, and in the Occupational Therapy room in the geriatric ward, were any positive interactions between staff and residents observed more than 30% of the time. Positive interactions were viewed as staff answering resident's requests, or showing affection for the resident.

Providing care to a group instead of to the individual defies the rights of the individual and depersonalizes the treatment, but may also promote acceptance of dehumanizing and infantilizing treatment. Providing services without any caring, such as force feeding someone, are also considered to be dehumanizing (Kayser-Jones, 1981; Clark and Bowling, 1990). Practices such as ignoring the need for privacy and exposing genitals, allowing people to urinate in public, and showering males and females in the same room, are all considered unacceptable by today's societal norms, and all have been frequently observed by researchers in nursing homes (Kayser-Jones, 1981; Clark and Bowling, 1990). Alternatively, in the family model of the nursing home (Nystrom and Segeston, 1996) practices such as open toileting were viewed not as dehumanizing, but rather as a sign of openness, and of intimacy.

Another way of depersonalizing care is to treat an adult as a child, or infantilization of care. Observed infantilization of care of people in nursing homes includes dressing adults as children, scolding them, and providing childlike activities for leisure (Kayser-Jones, 1981). Although Nystrom and Segesten (1996) used the structure of family in a positive light with the resident or child being the center of activity, treating an adult as a child can also be considered to be depersonalizing. Treating someone as a child also implies that they are unable to do for themselves, allowing for passive treatment and the formation of a power structure between the caregiver and the cared for (Kayser-Jones, 1981; Diamond, 1986). This power structure has also led to frequent reports of the resident's fear of their caregivers, and fear of repercussion should they speak out against the authority figure (Clark and Bowling, 1990; Diamond, 1986).

The other major characteristic of life in a nursing home described throughout the literature relates to the experience of detachment in which a person displays decreased participation and interest in social activities. Detachment includes withdrawal not only from activities, but also from the people in the surrounding environment. Living among others, yet being alone, characterizes desocialization. Disengaging or detaching has been hypothesized to be part of the normal process of aging, as this allows the elderly person to begin the process of withdrawal from society. Signs of complete detachment or disengagement from the environment have been observed in nursing homes. Bowling and Clark (1990) observed that during all observation time, at least one person was completely detached from the situation (uninvolved, unemotional, or uninterested) 81% to 90% of the time. These authors noted that although disengagement is considered to be a normal part of the aging process, that resident's happiness and engagement to the situation were improved with activity and stimulation around them. Disengagement in the nursing home population may therefore simply be from boredom and lack of stimulation.

Disengagement from pursuing relationships within the nursing home has also been the subject of investigation. Several authors have reported that nursing home residents are more likely to talk to staff than to other residents. Staff are seen as a link to the outside world, yet in several investigations (Morse and Intrieri, 1997; Powers, 1992) staff communication was primarily related to care needs and did not link the resident to the outside world. Poor relationships between residents in a nursing home could be in part due to the poor physical and mental functioning of the residents. Other explanations include the possibility that residents don't spend the energy getting to know other residents in such a transient environment (Nystrom and Segesten, 1996; Kayser-Jones, 1981), or that there simply is no one to talk to, or anything to talk about (Kaakinen, 1992). In a phenomenological study of communication in a nursing home, 72 participants were interviewed to determine what communication rules existed within the facility (Kaakinen, 1992). The most frequent response was to ignore senile residents, and to talk to residents who talk to you. Other rules included not complaining, not talking to the opposite sex, not talking about death and dying, and not talking too much. Learning to live with senile residents was the source of further phenomenological investigation by Gorman (1996). Ignoring or avoiding senile residents was found to be the most frequent strategy for those without cognitive deficits to be able to tolerate living in an environment with some people with senility. In trying to avoid others, residents reported expending large amounts of energy, guilt, as well as sensing loss of control over their own environment, and fears that they too would become senile (Gorman, 1996). From the literature, it appears that few relationships thrive between nursing home residents for various reasons, and therefore socialization rarely provides stimulation, comfort, and enjoyment.

Several investigations have sought to determine how people in nursing homes feel about living in this environment, and how quality of life is defined in the institution. Being an individual was reported as being the most important for a good quality of life to a group of 10 residents from 3 institutions in an exploratory, descriptive study. Being an individual meant having autonomy in decision making, feeling a sense of self worth, having privacy, and having personal possessions. Other factors important to obtaining a high quality of life for these residents included being connected to the outside world, and being able to function at their own optimum level (Oleson, Heading, McGlynn, Shadick, and Bistodeau, 1994). In a phenomenological investigation with 5 women living in long-term care, quality of life was found through dwelling in remembering in order to bring meaning to life at present, as well as feeling connected to others within the environment (Heliker, 1997). Similarly, Nystrom and Segesten (1996) reported that quality of life for residents of nursing homes meant having an acceptable level of functioning in day-to-day life, and a worry-free environment. A worry-free environment has been interpreted as feeling physically safe, but also not having to worry economically (Diamond, 1986). Aller and Van Ess Coeling (1996) reported that in 8 subjects questioned about quality of life, the three main themes that emerged were being able to communicate with others, being able to care for one's self, and being able to help others.

The themes found in the investigations of quality of life in a nursing home can all be related to the findings of the observational studies in the literature. Residents want privacy, personal possessions, and autonomy in decision making. Residents want to be able to do as much for themselves as possible, and have their individual needs recognized and respected. All of these findings relate to the theme of personalization of care. The other main theme throughout these quality of life studies was one of being connected to the environment and those within that environment. Residents want to be engaged in the present and sociable within their living environments. Further investigations are required to provide strategies to prevent depersonalization and detachment within the nursing home environment.

Multiple Sclerosis

Multiple sclerosis (M.S.) is a chronic, degenerative disease of the central nervous system. M.S. is typically diagnosed in the third decade of life, with a 2:1 predominance of women to men having the disease (Canadian Burden of Illness Study Group, 1998). Canada is considered a high frequency area for the development of M.S. with a prevalence rate of 55 to 202 cases (depending on the geographical location) per 100,000 persons in the population (Canadian Burden of Illness Study Group, 1998). The cause of M.S. remains uncertain; however, current hypotheses suggests "an autoimmune cause possibly triggered by viral infection in a genetically susceptible host" (Canadian Burden of Illness Study Group, 1998: 23). The disease process involves multiple plaques, or areas of sclerosis, damaging the myelin surrounding the nerves, resulting in decreased nerve conduction and subsequent impairment in sensory, motor, and autonomic functioning.

The disease process itself is widely varied, and unpredictable. The most common manifestations include a progressive disease course with gradual and continual worsening, or an exacerbating, remitting disease course with bouts of acute activity, followed by periods of remission (Frankel, 1985). To date, prognostic indicators for progression of the disease have not been determined. Life expectancy is also widely varied, depending on the cause of death. Almost half of the people with M.S. die of complicating factors such as pneumonia, one quarter die through suicide, and one quarter die of miscellaneous causes that cannot be attributed to M.S. (Murphy Miller and Hens, 1993).

Living with Multiple Sclerosis

The level of disability resulting from the multiple areas of sclerosis is widely varied, depending on the areas and extent of damage to the nerves (Frankel, 1985). Physical impairment may result in motor weakness, fatigue, and spasticity. Sensory impairment may result in numbness, neuralgic pain, and alterations in balance. Other physical impairments include visual symptoms such as blurred or double vision and optic neuritis. Bladder, bowel, and sexual function may also be affected.

If plaques are found in the brain, various cognitive impairments may result. Memory and attention deficits, conceptual reasoning, visuospatial perception difficulties, and personality changes may occur (Murphy Miller and Hens, 1993). Cognitive deficits are more often found in progressive M.S., rather than in relapsing, remitting types of the disease. Euphoria has also been reported as a sequela of M.S. in 5% to 26% of persons (Hainsworth, 1994) and is found most often in those persons with other cognitive deficits, and long-term progressive disease (Murphy Miller and Hens, 1993). Reports of depression in persons with M.S. range from an incidence of 6% to 27%, again with the highest incidence of depression being in those persons with other cognitive deficits (Hainsworth, 1994). Depression can also be seen as a reaction to the disease due to the associated uncertainty, fatigue, and anticipated disability (Murphy Miller and Hens, 1993).

Various studies have attempted to determine which factors predict health-related quality of life in persons with M.S. Consensus exists throughout the literature that the ability to perform activities of daily living, without the use of assistive devices, is a strong predictor of improved quality of life (Brunet, Hopman, Singer, Edge, and MacKenzie, 1996; Canadian Burden of Illness Study Group, 1998). Vision has also been strongly correlated with quality of life. The experience of living with M.S. does involve coping with the disability and handicap imposed by the physical, sensory, and cognitive changes that result from the multiple sclerotic plaques. Further to this, living with M.S. also relates to living with a chronic, unpredictable disease.

The experience of living with M.S. has been described by various authors using various research methodologies. The chronic, unpredictable nature of the disease may lead to learned helplessness and chronic sorrow. Learned helplessness has been described as the cognitive set in which a person believes that outcomes occur independent of their own actions. In the case of M.S., learned helplessness is thought to occur because of the unpredictable nature of the disease, regardless of any personal attempts to take control over one's own body (McGuiness, 1996). In a convenience sample of 72 individuals with M.S. living in Southern Alberta, McGuiness (1996) found that learned helplessness was associated with more severe and active forms of the disease, and its associated increased functional and social disability. Learned helplessness contributes to a more passive approach toward one's own health, as well as loneliness and depression. Presumably a passive approach to health, or depression and loneliness may also lead to a further decrease in functioning. Due to the cross-sectional nature of the study design, it is difficult to know whether the relationship between decreased functioning and learned behaviors is causal or not. Also related to loss of control over the body, and the mourning over the loss of that control, is the experience of chronic sorrow. Chronic sorrow is a pervasive sadness that is permanent, periodic, and progressive (Hainsworth, 1994). In an investigation with 10 participants using the Burke Chronic Sorrow Questionnaire, 8 of the 10 interviewed were reported as having chronic sorrow in their lives. Whether or not these results can be generalized to the entire population of persons with M.S. is questionable due to the small number of persons in the sample.

Describing the experience of M.S. leads also to the description of how people cope living with this unpredictable, chronic disease. Coping has been related to four factors: knowledge of illness, coping resources available, problem-solving ability, and personal mastery (Murphy Miller, 1993). The sense of hope has also been described as an important feature in dealing with chronic illness, as hope gives a sense of well being, as well as enabling a person to live life as fully as possible (Foote, Piazza, Holcombe, Penelope, and Daffin, 1990). In a descriptive study of 40 persons with M.S., investigating the relationship between hope, self-esteem, and social support in persons with M.S., hope, self-esteem, and social support were all found to be related. In a phenomenological study of the lived experience of people with relapsing remitting M.S., themes centered around the concepts of coping, hope–hopelessness, uncertainty, loss, fear, and control and were related to previous findings in the literature. New findings, not reported in other reviewed studies, included getting to know M.S., or learning more about M.S., and finding health care professionals who know about M.S. Other findings not previously reported in the literature include conflict with the medical profession, and revealing or concealing their diagnosis from people who don't understand M.S.

Living in a Nursing Home with Multiple Sclerosis

As with the elderly population, people with M.S. enter into nursing homes when their care needs can no longer be met in the community, due to a lack of social, family, or financial resources available. Although the reasons for entering into a nursing home may be seen as similar to the geriatric population, the needs for people with M.S. in long-term care can be seen as distinctly different. The needs of people with M.S. are different due to the younger age of this population, as well as the high physical, social, and psychological care needs. A survey of experts in the care of persons with M.S. was undertaken to determine what services were required for this population residing in long-term care (Buchanan and Lewis, 1997). Although many of the services were similar to those required for the general nursing home population, such as rehabilitation and outings, specialized services for a younger population were also identified. These included education programs, computer training, and vocational planning. Services specific to M.S. were also defined, such as education programs about the disease process, as well as individual and family counseling.

Care staff have also recognized that the needs of people with M.S. in long-term care are different compared with those of the geriatric population, and have reported that looking after people with M.S. is difficult (Buchanan and Lewis, 1997). Staff who are used to looking after the geriatric population report that they feel unable to meet the psychological and social needs of persons with M.S. Due to the high care needs, the young disabled population is also not desirable to hospital administrators due to the high costs of care (Buchanan, 1993). Of the limited literature about people with M.S. living in long-term care, half of this documentation was found in the "difficult cases" section of nursing journals. The case of "Gwen" gives some insight as to why the person with M.S. is more difficult to look after:

> she seemed particularly venomous to young, attractive, nursing assistants. Perhaps they reminded her of herself—and of all she'd lost (Schmitt, 1989:55).

Staff surveyed in 100 nursing homes in Massachusetts reported that the biggest areas of concern for people with M.S. living in long-term care were difficulty for the person and their family in adjusting to the placement, and signs of serious depression (Frankel, 1984).

Although studies outlining the "expert" opinion on what services are required for persons in long-term care, no studies have taken place regarding the self-perceived needs of people with M.S. living in long-term care. One study was undertaken by Donohue, Wineman, and O'Brien, 1996 to determine what alternative long-term care facilities people with M.S. believed that they would need in the future, and what they would be willing to use. All of those surveyed stated that nursing home placement was the last option.

People with M.S. themselves also feel that they are different from the rest of the nursing home population. From the few case reports in the literature, it appears that this self-perceived difference is due to the large age difference, rather than the difference in levels of ability and greater amount of care required. Gwen, a 27-year-old woman with M.S., describes entering into a care home as "living in a warehouse for old people" (Schmitt, 1989:55). Other case studies document the young person believing he has entered into the nursing home to die, due to the high prevalence and exposure to death surrounding that person (Parke, 1997).

Both staff and the person with M.S. perceive their needs as being different. Both staff and persons with M.S. feel as though they do not belong in the nursing home environment. Such feelings of being different, as being treated differently, could be described as being stigmatized. Stigma refers to the negative or adverse response to someone who is considered a deviant. A deviant is one who is perceived to be different from what is expected of him, and that difference is considered to be bad, or less desirable (Goffman, 1963). Whether or not people with M.S. living in long term care are a stigmatized population or not is uncertain from the scant literature available. The few "difficult patient" reports may be unusual and for this reason have been reported in the literature, rather than being the norm for this population. Whether or not a population is actually stigmatized is important. If staff knowingly or unknowingly label a patient as "different," the care provided to that patient will be different.

> providing care for stigmatized populations is fraught with numerous complex issues, including an often insensitive social system . . . Providers, however, are members of their own social or cultural groups, and are thus subject to the same socialization processes. As a result, they may unknowingly perpetuate labels that stigmatize their patients. Whatever the cause, stigmatized populations may receive differential care and potentially be under served and vulnerable (Roper and Anderson, 1994:294).

Things or experiences which are unusual, different, or uncertain are avoided (Roper and Anderson, 1994; Fitzpatrick, Hinton, Newmann, Scambler, and Thompson 1984). Thus, if a person with M.S. who lives in a nursing home is seen as "different," then there is the potential that interactions with this person will be avoided, or cut short. This may in turn affect their quality of care, and their subsequent quality of life, if other people in the nursing home avoid interacting with people with M.S.

There is also the potential that living in a nursing home can minimize the stigma of a disabled population. The two groups of people who are believed to be able to minimize a stigma are those who share the stigma (other nursing home residents), and the "wise" (those who work in the nursing home) (Goffman, 1963). Thus, whether living in a nursing home results in people with M.S. being stigmatized, or if it has the effect of minimizing stigma is unknown, but worthy of investigation.

Whether or not a younger person living in a nursing home would have the same experiences as an older person is not known. Perhaps because of their higher care needs, the person with M.S. will not be depersonalized. Or conversely, perhaps because they have higher care needs, staff will find it easier to dehumanize the recipient of that care. Whether the younger person will have more energy to engage in activities or social relationships, or whether they too will become desocialized is not known. It is also not known if living in a nursing home will change the experiences of living with M.S. For example, does living in a nursing home increase hope—as hope has been related to more social support, and more opportunities for social support—or does it decrease hope due to the obvious face of death? Do people with M.S. have to work less hard to conceal their illness, or does this not change? The answers to these questions cannot be found in the literature, and therefore there is a need to investigate the experience of persons with M.S. living in nursing homes.

II. THE PURPOSE OF THE STUDY

The purpose of this study is to explore and describe the experiences of people with M.S. living in nursing homes in Edmonton.

III. DEFINITION OF TERMS

Experiences refers to the life events of an individual that either the individual or another person acknowledges happened as ascertained through interview, records, and participant observation.

Nursing home refers to an institution which provides 24-hour total care by qualified nursing and allied health care personnel to persons with chronic, long-term health problems requiring professional assistance.

Living in refers to the daily process of adapting and redefining one's existence within the experience of institutional life.

IV. RESEARCH DESIGN

A focused ethnography will be used to explore and describe the experiences of living in a nursing home according to people with M.S.

1. Sample

The incidence of M.S. in Edmonton is currently the highest in Canada, with 202 cases per 100,000 persons (Canadian Burden of Illness Study Group, 1998). The exact number of people with M.S. living in nursing homes in Edmonton is not known, but 238 people with M.S. were living in nursing homes in Alberta in 1992 (Smith et al., 1991). In Edmonton, Capital Care is a group of seven public nursing home facilities throughout the city. Historically, people with M.S. who required long-term care in Edmonton were admitted to one of the Capital Care group facilities.

The selected sample will be one ward from within the group of Capital Care facilities. Once institutional approval has been gained, the census statistics for the Capital Care Group will be reviewed in order to determine on which wards five or more persons with M.S. reside. When wards on which five or more persons with M.S. reside have been identified, a letter will be sent to the resident care manager (RCM) of that ward outlining the purpose of the investigation and seeking approval for the investigation to take place on the ward, should enough of the residents with M.S. agree to participate in the investigation. The information letters for the potential subjects on that ward will also be sent to the RCM at the same time. The procedure for recruitment and completion of the informed consent can be found in Appendix A, Protection of Human Subjects.

The ward which will then be chosen to participate in the investigation will fulfill the requirement that five persons with M.S. reside on the unit who fit the inclusion and exclusion criteria as follows:

Inclusion Criteria:

1. A definitive diagnosis of M.S. as documented in the medical records.
2. Age up to and including 55 years of age at the commencement of the investigation.
3. Having lived in a nursing home for more than 6 months.
4. English speaking.
5. Agreeing to participate in the study.

Exclusion Criteria:

1. No definitive diagnosis of M.S. as documented in the medical records.
2. Age more than 55 years of age at the commencement of the investigation.
3. Having lived in a nursing home for less than 6 months.
4. Documented cognitive deficits which affect daily functioning, as documented in the medical records.
5. Non-English speaking.
6. Not agreeing to participate in the study.

From the ward sample, a purposive sample of three people with M.S. will be selected to be the main informants for the study. These informants will be selected according to the length of time they have lived on the ward, their knowledge of the people and processes on the ward, and their ability and willingness to discuss their experiences with the researcher. By choosing a ward on which a minimum of five persons with M.S. live, determination of three key informants will be more probable, and will allow leeway for attrition in the study sample.

All of the residents who live on the ward, as well as the care staff and non–direct care staff who work on the ward, are also considered to be part of the study sample. Informed consent will not be sought from these persons as they will not be participating in formal interviews for the investigation.

The strength of this purposive sampling is the assurance that the ward that is selected will have the appropriate number of persons with M.S. who are eligible to participate. The weakness of this particular type of sampling is that, by choosing informants only from one ward, their experiences only represent the experiences of those persons on that unit, and may not be indicative of other people's experiences. The purpose of this qualitative research, however, is not to generalize the results, but rather to explore and describe the experiences of those who do participate in the investigation in order to provide direction for further investigations.

2. Methods

The method of data collection will be participant observation. Participant observation allows for the collection of data from multiple sources including observing behaviors, informal and formal interviews, and review of existing documents (Roper and Shapira, 2000). Observational methods have been described as the ideal where the everyday life experiences of people are not known and difficult to measure (Clark and Bowling, 1990). Using only questionnaires or interviews with elderly persons in nursing homes is not the research method of choice. Residents are fearful of repercussion if they express any criticism toward those who are looking after them (Clark and Bowling, 1990; Kaakinen, 1992). People with M.S. living in nursing homes may also be afraid of expressing their true feelings about life within the institution, and therefore a focused ethnography is the research methodology of choice.

In order to set up the role of researcher as participant observer, the advice of the RCM will direct the way in which the information is provided to the staff and residents of the ward. The purpose of this meeting will be to outline the purpose of the investigation, the role of the researcher, the length of time and schedule for the project, and what the findings of the research will be used for. Further to the meeting, a notice sheet outlining the purpose and procedures for the study will also be posted on the ward, to remind staff and residents of the researcher's role throughout the project, as well as to inform those persons who were not in attendance at the original meeting (Appendix A9).

Participant observation will occur for a total period of 3 months. The schedule for data collection will include day and evening shifts, as well as weekday and weekend shifts in order to provide a representative sample of the various experiences of a person living in a nursing home. The proposed schedule is as follows, with weeks A and B being alternated for the duration of the data collection:

Week A
Monday: 15:30–20:30

Wednesday: 7:30–15:30

Saturday: 15:30–20:30

Week B
Tuesday: 15:30–20:30

Thursday: 7:30–15:30

Sunday: 7:30–15:30

The major daily activities in institutional life include mealtime, social and recreational activities, provision of personal care, and attendance of visitors (Kayser-Jones, 1981). The proposed strategy for participant observation will ensure all of the major activities are included, and will provide a holistic view of what life is like for people with M.S. living in a nursing home. In Capital Care facilities, mealtime, social and recreational activities, and some visiting all occur in the same area, known as the dayroom. Personal care occurs in the residents' rooms, as well as in showers and bathrooms.

For the first 6 weeks of data collection, the researcher will spend all time in the dayroom. Sampling of the events in the dayroom will allow the researcher to explore what experiences the person with M.S. has in the social environment of the nursing home. An understanding of how the person with M.S. "fits in" will be observed and recorded by description of the interactions with others (staff and residents). Behaviors are recorded, and informal interviews occur in order to clarify the meaning of the behaviors that have been observed (Roper and Shapira, 2000). This initial period in the dayrooms will provide the investigator with a broad picture of the daily functioning of the ward, and allow the identification of who the most appropriate key informants will be.

Once the key informants have been identified, the strategy for data collection will change. During the next 6 weeks, the researcher will undertake participant observation with each of the key informants spending two periods of one week with each of the three key informants. The duration of the participant observation with each individual will be split up into two separate weeks in order to allow them time on their own. The proposed schedule for participant observation with the key informants will therefore be as follows:

Schedule of Participant Observation

Week 7: Informant a

Week 8: Informant b

Week 9: Informant c

Week 10: Informant a

Week 11: Informant b

Week 12: Informant c

Participant observation with each of the key informants will involve spending the day with the person with M.S., in order to observe and participate in the experiences that constitute daily existence. During half of the day, the key informant should be inactive, and during this time the researcher will complete the field notes and begin transcriptions. During the weeks of participant observation with a particular key informant, formal interviews will occur with that person. The purpose of the interview is to gain a deeper insight into the experience of life in a nursing home for the person with M.S., through open-ended questions that may not be answerable from observation or informal interviews alone. Formal interviews will be audio tape recorded to ensure full representation of the response. Transcription will then be performed on a computer after the interview.

Formal interviews will include the following schedule of open-ended questions:

1. What is it like for you living in a nursing home?
2. How is it different for you living in a nursing home, compared to your life before entering into the nursing home?
3. What have been the best experiences you have had since living in a nursing home?

4. What have been the hardest experiences you have had since living in a nursing home?

5. What are the experiences which you have had since being here that make you feel as though you belong here?

6. What are the experiences you have had since being here that make you feel as though you don't belong here?

In the event of a resident becoming distressed during an interview, all efforts will be made to minimize the distress immediately. The interview will be stopped if necessary, and the researcher will allow the participant to debrief without the discussion being part of the data collected. The head nurse will be informed if the resident appears to have suicide ideation so that staff will monitor the psychological state of the resident. The resident will be provided with a visit from a chartered psychologist (on contract to the project) if necessary and agreed to. The psychologist will be provided with only the information which is essential for the required intervention, and only with the agreement of the person with M.S.

Data will be recorded in a field note format, which is a running diary of the events of the day (Appendix B). Brief notes will be written during actual observation, which will then be expanded upon by the researcher later. The field note has half of the page with a running diary of the events that occur, and the other half of the page is left for the researchers' interpretation of the events of the day, such as what inferences can be drawn and what moods were evident. Trying to write a minimal amount while observing, yet recording enough to be accurate and paint a complete picture, is essential. Excessive writing during periods of observation may be distracting to those being observed, and result in changes in behavior. Therefore, after each period of observation, the researcher will spend time completing the fieldwork notes. A description of the events, people, conversations, and feelings will all be recorded (Roper and Shapira, 2000).

At the end of each day, the researcher will also write a personal diary, outlining personal reflections on the experience of the day. Writing an end-of-day reflection helps to determine what direction the research should take, and may help to outline what personal biases may be evident on the part of the researcher.

On the alternate days in which the investigator is not in the field, the fieldwork notes will be transferred from pen and paper copy to the computer in preparation for data analysis. By completing field work notes daily and entering the information into the computer shortly thereafter, assurances can be made that the information will be meaningful, and less information lost or forgotten.

When no participants are present in the dayroom, this time will be used for completing field notes, as well as review of the existing available documents. There may be no one in the dayroom approximately half of the time. During this time, residents will be having their care needs attended to, sleeping, or on other parts of the ward. This allows for the other half of the time to be used for data transcription and coding.

The medical records will be reviewed for description of the characteristics and experiences of people with M.S. living in a nursing home from the perspective of the nursing and allied health personnel. The chart will be reviewed first for demographic information such as age, marital status, length of stay, and classification level of amount of care required (Appendix A3). The contents of the chart will be reviewed for descriptors of the activities, moods, and behaviors of the person with M.S. Data from the medical records will be recorded in field note style.

3. Reliability and Validity

In order to ensure that the results obtained are accurate recordings of "the truth," several strategies will be employed. Allowing the researcher time to complete field notes after periods of observation and use of audio recordings during formal interviews will ensure complete and accurate documentation. Inputting the data into the computer within 24 hours also checks the data to ensure an accurate and complete recall of the information. To ensure data collection procedures are appropriate and working prior to the investigation, a pilot study will take place for one week, before commencement of the research project. The pilot study will occur on a ward which did not fulfill the inclusion criteria for the study (a total of fewer than five people with M.S. resided on the unit). A pilot study will ensure that data collection materials are appropriate and working and provide preliminary results, from which a coding list can be started for the data analysis.

Ethnography provides information from a number of perspectives. Behaviors are observed and recorded and inferences about that behavior can be validated through informal questioning immediately after the behavior occurs. By collecting data from multiple sources, in terms of observation, questioning, and with a number of people, data is ensured to be valid. Collecting data on the same content from a number of different methods gives more assurance that the truth is being reported than does collection of data with only one method or from only one person (Roper and Shapira, 2000). By selecting key informants who are considered to be experts and knowledgeable about the topic also ensures validity of the information gathered. Asking open-ended questions provide the informant with a venue to tell the truth from his or her perspective. Answering closed-ended questions which the researcher has derived may influence the informant, resulting in an invalid response.

4. Methods of Data Analysis

The purpose of this investigation is to explore and describe the experience of persons with M.S. living in a nursing home in Edmonton. The data collected provides information on behaviors as well as thoughts and feelings about the experience, and therefore analysis of both the behavior and the spoken and written word is imperative. Data analysis will occur using the software package Ethnograph (Qualis Research Associates).

Data analysis begins almost immediately in ethnography. By completing the field notes daily and inputting this into the computer, and writing perceptions, moods, and inferences alongside the actual observation and interview notes, data analysis has commenced. The daily diary of the researcher's perceptions, moods, and inferences will also be used to identify possible codes or categories.

A preliminary list of codes will be determined from analysis of the pilot test data. Codes will be developed according to different domains, as outlined in Lofland's (cited in Miles and Huberman, 1994:61) schema, as follows:

1. *Acts*: action in a situation that is temporally brief, consuming only a few seconds, minutes, or hours
2. *Activities*: actions in a setting of more major duration—days, weeks, months—constituting a significant element of people's involvements
3. *Meanings*: the verbal productions of participants that define and direct action
4. *Participation*: people's holistic involvement in or adaptation to a situation or setting under study

    5. *Relationships*: interrelationships among several persons considered simultaneously

    6. *Settings*: the entire setting under study conceived as the unit of analysis

Codes will be developed along the way, in order to prevent any possible bias by predetermining what categories or codes will exist. A list of codes will be compiled, along with operational definitions of the codes, to ensure consistency in the data analysis. By the immediate review and rereading of the data prior to entering into the computer, the data are checked to ensure that no important data are missing. Initial coding and analysis of data for each of the different types of data (chart review, observations, formal and informal interviews) will occur separately. Coding of all data will include coding for content, as well as providing codes for the persons involved in the description, so that cross-referencing can occur, according to content or according to person. Codes will be used for all persons with M.S., for other persons on the ward, and for all staff involved. A list of codes identifying particular individuals will be kept separately to ensure confidentiality of the data.

For analysis of the chart reviews, descriptive statistics will be performed on the demographic information to provide an overview of the persons involved in the study. Coding of the data collected line by line from the written health records will be performed using Ethnograph software.

The field notes include description of behaviors, as well as informal interviews. Coding of the field notes will therefore include coding of types of behavior, as well as coding of the spoken word. Behaviors will be coded according to the type of observed behavior, and frequency counts of the behavior will be performed to determine how often a behavior occurs. Informal interviews will be coded line by line for content. Formal interviews will also occur line by line for content.

Analysis will then be grouped according to persons with M.S. to see if there are differences in the experiences of the different key informants. Analysis of the behavioral information will be compared to the descriptive information to see if consistencies or differences are evident.

To determine whether or not the results are true and not biased, clear and comprehensive notes will be kept during data analysis to document the direction the analysis is taking. Such an "audit trail" allows others to review the data analysis procedure to check whether or not researcher bias has influenced the data analysis (Morse and Field, 1995).

When data analysis has been completed, the findings will be reported back to the ward in a review meeting.

5. Protection of Human Subjects

The proposal will be reviewed by the Human Ethics Committee, Part B at the University of Alberta, and the ethics committee of the Capital Care Group. Subject to their approval, each subject will then be approached with a letter outlining the objectives of the study and the commitments required. Should the subject choose to participate in the study, he or she will be asked to sign a consent form (Appendix A). All of those persons who participate in the study will be identified by code only, and all published data will preserve the confidentiality of all participants. All data will be kept in a locked and secure environment.

REFERENCES

Aller, L., & Van Ess Coeling, H. (1996). Quality of life: Its meaning to the long-term care resident. *Journal of Gerontological Nursing, February*: 20–24.

Brunet, D., Hopman, W., Singer, M., Edge, C., & MacKenzie, T. (1996). Measurement of health related quality of life in multiple sclerosis. *The Canadian Journal of Neurological Sciences, 23 (2)*: 99–103.

Buchanan, R. (1993). The difficulty placing younger medicaid beneficiaries in nursing facilities. *American Journal of Physical Medicine and Rehabilitation, 72 (4)*: 226–227.

Buchanan, R., & Lewis, P. (1997). Services that nursing facilities should provide to residents with MS: Survey of health professionals. *Rehabilitation Nursing, 22 (2)*: 67–72.

Canadian Burden of Illness Study Group. (1998). Burden of illness of multiple sclerosis: Part I: Cost of illness. *Canadian Journal of Neurological Sciences, 25*: 23–30.

Canadian Burden of Illness Study Group. (1998). Burden of illness of multiple sclerosis: Part II: Quality of life. *Canadian Journal of Neurological Sciences, 25*: 31–38.

Clark, P., & Bowling, A. (1990). Quality of everyday life in long stay institutions for the elderly. An observational study of long stay hospital and nursing home care. *Social Science and Medicine, 30 (11)*: 1201–1210.

Diamond, T. (1986). Social policy and everday life in nursing homes: A critical ethnography. *Social Science and Medicine, 23 (12)*: 1287–1295.

Donohoe, K., Wineman, M., & O'Brien, R. (1996). Are alternative long-term care programs needed for adults with chronic progressive disability? *Journal of Neuroscience Nursing, 28 (6)*: 373–380.

Fitzpatrick, R., Hinton, J., Newman, S., Scambler, G., & Thompson, J. (1984). *The Experience of Illness*. New York: Tavistock Publications.

Foote, A., Piazza, D., Holcombe, J., Penelope, P., & Daffin, P. (1990). Hope, self-esteem and social support in persons with multiple sclerosis. *Journal of Neuroscience Nursing, 22 (3)*: 155–159.

Frankel, D. (1984). Long-term care issues in multiple sclerosis. *Rehabilitation Literature, 45 (9–10)*: 282–285.

Frankel, D. (1985). Multiple sclerosis. In D. Umphred, (ed.), *Neurological rehabilitation, Volume 3* (pp. 398–416). Toronto: C.V. Mosby Company.

Goffman, E. (1961). *Asylums*. New York: Doubleday.

Goffman, E. (1963). *Stigma. Notes on the Management of Spoiled Identity*. Englewood Cliffs, NJ: Prentice Hall.

Gorman, L. (1996). I'm on the edge all the time: Resident's experiences of living in an integrated nursing home. *Australian Journal of Advanced Nursing, 13 (3)*: 7–11.

Gubrium, J. (1993). *Speaking of Life. Horizons of Meaning for Nursing Home Residents*. New York: Aldine De Gruyter.

Hainsworth, M. (1994). Living with multiple sclerosis: The experience of chronic sorrow. *Journal of Neuroscience Nursing, 26 (4)*:237–240.

Heliker, D. (1997). A narrative approach to quality care in long-term care facilities. *Journal of Holistic Nursing, 15 (1)*: 68–81.

Jacelon, C. (1995). The effect of living in a nursing home on socialization in elderly people. *Journal of Advanced Nursing, 22*: 539–546.

Kaakinen, J. (1992). Living with silence. *The Gerontologist, 32 (2)*: 258–264.

Kayser-Jones, J. (1981). *Old, Alone and Neglected. Care of the Aged in the United States and Scotland*. Berkeley: University of California Press.

McGuinness, S. (1996). Learned helplessness in the multiple sclerosis population. *Journal of Neuroscience Nursing, 23 (3)*:163–170.

Miles, M., & Huberman, A. (1994). *Qualitative Data Analysis* (2nd ed.). Thousand Oaks: Sage Publications.

Morse, J., & Field, P. (1995). *Qualitative Research Methods for Health Professionals*. (2nd ed.). Thousand Oaks: Sage Publications.

Morse, J., & Intrieri, R. (1997). 'Talk to me' Patient communication in a long-term care facility. *Journal of Psychosocial Nursing, 35 (5)*: 34–39.

Murphy Miller, C., & Hens, M. (1993). Multiple Sclerosis: A literature review. *Journal of Neuroscience Nursing, 25 (3)*: 174–179.

Murphy Miller, C., (1993). Trajectory and empowerment theory applied to care of patients with multiple sclerosis. *Journal of Neuroscience Nursing, 25 (8)*:343–348.

Murphy Miller, C. (1997). The lived experience of relapsing multiple sclerosis: A phenomenological study. *Journal of Neuroscience Nursing, 29 (5)*:294–304.

Nystrom, A., & Segesten, K. (1996). The family metaphor applied to nursing home life. *International Journal of Nursing Studies, 33 (3)*: 237–248.

Oleson, M., Heading, C., McGlynn Shadick, K., & Bistodeau, J. (1994). Quality of life in long-stay institutions in England: Nurse and resident perceptions. *Journal of Advanced Nursing, 20*: 23–32.

Parke, B. (1997). The young adult as a nursing home client. The challenge of Karl's legacy. *Canadian Nursing Home, 8 (1)*: 27–28.

Pearson, A., Hocking, S., Mott, S., & Riggs, A. (1993). Quality of care in nursing homes: From the resident's perspective. *Journal of Advanced Nursing, 18*: 20–24.

Pitters, S. (1995). Long term care facilities. In Sawyer, E., & Stephenson, M. (ed.). *The Issues and Challenges for Long Term Care* (pp. 151–188). Ottawa: CHA Press.

Powers, B. (1992). The roles staff play in the social networks of elderly institutionalized people. *Social Science and Medicine, 34 (12)*: 1335–1343.

Roper, J., & Anderson, N. (1994). Stigma. Qualitative perspectives. *Clinical Nursing Research, 3 (4)*: 294–296.

Roper, J. M., & Shapira, J. (2000). *Ethnography in Nursing Research*. Thousand Oaks: Sage Publications.

Running, A. (1997). Snapshots of experience: vignettes from a nursing home. *Journal of Advanced Nursing, 25*: 117–122.

Schmitt, D. (1989). Helping Gwen to keep going. *Nursing, March*: 55–56.

Smith, D., Schalm, C., Shaw, S., Wellock, C., & Lyle, M. (1991). *Residents in Alberta's Long Term Care Facilities: A Descriptive Profile*. Edmonton: Long Term Care Branch. Alberta Health.

The Relationship Between Physical and/or Psychological Abuse and Health Status

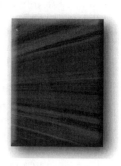

PAMELA A. RATNER

University of Alberta
Faculty of Nursing
Edmonton, Alberta, Canada

The abuse many women experience within their marital relationships recently has emerged as a recognized social problem. As a result, we have witnessed a large increase in social science literature on the subject. However, focusing on the social context within which wife abuse occurs diverts attention from the severity of the abuse many wives experience and results in a failure to recognize the extent of the physical and psychological injury associated with abuse (Hatty, 1987).

Several authors have suggested that health care professionals, in particular, have had their attention diverted and have failed to provide appropriate health care to women who are abused, perhaps because they are educated to deal with problems of physical or sometimes psychosomatic etiology and not of social etiology (Dobash & Dobash, 1979; Stark, Flitcraft, & Frazier, 1979; MacLeod, 1980). One consequence of this lack of attention is a dearth of knowledge of the health problems and health care utilization patterns of women who are abused.

Nurses and other health care professionals can play an important role in assisting abused women in obtaining optimal health. However, effective screening and intervention programs can only be developed and implemented if a sound understanding is acquired of the health problems and health care utilization patterns of women who are abused.

PREVALENCE OF WIFE ABUSE IN CANADA

The prevalence of wife abuse in Canada frequently is reported as involving one woman in ten, married or living with a male partner (House of Commons Standing Committee on Health, Welfare and Social Affairs, 1982; Lewis, 1982; Morrison, 1988; Ontario Medical Association Committee on Wife Assault, 1988; Selkirk, 1987) and usually is attributed to the work of MacLeod (1980). This rate, however, appears to be an approximation based on the work of Handelman and Ward (1976) in which no actual victimization data were collected and at best is merely an estimate (Smith, 1987).

No national representative study of the prevalence of wife abuse in Canada appears to have been conducted and only three regional studies of the prevalence of wife abuse were identified. All three studies employed Straus's (1979) Conflict Tactics Scales (CTS), which allow for some degree of comparison. Kennedy and Dutton (1987, 1989) surveyed a representative sample of 1,045 Alberta residents and reported an overall wife abuse rate of 11.2%. This rate was found to be identical to the American rate determined by Straus and Gelles (1986), who employed similar research methods. However, severe violence was reported less frequently in Alberta than in the United States. The reported rate of severe violence, as determined by Kennedy and Dutton, was 2.3% in Alberta, compared to 3.0% in the United States. Beatings and threats with knives or guns were reported only 25% as frequently as in the American sample and the use of a knife or gun was not reported by the Alberta sample.

Smith (1987) conducted a telephone survey of 604 women in Toronto using a slightly modified version of the CTS. He found that 36.4% of the women had been abused by a husband, partner, boyfriend, or date on at least one occasion in their relationship, 14.4% had been physically abused by their present or ex-husband or partner during the survey year, and 5.1% had been severely abused.

Brinkerhoff and Lupri (1988) interviewed 562 couples in Calgary using self-administered questionnaires. They reported an overall wife abuse rate of 10.3% and a rate of 4.8% for severe violence. The proportion of husbands reported to have threatened their wives with a knife or gun was six times that reported by Kennedy and Dutton (1987, 1989).

Straus, Gelles, and Steinmetz (1980) reported that wife abuse rates in the United States were remarkably stable from region to region. Why then is there such variation in the three Canadian studies? As Smith (1987) pointed out, caution should be employed when comparing abuse rates from different surveys. Although the studies all used the same measurement instrument, there were several variations in the methods employed. First, the target populations differ (city versus province). Second, different interview techniques were used (face-to-face versus telephone). Finally, the CTS was administered in different ways (self-administered versus interviewer-administered) and to different subjects (males only versus females only versus an aggregate of males and females). These differences could account for some or all of the variations in the reported wife abuse rates.

HEALTH PROBLEMS OF WOMEN WHO ARE ABUSED

Physical Injuries

American and British investigators have reported that physically abused women suffer a wide array of injuries, including fractures, particularly to the nose, ribs, jaw, and arms; multiple contusions; lacerations; burns; and head injuries (Appleton, 1980; Drake, 1982; Rounsaville & Weissman, 1977–1978; Stark et al., 1981). An underlying trend that occurs in all of these investigations is that abused women sustain injuries around the head and neck area most frequently.

Stark et al. (1981) compared the physical injuries of abused women and non-abused women in a hospital emergency department (ED) setting. Based on the findings, the investigators concluded that abused women can be distinguished from non-abused women by the frequency, anatomic location, and type of injury. Abused women were reported to be injured three times as often as non-abused women. The physical sites of injury tended to cluster around the head, face, throat, chest, and abdomen. In contrast, non-abused women were reported to experience injuries to the extremities or hip area. Injuries caused by abuse were likely to be abrasions, contusions, or pains for which no physiological cause could be determined, whereas non-abusive injuries were likely to be sprains or strains. No significant difference was found in the frequency of fractures, dislocations, and lacerations between abused and non-abused women.

Kerouac, Taggart, Lescop, and Fortin (1986) and Nuttall, Greaves, and Lent (1985) studied samples of Canadian women who were abused. Nuttall et al. reported that, of 301 abused women, 37% reported bruising and approximately 20% reported injuries severe enough to require medical attention, although the nature of the injuries was not described. Kerouac et al. found that one-third of 130 abused women had suffered bruises, lacerations, and bone fractures. As a result of the paucity of Canadian research, it cannot be determined if Canadian women suffer injuries to the same degree of severity as their American counterparts. It should be noted, however, that neither of these groups of investigators reported injuries as severe as the American investigators.

Mental Health Problems

Physically abused women have been found to suffer from anxiety (Hillard, 1985; Jaffe, Wolfe, Wilson, & Zak, 1986; Kerouac et al., 1986), depression (Bergman, Larsson, Brismar, & Klang, 1987; Domino & Haber, 1987; Jaffe et al., 1986; Kerouac et al., 1986; Nuttall et al., 1985), somatization (Jaffe et al., 1986; Kerouac et al., 1986), hypochondriasis (Domino & Haber, 1987), and hysteria (Domino & Haber, 1987) with greater frequency than women who are free of abuse. However, most of the research in this area has been plagued with conceptual and methodological problems. For example, the representativeness of the samples is questionable as they have generally been small in number (20 to 130 women), nonprobability in nature, and often confined to hospital ED or emergency shelter settings. Further, the comparison groups employed in these studies often have differed significantly from the study samples, particularly in terms of demographic characteristics.

Despite the reported frequency of mental health problems associated with physical abuse, few investigators have studied whether abused women are at risk for suicide. Gayford (1975) reported that 50% of the abused women he interviewed had attempted suicide. However, Hillard (1985) reported a much lower prevalence of suicide attempts, with 20% of the women in her sample having attempted suicide. Only one identified study compared the suicide attempt rate of abused women with non-abused women. Stark et al. (1981) reported that 26% of abused women, compared to 3% of non-abused women, had attempted suicide.

Findings of studies of the frequency of alcohol and drug abuse in abused women generally are inconclusive. Neither Appleton (1980) nor Star (1978) found that abused women had an increased prevalence of alcoholism, compared to non-abused women. However, Hillard (1985), Bergman et al. (1987), and Stark et al. (1981) concluded that abused women had a significantly higher prevalence of alcohol abuse. The findings related to drug abuse also are equivocal. Hillard reported that the number of abused women addicted to illicit drugs was not significantly different from the number of drug-addicted non-abused women. In contrast, Bergman et al. and Stark et al. reported that abused women were significantly more likely to be drug addicts.

Chronic Health Problems

Little research has been conducted to examine the relationship between abuse and chronic health problems. Haber (1985) and Haber and Roos (1984) reported that 53% of 150 women who presented to a chronic pain centre had a history of physical and/or sexual abuse. All of the abused women's problems with pain—low back pain, headache, and abdominal pain—reportedly followed the first incident of abuse. Women with abdominal or vaginal pain of unknown etiology had the highest incidence of previous abuse.

Pregnancy

Researchers also have examined the association between pregnancy and abuse, and several have suggested that women experience abuse at unusually high rates during pregnancy. Almost one-quarter of the violent families Gelles (1975) interviewed reported abuse during pregnancy. Helton, McFarlane, and Anderson (1987) revealed that 8% of the women they studied reported abuse during their current pregnancy and 15% reported past histories of abuse; whereas the Hillard (1985) study revealed that 3.9% experienced abuse during their current pregnancy and 10.9% had experienced abuse in the past and were still in a relationship with the assailant. Pregnancy outcome was not investigated by Helton et al., but Hillard reported that no marked differences in outcomes were demonstrated in the women who were abused as compared to non-abused women.

Bullock and McFarlane (1989) examined the effect of abuse on pregnancy outcome in terms of birthweight. Significantly more low-birthweight infants were born to abused women than to non-abused women. Interestingly, the abused women reported less alcohol use than did the non-abused women, however, the abused women smoked more than the non-abused women.

In contrast to the majority of investigators who have examined abuse and pregnancy, Gelles (1988) concluded that the relationship is spurious when one controls for age. He found that women under the age of 25 were more likely to be both pregnant and abused. Thus, he concluded that although pregnant women are not an especially vulnerable group, pregnancy does not protect them from the abuse experienced by other young women.

HEALTH CARE UTILIZATION PATTERNS OF WOMEN WHO ARE ABUSED

No study was identified that focused specifically on the health care utilization patterns of abused women. However, several studies, when pieced together, can provide an emerging profile of the health care utilization patterns of abused women.

Bowker and Maurer (1987) surveyed an American national sample of abused women and found that 39% reported receiving help from physicians or nurses. They concluded that the severity of abuse was associated with an increased probability of health care utilization. Brismar, Bergman, Larsson, and Strandberg (1987) reported that abused women utilized health care services with considerably greater frequency than non-abused women. More abused women had been admitted to the hospital and utilized psychiatric care, including in-patient psychiatric clinics, than non-abused women.

Several groups of investigators have attempted to determine the proportion of abused women among women seeking hospital ED care with estimates ranging from 3.8% to 35% (Appleton, 1980; Goldberg & Tomlanovich, 1984; McLeer & Anwar, 1989; Rounsaville & Weissman, 1977–1978; Stark et al., 1981; Tilden & Shepherd, 1987). McLeer and Anwar noted that age was related to physical abuse: 42% of female trauma cases in the 18 to 20 year age group had a history of abuse, 35% of the women 21 to 30 years of age were abused, as were 18% of injured women 61 years of age and older. These studies, however, all faced the problem of how to accurately identify women as abused.

SUMMARY

The abuse of women is a problem that clearly warrants the attention of nurses and other health care professionals. The studies reviewed suggest that women who are abused suffer from multiple physical and psychological health problems. Further, there is evidence to suggest that abused women frequently utilize health care services. If effective identification and intervention programs for abused women are to be established, it is essential that an understanding of the health problems and health care utilization patterns of this group be ascertained.

Most of the existing research in this area has been descriptive or exploratory in nature and has generally occurred in emergency shelter or hospital ED settings. The researchers have focused solely on the consequences of physical abuse; the consequences of ongoing verbal or psychological abuse have not been examined. Finally, convenience sampling has been utilized widely with reference to comparison groups and representativeness of the sample rarely being considered. Clearly, additional research is required regarding the nature of abused women's health problems and health care utilization patterns, particularly within the Canadian context.

PURPOSE OF THE STUDY

The purpose of this study is to answer the question: Is there a significant relationship between the type of abuse women may experience and their health problems and health care utilization patterns? In addition, the following sub-questions will be addressed:

1. Do women who are physically abused suffer health problems with greater frequency than women who are not abused?

2. Do women who are physically abused utilize health care services with greater frequency than women who are not abused?

3. Do women who are psychologically abused suffer health problems with greater frequency than women who are not abused?

4. Do women who are psychologically abused utilize health care services with greater frequency than women who are not abused?

5. Is there a difference in the frequency of health problems between women who are physically abused and women who are psychologically abused?

6. Is there a difference in the frequency of utilization of health care services between women who are physically abused and women who are psychologically abused?

DEFINITION OF TERMS

Health problems: Those conditions that impede or threaten to impede the attainment of an optimal level of physical or psychological well-being. These deviations from health will be identified by the sample in response to a structured questionnaire (see Appendices A, B, and C).

Health care utilization patterns: Those activities that make use of health care professionals' services in order to gain help for health problems. These activities will be identified by the sample in response to a structured questionnaire (see Appendix A).

Type of abuse: Two types of abuse will be considered in this study: psychological abuse and physical abuse.

Psychological abuse: The use of verbal and nonverbal acts that symbolically hurt another, or the use of threats to hurt another (Straus, 1979).

Physical abuse: The use of violence in the form of bodily aggression; an act that threatens or causes physical injury to another person (Brinkerhoff & Lupri, 1988).

RESEARCH DESIGN

The design of this study is a cross-sectional survey, the purpose of which is to examine the relationship between the type of abuse women may experience (i.e., no abuse, physical abuse, and/or psychological abuse) and their reported health problems and health care utilization patterns.

THE SAMPLE

The population for this study will be women, 18 years of age or older, who are married (including common-law relationships) and living with, or lived with in the previous year, a male partner in the greater Edmonton area, who can be contacted by telephone direct-dialing, and who can speak and understand English.

A probability sample will be obtained using random-digit dialing. This approach allows every working telephone number in the population an equal probability of selection. A list of 2,000 telephone numbers with Edmonton area exchanges will be obtained from the Population Research Laboratory (PRL) at the University of Alberta. The PRL generates sample telephone numbers by combining the use of telephone directories with the random assignment of digits. The generation of the telephone numbers consists of three steps. First, all five-digit banks of telephone numbers, published in the Edmonton telephone directory, are identified and entered into a computer file. Second, a simple random sample (with replacement) of 2,000 numbers is selected. Finally, a two-digit random number between 00 and 99 is appended to each of the numbers to obtain a sample of seven-digit telephone numbers. Any duplicate numbers are removed. This approach allows unlisted as well as listed numbers an equal chance of being included in the sample (Lalu, 1991).

The sampling frame will most likely result in a 50% efficiency rate with 60% of the telephone numbers belonging to households with an eligible woman. Based on Kennedy and Dutton's (1987) experience, approximately 25% of the telephone numbers called will result in an inability to make contact, language problems, or refusals to participate. Calling will continue until 400 interviews are completed. Kennedy and Dutton reported that the incidence of wife abuse involving physical aggression was 14.1% in Edmonton. On this basis, of a sample of 400 women, 55 women will report that they are physically abused by their husbands. The incidence of psychological abuse is not known. However, the remaining 345 women interviewed will be either psychologically abused or free from abuse. The size of the subgroups will be sufficient to detect medium "effect sizes" with a significance criterion on a two-tailed test at the .05 level and power equal to .80 (Cohen, 1988).

The investigator will interview a woman at the residence of the telephone number selected if: (a) the dwelling unit is the woman's usual place of residence, (b) she lives with, or in the previous year has lived with, a male partner, (c) she is 18 years of age or older, (d) she speaks and understands English, and (e) she consents to the interview.

METHOD OF DATA COLLECTION

The investigator will use telephone interviews in which four questionnaires are administered. First, a questionnaire designed by the author to elicit the physical health problems, health care utilization patterns, and demographic characteristics of the sample will be administered (see Appendix A).

The General Health Questionnaire (GHQ) (Goldberg & Hillier, 1979) will be administered to measure the mental health status of the sample (see Appendix B). The 28-item GHQ, consisting of four subscales—somatic symptoms, anxiety and insomania, social dysfunction, and severe depression—is perhaps the most widely used screening test for psychiatric morbidity in the community. Each item can be scored as a multiple-response scale or "Likert scale" and have weights assigned to each position (e.g., 0 = not at all, 3 = much more than usual). The items are summed to give a total GHQ score.

The third questionnaire, known as the CAGE questionnaire for its key words (Cut down, Annoyed, Guilty, Eye-opener), is a brief alcoholism screening test (Ewing, 1984; Mayfield, McLeod, & Hall, 1974) (see Appendix C). It is generally recognized as the most widely used questionnaire in screening for alcoholism (Strang, Bradley, & Stockwell, 1989). The questionnaire consists of four questions of a nonincriminating nature and is a sensitive indication of covert problem drinking. A criterion of at least two positive responses will be accepted as an indicator of alcohol dependency.

Finally, the Straus (1979) Conflict Tactics Scales (CTS)—a self-report scale of psychological and physical aggression in conflicts with a partner—will be administered (see Appendix D). It consists of 19 items and is designed to measure the use of reasoning, verbal aggression, and physical aggression within relationships. The items range in order of presentation as follows: The first 3 items have to do with reasoning, the next 7 items deal with verbal aggression, and the remaining 9 items describe acts of physical aggression.

Raw scores represent frequency ranges for each item and vary from 0 ("never") to 6 ("more than 20 times"). Total scores for each of 3 subscales are derived by summing the raw scores for each of the items and can be used to identify whether a woman is psychologically abused, physically abused, or free from abuse by her husband.

The women in the sample will be telephoned and interviewed if consent is obtained. If initial contact is not made, the investigator will attempt to make contact at various times of the day and week. If the woman consents to an interview but finds the time of the initial contact inconvenient, a suitable time will be established, and the interview will be conducted at that time. An introductory statement, including information about anonymity and confidentiality, will be provided to the informants and then the interview will be conducted. The interviewer will read each question to the informant, allowing adequate time for response, and will restate questions as needed for clarification.

RELIABILITY AND VALIDITY

The interview schedule will be pretested on 25 women in the population, selected by random-digit dialing, who consent to pretest the questionnaire. The progression and clarity of the questions and the time required for interview completion will be evaluated by the investigator based on the comments of the respondents. The questionnaire will be revised as necessary with additional pretests conducted following each revision until the investigator is satisfied that the respondents understand what is required of them.

The questionnaire, designed to elicit information regarding physical health problems and health care utilization patterns, is assumed to have content validity because it arose from the research literature that is available. The GHQ has been found to have a sensitivity of 84% and a specificity of 82% (Bridges & Goldberg, 1989). The GHQ has been demonstrated to correlate with a number of other measures of psychiatric disturbance and has been shown to be a relatively effective psychiatric screening measure (Banks, 1983; Malt, 1989; Rabins & Brooks, 1981; Vieweg & Hedlund, 1983).

King (1986) assessed the validity of the CAGE questionnaire and found the sensitivity and specificity to be acceptable at 84% and 95% respectively. These results compare favorably with the findings of Bernadt, Mumford, and Murray (1984) who compared the CAGE against laboratory tests and found the sensitivity and specificity to be 91% and 77% respectively.

The CTS has been utilized in several studies of family violence (Brinkerhoff & Lupri, 1988; Campbell, 1986, 1989; Henton, Cate, Koval, Lloyd, & Christopher, 1983; Hornung, McCullough, & Sugimoto, 1981; Jaffe et al., 1986; Kennedy & Dutton, 1987, 1989; Smith, 1987; Straus, 1974) and four different investigators have established that the instrument measures three factorially separate variables (Barling, O'Leary, Jouriles, Vivian, & MacEwen, 1987; Jorgensen, 1977; Schumm, Martin, Bollman, & Jurich, 1982; Straus, 1979). Internal consistency of the CTS has been addressed by item to total score correlations (.70 to .87) and alpha coefficients for the three categories (Straus, 1979). Construct validity was established in studies that found associations with the CTS consistent with predictions (Kalmuss & Straus, 1982; Straus, Gelles, & Steinmetz, 1980). Validity data also have been generated by comparing reports of different family members (Browning & Dutton, 1986; Straus, 1974) and comparing scores with indepth interviews (Gelles, 1972). The CTS physical aggression scale has shown significant inter-partner reliability (Jouriles & O'Leary, 1985).

One concern regarding the measurement of abuse of women is whether informants will report abuse to an anonymous interviewer. Some under-reporting may occur; however, Straus et al. (1980) reported that respondents refused to answer questions about abuse no more frequently than respondents in telephone surveys in general. Further, Arias and Beach (1987) found that socially desirable response set is not related to the willingness of women to report abuse.

DATA ANALYSIS

The analysis of data obtained in this study will include graphic representations of the data. First, tables displaying the three groups—physically abused, psychologically abused, and non-abused women by age, length of relationship, marital status, number of children, employment status, income, and education—will be presented. As the measures of type of abuse, health problems, and health care utilization patterns are nominal in nature, cross-tabulations will be used to organize the data. The frequencies with which health problems occur and services are utilized are unlikely to be normally distributed. Accordingly, the frequencies will be categorized, and in order to demonstrate the relationship between variables, Chi-square analysis will be carried out. Significance will be set at $p < .05$.

Hierarchical regression will be employed to determine if physical abuse status predicts GHQ scores following that afforded by various demographic data. Analysis of variance (ANOVA) will be utilized to analyze the relationship between GHQ scores and psychological abuse. Post hoc analysis using the Scheffé (1953) test will be carried out to counteract inflation of the Type I error rate caused by multiple comparisons (Tabachnick & Fidell, 1989). The odds ratio with 95% confidence limits will be calculated for alcohol dependence. Kruskal-Wallis ANOVA will be employed for the analysis of the backache and headache data. Finally, Chi-square analysis will be employed for the analysis of medication use, the number of spontaneous abortions, and health care utilization.

PROTECTION OF HUMAN SUBJECTS

The proposal will be reviewed by the Ethics Committee of the Faculty of Nursing at the University of Alberta. Several strategies will be utilized to protect the rights of the women who agree to participate in this study. First, oral consent of the women will be obtained prior to the administration of the questionnaire. The women will be informed of the purpose of the study, that participation is voluntary, and that they have the right to refuse to participate. Further, the women will be told that they can refrain from answering any questions and can terminate the interview at any time. Anonymity of the women will be maintained at all times. Data will be organized by subject codes, and the investigator will keep the telephone numbers of the women in a separate locked file. The names and addresses of the women will remain unknown to the investigator.

In the event that the women ask questions regarding their health, the investigator will provide answers to the best of her ability following the completion of the data collection. If the investigator is unsure of appropriate responses, she will refer the woman to resource personnel. The investigator will have a list of appropriate resource personnel and telephone numbers available at all times.

REFERENCES

Appleton, W. (1980). The battered woman syndrome. *Annals of Emergency Medicine, 9:*84–91.

Arias, I., & Beach, S. R. H. (1987). Validity of self-reports of marital violence. *Journal of Family Violence, 2:*139–149.

Banks, M. H. (1983). Validation of the General Health Questionnaire in a young community sample. *Psychological Medicine, 13:*349–353.

Barling, J., O'Leary, K. D., Jouriles, E. N., Vivian, D., & MacEwen, K. E. (1987). Factor similarity of the Conflict Tactic Scales across samples, spouses, and sites: Issues and implications. *Journal of Family Violence, 2:*37–54.

Bergman, B., Larsson, G., Brismar, B., & Klang, M. (1987). Psychiatric morbidity and personality characteristics of battered women. *Acta Psychiatrica Scandinavica, 76:*678–683.

Bernadt, M. W., Mumford, J., & Murray, R. M. (1984). A discriminant-function analysis of screening tests for excessive drinking and alcoholism. *Journal of Studies on Alcohol, 45:*81–86.

Bowker, L. H., & Maurer, L. (1987). The medical treatment of battered wives. *Women and Health, 12*(1):25–45.

Bridges, K., & Goldberg, D. (1989). Self-administered scales of neurotic symptoms. In C. Thompson (ed.), *The instruments of psychiatric research* (pp. 157–176). Chichester, England: John Wiley.

Brinkerhoff, M. B., & Lupri, E. (1988). Interspousal violence. *Canadian Journal of Sociology, 13:*407–434.

Brismar, B., Bergman, B., Larsson, G., & Strandberg, A. (1987). Battered women: A diagnostic and therapeutic dilemma. *Acta Chirurgica Scandinavica, 153:*1–5.

Browning, J., & Dutton, D. (1986). Assessment of wife assault with the Conflict Tactics Scale: Using couple data to quantify the differential reporting effect. *Journal of Marriage and the Family, 48:*375–379.

Bullock, L. F., & McFarlane, J. (1989). Birth-weight/battering connection. *American Journal of Nursing, 9:*1153–1155.

Campbell, J. C. (1986). Nursing assessment for risk of homicide with battered women. *Advances in Nursing Science, 8*(4):36–51.

Campbell, J. C. (1989). A test of two explanatory models of women's responses to battering. *Nursing Research, 38:*18–24.

Cohen, J. (1988). *Statistical power analysis for the behavioral sciences* (2d ed.). Hillsdale, NJ: Lawrence Erlbaum.

Dobash, R. E., & Dobash, R. (1979). *Violence against wives: A case against the patriarchy.* New York: Free Press.

Domino, J. V., & Haber, J. D. (1987). Prior physical and sexual abuse in women with chronic headache: Clinical correlates. *Headache, 27:*310–314.

Drake, V. K. (1982). Battered women: A health care problem in disguise. *Image, 14*(2):40–47.

Ewing, J. A. (1984). Detecting alcoholism: The CAGE questionnaire. *JAMA, 252:*1905–1907.

Gayford, J. J. (1975). Wife battering: A preliminary survey of 100 cases. *British Medical Journal, 1:*194–197.

Gelles, R. (1972). *The violent home: A study of physical aggression between husbands and wives.* Beverly Hills, CA: Sage.

Gelles, R. (1975). Violence and pregnancy: A note on the extent of the problem and needed services. *Family Coordinator, 24:*81–86.

Gelles, R. J. (1988). Violence and pregnancy: Are pregnant women at greater risk of abuse? *Journal of Marriage and the Family, 50:*841–847.

Goldberg, D. P., & Hillier, V. P. (1979). A scaled version of the General Health Questionnaire. *Psychological Medicine, 9:*139–145.

Goldberg, W. G., & Tomlanovich, M. C. (1984). Domestic violence victims in the emergency department: New findings. *JAMA, 251:*3259–3264.

Haber, J. (1985). Abused women and chronic pain. *American Journal of Nursing, 85:*1010, 1012.

Haber, J., & Roos, C. (1984). Effects of spouse abuse and/or sexual abuse in the development and maintenance of chronic pain in women. *Pain, 20*(suppl. 2):S187.

Handelman, M., & Ward W. (1976). *Battered women, emergency shelter and the law.* Windsor, Ontario: University of Windsor.

Hatty, S. (1987). Woman battering as a social problem: The denial of injury. *Australian and New Zealand Journal of Sociology, 23:*36–46.

Helton, A. S., McFarlane, J., & Anderson, E. T. (1987). Battered and pregnant: A prevalence study. *American Journal of Public Health, 77:*1337–1339.

Henton, J., Cate, R., Koval, J., Lloyd, S., & Christopher, S. (1983). Romance and violence in dating relationships. *Journal of Family Issues, 4:*467–482.

Hillard, P. J. A. (1985). Physical abuse in pregnancy. *Obstetrics and Gynecology, 66:*185–190.

Hornung, C. A., McCullough, B. C., & Sugimoto, T. (1981). Status relationships in marriage: Risk factors in spouse abuse. *Journal of Marriage and the Family, 43:*675–692.

House of Commons Standing Committee on Health, Welfare and Social Affairs. (1982). *Inquiry into violence in the family.* Ottawa, Ontario: Queen's Printer of Canada.

Jaffe, P., Wolfe, D. A., Wilson, S., & Zak, L. (1986). Emotional and physical health problems of battered women. *Canadian Journal of Psychiatry, 31:*625–629.

Jorgensen, S. R. (1977). Social class heterogamy, status striving, and perceptions of marital conflict: A partial replication and revision of Pearlin's contingency hypothesis. *Journal of Marriage and the Family, 39:*653–661.

Jouriles, E. N., & O'Leary, K. D. (1985). Interspousal reliability of reports of marital violence. *Journal of Consulting and Clinical Psychology, 53:*419–421.

Kalmuss, D. S., & Straus, M. A. (1982). Wife's marital dependency and wife abuse. *Journal of Marriage and the Family, 44:*277–286.

Kennedy, L. W., & Dutton, D. G. (1987). *The incidence of wife assault in Alberta* (Edmonton area series rep. No. 53). Edmonton, Alberta: University of Alberta, Population Research Laboratory and Department of Sociology.

Kennedy, L. W., & Dutton, D. G. (1989). The incidence of wife assault in Alberta. *Canadian Journal of Behavioural Science, 21*(1):40–54.

Kerouac, S., Taggart, M., Lescop, J., & Fortin, M. (1986). Dimensions of health in violent families. *Health Care for Women International, 7:*413–426.

King, M. (1986). At risk drinking among general practice attenders: Validation of the CAGE questionnaire. *Psychological Medicine, 16:*213–217.

Lalu, N. M. (1991). *Sampling methods for telephone surveys* (Research Discussion Paper No. 74). Edmonton: University of Alberta, Department of Sociology.

Lewis, D. J. (1982). *A brief on wife battering with proposals for federal action.* Ottawa, Ontario: Canadian Advisory Council on the Status of Women.

MacLeod, L. (1980). *Wife battering in Canada: The vicious circle.* Ottawa, Canada: Canadian Advisory Council on the Status of Women.

Malt, U. F. (1989). The validity of the General Health Questionnaire in a sample of accidentally injured adults. *Acta Psychiatrica Scandinavica, 80*(suppl. 355):103–112.

Mayfield, D., McLeod, G., & Hall, P. (1974). The CAGE questionnaire: Validation of a new alcoholism screening instrument. *American Journal of Psychiatry, 131:*1121–1123.

McLeer, S. V., & Anwar, R. (1989). A study of battered women presenting in an emergency department. *American Journal of Public Health, 79:*65–66.

Morrison, L. J. (1988). The battering syndrome: A poor record of detection in the emergency department. *Journal of Emergency Medicine, 6:*521–526.

Nuttall, S. E., Greaves, L. J., & Lent, B. (1985). Wife battering: An emerging problem in public health. *Canadian Journal of Public Health, 76:*297–299.

Ontario Medical Association Committee on Wife Assault. (1988). *Ontario Medical Association reports on wife assault.* Ottawa, Ontario: National Clearinghouse on Family Violence, Health and Welfare Canada.

Rabins, P. V., & Brooks, B. R. (1981). Emotional disturbance in multiple sclerosis patients. Validity of the General Health Questionnaire (GHQ). *Psychological Medicine, 11*:425–427.

Rounsaville, B., & Weissman, M. M. (1977–1978). Battered women: A medical problem requiring detection. *International Journal of Psychiatry in Medicine, 8*:191–202.

Scheffé, H. H. (1953). A method of judging all contrasts in the analysis of variance. *Biometrika, 40*:87–104.

Schumm, W. R., Martin, M. J., Bollman, S. R., & Jurich, A. P. (1982). Classifying family violence: Whither the woozle? *Journal of Family Issues, 3*:319–340.

Selkirk, D. (1987). Family violence: Opportunity for change. *Axon, 9*(2):3–8.

Smith, M. D. (1987). The incidence and prevalence of woman abuse in Toronto. *Violence and Victims, 2*:173–187.

Star, B. (1978). Comparing battered and non-battered women. *Victimology, 3*(1–2):32–44.

Stark, E., Flitcraft, A., & Frazier, W. (1979). Medicine and patriarchal violence: The social construction of a "private" event. *International Journal of Health Services, 9*:461–493.

Stark, E., Flitcraft, A., Zuckerman, D., Grey, A., Robison, J., & Frazier, W. (1981). *Wife abuse in the medical setting: An introduction for health personnel* (Domestic Violence Monograph No. 7). Rockville, MD: National Clearinghouse on Domestic Violence.

Strang, J., Bradley, B., & Stockwell, T. (1989). Assessment of drug and alcohol use. In C. Thompson (ed.), *The instruments of psychiatric research* (pp. 211–237). Chichester, England: John Wiley.

Straus, M. A. (1974). Leveling, civility, and violence in the family. *Journal of Marriage and the Family, 36*:13–29.

Straus, M. A. (1979). Measuring intra-family conflict and violence: Conflict Tactics (CT) Scales. *Journal of Marriage and the Family, 41*:75–88.

Straus, M. A., & Gelles, R. J. (1986). Societal change and change in family violence from 1975 to 1985 as revealed by two national surveys. *Journal of Marriage and the Family, 48*:465–479.

Straus, M. A., Gelles, R. J., & Steinmetz, S. K. (1980). *Behind closed doors: Violence in the American family.* New York: Anchor Books.

Tabachnick, B. G., & Fidell, L. S. (1989). *Using multivariate statistics* (2d ed.). New York: Harper and Row.

Tilden, V. P., & Shepherd, P. (1987). Increasing the rate of identification of battered women in an emergency department: Use of a nursing protocol. *Research in Nursing and Health, 10*:209–215.

Vieweg, B. W., & Hedlund, J. L. (1983). The General Health Questionnaire (GHQ): A comprehensive review. *Journal of Operational Psychiatry, 14*(2):74–81.

APPENDIX A

Interview Schedule

INTERVIEWER INSTRUCTIONS: If a man answers, ask if you may speak to his wife. If a woman answers (or when the woman comes to the phone), state: Hello, my name is _____, and I am a researcher in the Faculty of Nursing at the University of Alberta. We are presently conducting research regarding the problems women may experience in their marriages and with their health. If you are over 18 years of age and presently married or living in a common-law relationship, or have been in the past year, I hope you will agree to participate in this research. Your phone number was selected randomly and I do not know your name or address. All that is required of you is that you answer some questions over the telephone about your marriage, particularly about how your husband handles conflict, and about your health. It will only take about 10 to 15 minutes. If there are questions that you would prefer not to answer, please say so at any time during the interview.

1. a. What is your current marital status?

> Married 01
> Common-law 02
> Separated. 03
> Divorced 04
> Widowed 05
> Other (Specify) . . . . 06 _____
> Don't know (DK) 98
> No response (NR) 99

2. a. In the past year have you had an appointment with a family doctor? (If separated/divorced, for the year in which couple was last together)

> No . . . . 01 (go to 3)
> Yes 02
> Don't know 98
> No response 99

   b. How many appointments did you have?

> Actual number . . . . _____
> Don't know 998
> No response 999

3. a. In the past year have you had to go to a hospital emergency room for a problem of your own?

> No . . . . 01 (go to 4)
> Yes 02
> Don't know 98
> No response 99

   b. How many times did you go to an emergency room?

> Actual number . . . . _____
> Don't know 998
> No response 999

4. a. In the past year have you gone to a medi-centre for a problem of your own?

> No . . . . 01 (go to 5)
> Yes 02
> Don't know 98
> No response 99

b. How many times did you go to a medi-centre?

Actual number . . . . _____

Don't know 998

No response 999

5. a. Have you spoken with a public or community health nurse about your health in the past year?

No . . . . 01 (go to 6)

Yes 02

Don't know 98

No response 99

b. How many times did you speak with a public or community health nurse?

Actual number . . . . _____

Don't know 998

No response 999

6. a. In the past year have you had an appointment with a psychiatrist?

No 01

Yes 02

Don't know 98

No response 99

7. a. In the past year have you been hospitalized?

No . . . . 01 (go to 8)

Yes 02

Don't know 98

No response 99

b. How many days were you hospitalized?

Actual number . . . . _____

Don't know 98

No response 99

8. a. Have you used any of the following in the past year?

	No	Yes	DK	NR
Chiropractor	01	02	98	99
Pain clinic	01	02	98	99
Psychologist	01	02	98	99
Acupuncture	01	02	98	99
Other health care services	01	02	98	99

(Specify): _____

9. a.   Have you had a broken bone or bones in the past year?

   No . . . . 01 (go to 10)

   Yes 02

   Don't know 98

   No response 99

   b.   On how many different occasions have you had a bone or bones broken in the past year?

   Actual number . . . . _____

   Don't know 98

   No response 99

   c.   Where on your body did this happen? (May answer more than once) (Circle up to three)

   Hands or arms 01

   Legs or feet 02

   Hips 03

   Ribs 04

   Spine (back). 05

   Nose 06

   Skull. 07

   Other (Specify) . . . . 08 _____

   _____

   Not applicable 97

   Don't know 98

   No response 99

10. a.   Have you had a large bruise or bruises on your body in the past year?

    No . . . . 01 (go to 11)

    Yes 02

    Don't know 98

    No response 99

    b.   On how many different occasions have you had a bruise or bruises in the past year?

    Actual number . . . . _____

    Don't know 998

    No response 999

c.   Where on your body did this happen? (May answer more than once) (Circle up to three)

Hands or arms 01

Legs or feet 02

Abdomen (stomach) 03

Chest 04

Back 05

Neck 06

Face 07

Head 08

Other (Specify) . . . . 09 _____

_____

Not applicable 97

Don't know 98

No response 99

11. a.   Have you had a cut that needed stitches in the past year?

No . . . . 01 (go to 12)

Yes 02

Don't know 98

No response 99

b.   On how many different occasions have you had a cut that needed stitches in the past year?

Actual number . . . . _____

Don't know 998

No response 999

c.   Where on your body did this happen? (May answer more than once) (Circle up to three)

Hands or arms 01

Legs or feet 02

Abdomen (stomach) 03

Chest 04

Back 05

Neck 06

Face 07

Head 08

Other (Specify) . . . . 09 _____

_____

Not applicable 97

Don't know 98

No response 99

12. a. Have you had a sprain or strain in the past year?

No . . . . 01 (go to 13)

Yes 02

Don't know 98

No response 99

b. On how many different occasions have you had a sprain or strain in the past year?

Actual number . . . . _____

Don't know 998

No response 999

c. Where on your body did this happen? (May answer more than once)

(Circle up to three)

Hands or arms 01

Legs or feet 02

Abdomen (stomach) 03

Chest 04

Back 05

Neck 06

Other (Specify) . . . . 07 _____

_____

Not applicable 97

Don't know 98

No response 99

13. a. Have you had a head injury in the past year?

No . . . . 01 (go to 14)

Yes 02

Don't know 98

No response 99

b. What kind of head injury was it? (Describe) (Up to two injuries)

Not applicable 97

Don't know 98

No response 99

14. a. Have you had a ruptured ear drum in the past year?

No 01

Yes 02

Don't know 98

No response 99

15. a. Have you had any other injuries in the past year?

No . . . . 01 (go to 16)

Yes 02

Don't know 98

No response 99

b. What kind of injuries have you had? (Describe type and location of injury) (May describe up to three injuries)

Not applicable 97

Don't know 98

No response 99

16. a. How often do you have headaches?

Never . . . . 01 (go to 17)

Rarely. 02

Occasionally. 03

Frequently 04

Every day. 05

Don't know 98

No response 99

b. Would you describe the intensity of the headache that you usually have as:

Very slight 01

Mild 02

Moderate 03

Severe 04

Excruciating. 05

Not applicable 97

Don't know 98

No response 99

c. How often does your headache cause you to limit your physical activity?

Never 01

Rarely. 02

Occasionally. 03

Frequently 04

Almost always 05

Always 06

Not applicable 97

Don't know 98

No response 99

17. a.   How often do you have backaches?

  Never . . . . 01 (go to 18)

  Rarely 02

  Occasionally 03

  Frequently 04

  Every day 05

  Don't know 98

  No response 99

 b.   Would you describe the intensity of the backache that you usually have as:

  Very slight 01

  Mild 02

  Moderate 03

  Severe 04

  Excruciating 05

  Not applicable 97

  Don't know 98

  No response 99

 c.   How often does your backache cause you to limit your physical activity?

  Never 01

  Rarely 02

  Occasionally 03

  Frequently 04

  Almost always 05

  Always 06

  Not applicable 97

  Don't know 98

  No response 99

18. a.   Have you had a miscarriage since you have been living with your present partner? (If divorced or separated, while living with former partner)

  No . . . . 01 (go to 19)

  Yes 02

  Don't know 98

  No response 99

b. How many miscarriages have you had since living with your present partner? (If divorced or separated, while living with former partner)

Actual number . . . . _____

Don't know 998

No response 999

19. a. How many different kinds of prescription medicines have you used in the
past month?

Actual number . . . . _____

Don't know 998

No response 999

20. a. Have you taken any of the following medicines in the past month?

	No	Yes	DK	NR
Pain killers (non-prescription)	01	02	98	99
Prescription pain killers	01	02	98	99
Sleeping pills	01	02	98	99
Antidepressants	01	02	98	99
Tranquilizers	01	02	98	99
Any other medication	01	02	98	99

(Specify) _____

_____

_____

21. a. How old did you turn on your last birthday?

Actual age . . . . _____

Don't know 998

No response 999

22. a. How long have you lived with your present partner? (If divorced or separated, how long with former partner)

Actual number. . . . . _____

Don't know 98

No response 99

23. a.   How many children do you have?

Actual number .... _____

Don't know 98

No response 99

24. a.   How many children are currently living with you?

Actual number .... _____

Don't know 98

No response 99

25. a.   Are you presently working full-time, part-time, going to school, keeping house, or something else? (If divorced or separated: What were you doing while with former partner?)

Employed full-time 01

Employed part-time 02

Unemployed 03

Retired 04

In school 05

Keeping house......... 06

Other (e.g., disabled).... 07

Don't know 98

No response.......... 99

26. a.   Is your partner presently working full-time, part-time, going to school, keeping house, or something else? (If divorced or separated: What was former partner doing when living together?)

Employed full-time 01

Employed part-time 02

Unemployed 03

Retired 04

In school 05

Keeping house......... 06

Other (e.g., disabled).... 07

Don't know 98

No response.......... 99

27. a.   What is the highest level of education that you completed?

   No schooling 01

   Elementary

      Incomplete. 02

      Complete 03

   Junior high

      Incomplete. 02

      Complete 03

   High school

      Incomplete. 06

      Complete 07

   Non-university (voc/tech, nursing)

      Incomplete. 08

      Complete 09

   University

      Incomplete. 10

      Diploma/certificate . . . 11

      Bachelor's degree 12

      Professional degree . . . 13

      Master's degree 14

      Doctorate 15

   Don't know 98

   No response 99

28. a.   What is the highest level of education that your (former) partner completed?

   (Code same as previous question) ⸺⸺⸺

29. a.   What was the total income of you and your husband for this past year before deductions and taxes? (If divorced or separated: . . . the last year you were together.) I do not need the exact amount, just the general category. Would it be:

   Less than $10,000 01

   Between $10,000 and $19,999 02

   Between $20,000 and $29,999 03

   Between $30,000 and $39,999 04

   Between $40,000 and $49,999 05

   Between $50,000 and $59,999 06

   Between $60,000 and $69,999 07

Between $70,000 and $79,999 08

More than $80,000 09

Don't know 98

No response 99

30. a. How much of this total income did you contribute in this past year (or last year of marriage or relationship) before deductions and taxes?

Less than $10,000 01

Between $10,000 and $19,999 02

Between $20,000 and $29,999 03

Between $30,000 and $39,999 04

Between $40,000 and $49,999 05

Between $50,000 and $59,999 06

Between $60,000 and $69,999 07

Between $70,000 and $79,999 08

More than $80,000 09

Don't know 98

No response 99

Appendix B

GENERAL HEALTH QUESTIONNAIRE

Interviewer Script

I would like to know if you have had any medical complaints, and how your health has been in general, over the past year. Please answer all the questions by saying "better than usual," "same as usual," "worse than usual," or "much worse than usual." I am interested in your complaints over the past year, not those that you had prior to that.

Interviewer Code

Better than usual 01

Same as usual 02

Worse than usual 03

Much worse than usual 04

Don't know 98

No response 99

In the past year have you:

1. Been feeling perfectly well and in good health?
   01   02   03   04   98   99

2. Been feeling in need of some medication to pick you up?
   01   02   03   04   98   99

3. Been feeling run down and out of sorts?
   01   02   03   04   98   99

4. Felt that you are ill?
   01   02   03   04   98   99

5. Been getting any pains in your head?
   01   02   03   04   98   99

6. Been getting a feeling of tightness or pressure in your head?
   01   02   03   04   98   99

7. Been having hot or cold spells?
   01   02   03   04   98   99

8. Lost much sleep due to worry?
   01   02   03   04   98   99

9. Had difficulty staying asleep?
   01   02   03   04   98   99

10. Felt constantly under strain?
    01   02   03   04   98   99

11. Been edgy and bad-tempered?
    01   02   03   04   98   99

12. Been getting scared or panicky for no good reason?
    01   02   03   04   98   99

13. Found everything getting on top of you?
    01   02   03   04   98   99

14. Been feeling nervous and uptight all the time?

    01   02   03   04   98   99

15. Been managing to keep yourself busy and occupied?
    - [ ] More so than usual
    - [ ] Rather less than usual
    - [ ] Same as usual
    - [ ] Much less than usual

16. Been taking longer over the things you do?
    - [ ] Quicker than usual
    - [ ] Longer than usual
    - [ ] Same as usual
    - [ ] Much longer than usual

17. Felt on the whole you were doing things well?
    - [ ] Better than usual
    - [ ] Less well than usual
    - [ ] About the same
    - [ ] Much less well than usual

18. Been satisfied with the way you've carried out your task?
    - [ ] More satisfied
    - [ ] Less satisfied than usual
    - [ ] About same as usual
    - [ ] Much less satisfied than usual

19. Felt that you are playing a useful part in things?
    - [ ] More so than usual
    - [ ] Less useful than usual
    - [ ] Same as usual
    - [ ] Much less useful than usual

20. Felt capable of making decisions about things?
    - [ ] More so than usual
    - [ ] Less so than usual
    - [ ] Same as usual
    - [ ] Much less capable than usual

21. Been able to enjoy your normal day-to-day activities?
    - [ ] More so than usual
    - [ ] Less so than usual
    - [ ] Same as usual
    - [ ] Much less than usual

22. Been thinking of yourself as a worthless person?
    - [ ] Not at all
    - [ ] Rather more than usual
    - [ ] No more than usual
    - [ ] Much more than usual

23. Felt that life is entirely hopeless?
    - [ ] Not at all
    - [ ] Rather more than usual
    - [ ] No more than usual
    - [ ] Much more than usual

24. Felt that life isn't worth living?
    - ☐ Not at all
    - ☐ No more than usual
    - ☐ Rather more than usual
    - ☐ Much more than usual

25. Thought of the possibility that you might do away with yourself?
    - ☐ Definitely not
    - ☐ I don't think so
    - ☐ Has crossed my mind
    - ☐ Definitely have

26. Found at times you couldn't do anything because your nerves were too bad?
    - ☐ Not at all
    - ☐ No more than usual
    - ☐ Rather more than usual
    - ☐ Much more than usual

27. Found yourself wishing you were dead and away from it all?
    - ☐ Not at all
    - ☐ No more than usual
    - ☐ Rather more than usual
    - ☐ Much more than usual

28. Found that the idea of taking your own life kept coming into your mind?
    - ☐ Definitely not
    - ☐ I don't think so
    - ☐ Has crossed my mind
    - ☐ Definitely has crossed my mind

Appendix C

CAGE

1. Have you ever felt you ought to **C**ut down on your drinking in the past year?

   No. 01
   Yes 02
   Don't know 98
   No response 99

2. In the past year have people **A**nnoyed you by criticizing your drinking?

   No. 01
   Yes 02
   Don't know 98
   No response 99

3. In the past year have you felt bad or **G**uilty about your drinking?

    No. 01

    Yes 02

    Don't know 98

    No response 99

4. In the past year have you had a drink first thing in the morning to steady your nerves or get rid of a hangover (**E**ye-opener)?

    No. 01

    Yes 02

    Don't know 98

    No response 99

Appendix D

THE CONFLICT TACTICS SCALES

Interviewer Script

No matter how well a couple gets along, there are times when they disagree on major decisions, get annoyed about something the other person does, or just have spats or fights because they're in a bad mood or tired for some reason. They also use many different ways of trying to settle their differences. I'm going to read a list of some things that your husband (partner) might have done when you had a dispute, and would like you to tell me for each one how often he did it in the past year.

Interviewer (Circle each item)

    Never 00

    Once. 01

    Twice 02

    3–5 times 03

    6–10 times 04

    11–20 times 05

    More than 20 times 06

    Don't know 98

    No response 99

1. Discussed the issue calmly . . .

       00   01   02   03   04   05   06   98   99

2. Got information to back up his side of things . . .

       00   01   02   03   04   05   06   98   99

3. Brought in or tried to bring in someone to help settle things . . .

       00   01   02   03   04   05   06   98   99

4. Insulted or swore at you . . .

       00   01   02   03   04   05   06   98   99

5. Sulked and/or refused to talk about it . . .

       00   01   02   03   04   05   06   98   99

6. Stomped out of the room or house (or yard) . . .

       00   01   02   03   04   05   06   98   99

7. Cried . . .

       00   01   02   03   04   05   06   98   99

8. Did or said something to spite you . . .

       00   01   02   03   04   05   06   98   99

9. Threatened to hit or throw something at you . . .

       00   01   02   03   04   05   06   98   99

10. Threw or smashed or hit or kicked something . . .

        00   01   02   03   04   05   06   98   99

11. Threw something at you . . .

        00   01   02   03   04   05   06   98   99

12. Pushed, grabbed, or shoved you . . .

        00   01   02   03   04   05   06   98   99

13. Slapped or spanked you . . .

        00   01   02   03   04   05   06   98   99

14. Kicked, bit, or hit you with a fist . . .

        00   01   02   03   04   05   06   98   99

15. Hit or tried to hit you with something . . .

        00   01   02   03   04   05   06   98   99

16. Beat you up . . .

        00   01   02   03   04   05   06   98   99

17. Choked you . . .

        00   01   02   03   04   05   06   98   99

18. Threatened you with a knife or a gun . . .

        00   01   02   03   04   05   06   98   99

19. Used a knife or a gun . . .

        00   01   02   03   04   05   06   98   99

20. Are there any other things that your husband did when you had a dispute? (Describe) (Record up to three tactics)

I really appreciate the time you have taken to complete this survey. I'd like to assure you that everything you have told me will remain strictly confidential. As you have gathered from the questions, we are interested in how couples deal with conflict in their relationships, and how this might affect a woman's health. Now that you have had a chance to think about the topic, is there anything you would like to add to what we have discussed? (Describe):

Umbilical Cord Care

JENNIFER MEDVES

ABSTRACT

Umbilical cord care in the normal full-term neonate differs around the world; from benign neglect in the third world to highly complicated cleaning regimes in the developed world. The rationale for cleaning is to prevent infection, minimize colonization, promote healing, and hasten separation of the cord. However, umbilical separation is presumed to take place through a process of dry gangrene, thus cleaning with an antibacterial agent is illogical.

The proposed research will be a randomized trial of term, well infants with two different cleaning regimes to determine the treatment that promotes the quickest time in days to separation. The treatment group will have their cords cleaned at every diaper change with clean water, the control group will have their cords cleaned with alcohol swabs. Randomization of treatment will take place in the labor and delivery suite of a tertiary care hospital.

Umbilical cord swabs will be taken at 3 hours, 3 days, and day of cord separation to compare colonization of bacterial organisms within groups and between groups. The t-test statistic will be used to analyze the data. Demographic data will be analyzed to determine that the groups are similar using percentages. Power analysis reveals that 50 infants will be required for each group, for an alpha of 0.05 and a power of 0.8, and a medium effect (d = 0.5). Colonization will be designated nil, small, medium, or large growth of bacteria.

UMBILICAL CORD CARE

From the moment a normal, full-term baby is born the umbilical cord is no longer required for gaseous exchange and nutrition; however, for the premature baby, the access of a patent umbilical vein and arteries may be paramount. The precise mechanism of cord separation is not known, but drying, infection, bacterial contamination, and granulocytosis may influence the time in days to separation (Wilson, Ochs, Almquist, Dassel, Mauseth, & Ochs, 1985). The cord usually separates within the first two weeks of life (Arad, Eyal, & Fainmesser, 1981).

The normal practice in North America is, at birth, to divide and cut the cord and to put on a Hollister clamp for the first few days until the cord blackens and withers. In the following days a variety of treatments are recommended to promote healing and separation of the umbilical cord stump, these treatments vary as does the time to separation. At a time when women are being discharged earlier to their homes, an argument can be made to minimize the "treatments" a mother needs to give to her normal newborn. The randomized experiment proposed is designed to compare two methods of cleaning the umbilical cord stump in order to discover the method that promotes drying, healing, and most rapid separation without umbilical infection.

UMBILICAL CORD COLONIZATION AND UMBILICAL CORD CARE

A literature review of umbilical cord studies undertaken reveals the maternal concerns in treating the cord, the colonization and infection associated with the newborn umbilicus, the different methods of cleaning, and the different lengths of time to cord separation. By reviewing the extant literature a clear delineation between researchers is revealed. Medical doctors are not convinced that the problem of infection has been minimized and urge that an antibacterial regime should be continued, while midwives and nurses question the rationale and suggest a minimalist regime is more appropriate.

A consequence of encouraging women, in the late nineteenth and twentieth centuries, to have their babies in hospital has been the occasional outbreak of infection in nurseries, with sometimes dire consequences (Elias-Jones, Gordon, & Whittaker, 1961; Jellard, 1957). Since the 1960's "rooming-in" has been encouraged and this has led to a reduction in infection rates because babies spend their time with their mothers and not in large nurseries (Barclay, Harrington, Conroy, Royal, & Laforgia, 1994; Mansell, 1990). With the advent of even shorter stays in hospital for women and their newborns, the risk of cross-infection and acquisition of nosocomial infections will be reduced. At a time in England when many babies were born at home, Elias-Jones et al. noted that babies born at home did not colonize organisms at the same rate as babies born in hospital, and recommended that women confined to hospital for delivery be transferred home for postpartum care (1961).

In view of shorter stays, it may be time to stop treating the umbilical cord and allow nature to take its course. The seminal piece of research was a study by Barr (1984) who concluded that cleaning cords with alcohol delayed cord separation longer than cords cleaned with water. The research was conducted in Northern Ireland where midwives visit daily until the cord separates, so it is of monetary concern if cord separation is delayed. The number of babies in the study was small and so the reliability and validity of this work may be challenged.

Maternal Concerns

Although mothers and babies are likely to spend less time in hospital, teaching mothers handwashing techniques and to observe and report abnormalities to health care providers are probably more important than complicated cord cleaning methods.

New mothers have expressed concern when the cord fails to separate (Arad et al., 1981). Mothers have demonstrated their reluctance to clean the cord and occasionally have indicated revulsion (Salariya & Kowbus, 1988). When Grunau, Johnston, and Craig (1990) used umbilical cord care as a control in a pain study, 11 out of 36 babies cried following application of triple dye to their cords. Cord care may not be painful, but it may well be cold and uncomfortable. During the Grunau et al. study, they noted that the umbilical site was treated gently "perhaps demonstrating implicit beliefs that this is a sensitive area" (1990, p. 304). Naor, Merlob, Litwin, and Wielunsky (1989) noted the repulsive odor associated with cleaning the cord with alcohol. Alcohol has been implicated in a case of intoxication that occurred by absorption of the isopropyl alcohol through the umbilical area (Vivier, Lewander, Martin, & Linakis, 1994). Perry (1982) reminds nurses and midwives that any umbilical cord care practice must take into account the particular cultural beliefs of a mother, so that alcohol intoxication and the like is avoided. Mugford, Somichiwong, and Waterhouse (1986) demonstrated that a delay in the cord separation times required an extra full time-community midwife for every 3000 births per year.

Separation in Time in Days

Time of separation of the umbilical cord varies around the world. Studies show a longer time in days for cord separation in North America than Europe, Australia, and India. The reason for differences in time to cord separation may be due in part to the type of treatment recommended to enhance cord separation and minimize infection (Barr, 1984; Bhalla, Nafis, Rohatgi, & Singh, 1975). Average time in India was 5.8 days (Bhalla et al., 1975), Finland 6.3 days (Tötterman & Autio, 1970), Israel 6.4 days (Arad et al., 1981) and 6.3 days (Naor et al., 1989), Norway 6 days (Meberg and Schøyen, 1990), Holland 6 days (Oudesluys-Murphy, De Groot, and Eilers, 1986), Northern Ireland 6.2 days (Barr, 1982), and Australia (Bourke, 1990) 8.8 days (Barclay et al., 1994).

North American studies indicate time of separation from 10.9 in a Texas study (Rais-Bahrami, Schulte, & Naqvi, 1993), 10.7 days in a U.S. military study (Schuman & Oksol, 1985), and 15 days in a Seattle study (Wilson et al., 1985). In a randomized study, there is no correlation between early clamping and late clamping of the cord on the time of cord separation (Oxford Midwives' Research Group, 1991).

Umbilical cord separation time may be delayed in babies delivered by caesarian section (Rais-Bahrami et al., 1993; Novack, Mueller, & Ochs, 1988). This may be due, in part, to a delay in colonization of the skin by normal vaginal bacterial flora (Anonymous, 1994).

Colonization and Infections

Newborn infants are known to colonize *Staphyloccus aureus* in the umbilicus and nose (Meberg & Schøyen, 1990). The organisms most often cited as responsible for neonatal umbilical infections are *Staphyloccus aureus* (Elias-Jones et al., 1961; Gooch & Britt, 1978; Jellard, 1957; Paes & Jones, 1987; Pildes, Ramurthy, & Vidyasgar, 1973; Speck, Driscoll, Polin, O'Neill, & Rosenkrantz, 1977; and Watkinson & Dyas, 1992) and group B β-*hemolytic streptocci* (Wald, Merrill, Snyder, & Gutberlet, 1977). Medical doctors have therefore recommended "treating" the umbilical cord in order to reduce the incidence of colonization and infection (Tötterman and Autio, 1970; Andrich and Golden, 1984). The treatments recommended have included triple dye (Andrich and Golden, 1984), silver sulfadiazine (Barrett, Mason, & Fleming, 1979), methylated spirits (Mansell, 1990), betadine (Tötterman & Autio, 1970), and no treatment (Oudesluys-Murphy, De Groot, & Eilers, 1986). Ronchera-Oms et al. (1994) state that cords that colonize detached earlier than cords that did not colonize. Colonization rates varied in different studies and have been used as justification for treating the umbilical cord. Triple dye has been used in many hospitals to maintain a low colonization rate of *Staphylococcus aureus* (Pildes et al., 1973). Colonization rates do not, per se, indicate a potential or actual outbreak of infection (Gooch & Britt, 1978).

Serious Infections and Necrotizing Fasciitis

Occasionally umbilical cord separation had been delayed over three weeks and this may be associated with polymorphic neutrophil defects (Abramson et al., 1981). Novack et al. (1988) suggest that these babies should be followed for at least a year to determine the proportion of infants with delay in separation that subsequently develop neutrophil problems. A potentially lethal complication of delayed separation and infection can be necrotizing fasciitis, which is a rare complication of omphalitis (Samuel, Freeman, Vaishnav, Sajwany, & Nayar, 1994). During a ten-year study, in Washington state, 32 infants were admitted to a hospital with uncomplicated omphalitis; none had delay in cord separation, and all were treated successfully. At the same hospital, 7 other babies, 6 of whom had complicated omphalitis, developed necrotizing fasciitis with a 71% death rate (Sawin, Schaller, Tapper, Morgan, & Cahill, 1994). Chamberlin (1992) states that through an emergency department, in a children's hospital in Washington, District of Columbia, that had 57,000 visits and 11,500 admissions annually, 28 infants with omphalitis had been treated over 10 years. Chamberlin does not define the normal method of cleaning the cord but states that antibacterial agents are used in most United States institutions.

Cleaning Regimens

In the United States, the American Academy of Pediatrics (1974) recognized the different methods of cleaning umbilical cords and bathing and recommended minimal nontoxic and nonabrasive neutral methods; however, these recommendations are ignored in many institutions. The study found that many American hospitals were applying one of the following to babies unseparated cords: pHisohex, Betadine, Dial Soap, Hibiclens, Baby Magic, Gammophen, and Mennen's Baby Lotion. Cord care regimes also included triple dye, alcohol, iodophor, and bactricin ointment.

Design of Studies

Criticism of cord care studies to date has been the absence of colonization studies at the same time as the cord care methodology studies (Watkinson & Dyas, 1992; Russell,

1995). Several studies indicate that the use of antiseptic solutions reduces the bacterial colonization but delays cord separation (Bourke, 1990; Ronchera-Oms, Hernández, & Jimémez, 1994; Verber & Pagan, 1993). While infants who are admitted to neonatal units may have to have a different cord care regime, because they are at added risk for infection, the normal full-term infant may not require an antibacterial agent. English studies have recommended the continued use of Sterzac powder (Bain, 1994); and in Australia's NICUs alcohol or chlorhexidine (Yu, 1990).

The available studies of the effect of umbilical cord care on separation times reveal that none of the studies indicated that a power analysis was completed to determine sample size. The studies compared a variety of cleaning regimes. The medical doctors compared antibacterial agents in their research. Naor et al. (1989) compared alcohol and Rikospray, and there was no difference except that the alcohol group had smelly cords. Andrich and Golden (1984) and Arad et al. (1981) recommend triple dye instead of Bactricin ointment. Ronchera-Oms et al. (1994) compared four regimes and suggested further research into an antibacterial agent. Hexachlorophene powder as chlorhexidine solution is recommended in Verber and Pagan's 1992 study. A Norwegian study concluded that Sorbact and 0.5% chlorhexidine in 70% alcohol are equal in separation times (Meberg & Schøyen, 1990). The only North American randomized trial argues that alcohol promotes faster time in separation than triple dye (Schuman & Oksol, 1985). Watkinson and Dyas (1992) demonstrated that water alone is more effective in promoting earlier separation than alcohol and hexachlorophene powder, but implore the reviewers to continue to treat cords as the colonization levels are unacceptably high at a comparative odds ratio of 1.75%. Dr. Robert Rennie, a clinical microbiologist (personal communication, November 1, 1995) disagrees that an odds ratio of 1.75% is significant. Oudesluys-Murphy et al. (1986) described a daily bath and clean binder as the method of choice in Holland, with an average time to separation of 6.2 days.

In the research by, in whole or part, midwives and nurses, Mugford et al. (1986) showed comparative closeness in time of separation between various powders and solutions, but that even in the treatment group midwives tended to use alcohol swabs if they thought it to be necessary. Lawrence (1982) concluded that powder alone was more efficient than powder and steret swabs. Methylated spirits as against chlorhexidine solution is recommended by Mansell (1990). Salariya and Kowbus (1988) demonstrated that no treatment as against alcohol was quicker. Barclay et al. (1994) conducted a randomized trial and concluded that water alone versus chlorhexidine 0.5% in 70% alcohol was significantly quicker in promoting separation. Water alone is quicker than alcohol swabs in cord separation in two studies by Barr (184) and Bourke (1990).

In most Canadian hospitals, the method of choice of cleaning is alcohol swabs. Comparison between powders such as Sterzac and Rikospray are not possible as they are not readily available in Canada. Alcohol has been associated with a foul odor (Naor et al., 1989), and soft cords (Barr, 1984). If the purpose of cleaning is to speed up drying, then causing the cord to soften appears illogical (Barr, 1984). Several studies around the world have demonstrated that water alone promotes healing and separation faster than treatments such as alcohol. A study of practice in Canada has not been done to compare the practice of method of cleaning the umbilical cord and time in days to separation of the cord. In order to protect the babies against infection during the experiment and counter the medical concern of colonization and infection, swabs should be taken from the base of the umbilicus of each baby to monitor colonization and intervene in the unlikely event of omphalitis.

PURPOSE OF THE STUDY

The purpose of this study is to test the following hypothesis:

> Umbilical cord care that consists of water alone, in the normal full term newborn, will result in a significantly faster rate of cord separation and healing, than umbilical cord care that consists of alcohol swabs.

Umbilical cord separation will be measured in hours from birth and converted to units of 24 hours to produce time in days.

Alcohol treatment infants will have the umbilical cord and skin around the umbilicus cleaned at each diaper change with alcohol injection swabs until the cord separates.

Water treatment infants will have the cord and area cleaned at each diaper change with tap water on a cotton wool ball.

THE SAMPLE

Target Population

The sample will be newborn infants born at a tertiary care hospital. Randomization to control or experimental group will take place at time of birth, having obtained permission from the parents at admission to labor and delivery, a convenient time in labor, or post delivery.

Inclusion criteria for infants will be if they are born after at least 37 weeks gestation; Apgars 7 at 1 minute, 7 at 5 minutes; no obvious physical abnormality; no antibiotics received in the first ten days of life; and consent.

Excluded infants will be those who are admitted to the Neonatal Intensive Care Unit, infants born after premature rupture of membranes (longer than 24 hours before delivery), and infants of mothers who received antibiotics in the last month of pregnancy. Parents of the eligible infants will have to live within 50 km of the hospital because of the logistics of collecting umbilical cord swabs.

Demographic data will be obtained from the chart. The data collected will be time and date of delivery, delivery method, sex of infant, ethnicity, rank in family and age of mother.

Power Analysis

Power analysis for this study reveals that for a medium effect ($d = 0.5$), using a t test statistic, an alpha of 0.05, and power of 0.8; 50 infants for each group will be required for a total of 100 (Cohen, 1979). Post hoc tests using percentages will be used to analyze the demographic details to compare similarity between groups.

External Validity

Threats to external validity include interaction of selection and treatment, interaction of setting and treatment, and interaction of history and treatment (Cook and Campbell,

1979). The hospital to be used has 300 to 400 deliveries a month; admission to the trial will take two months at the most. The hospital admits women with both low-risk and high-risk pregnancies; in this way a cross section of women having babies in the Edmonton area should be admitted to the hospital. External validity will be achieved as there will be randomization of subjects; infants spend a very short time in hospital so it is unlikely that mothers will know which treatment promotes faster separation; mothers in classes prenatally are taught that they will treat the cord so there should be no Hawthorne effect; the study will take place over a short time so there should be no history effect; and the swab results will be kept confidential until after the subjects have been recruited into the study. The study findings should be generalizable to normal term neonates, but a further study will have to be conducted to study the effect of cleaning on the separation time in preterm and sick neonates.

METHODS AND INSTRUMENTS

Method of Admission to the Study

Prospective parents will be handed an explanation sheet by the nurse who admits them to the labor and delivery unit. Parents who wish to participate or who have questions will be seen by the principal investigator and a full explanation will be given. If the infant is to be admitted to the study, randomization will take place at 30 minutes post delivery using a random number chart. The consent form will be signed (Appendix B). Each mother will be taught cord care by the principal investigator or her designate. Newborn infants and their mothers will be discharged as the unit policy and the physician designate.

Method of Study

Three hours after delivery the first swab will be taken; the cord may or may not have been cleaned, but it is immaterial as the design is considering colonization. The second swab on day three will take place at home if necessary. Infants in the experimental group will have their cords cleaned with clean water on cotton wool balls at diaper changes or during a bath. The control group will have the cords cleaned with alcohol swabs at each diaper change.

The mother will be given the investigator's and supervisor's telephone number, and will be asked to ring the day that the cord separates. At that time the investigator will make a home visit to inspect the umbilicus and take a final swab.

Each mother will be handed a copy of the consent form, the investigator's contact telephone number, and a letter of explanation of the study and method of cleaning the cord when she agrees to participate in the study.

Method of Taking Swabs

Three swabs will be taken for each infant in the study. Swabs will be taken at the base of the cord in a rolled method as advocated by the urethral catheterization study (Maki, Ringer, & Alvardo, 1991). A template made of sterile gauze, which exposes 20 mm^3 of skin around the umbilicus, will be used. The Ames Swabs will be dipped in sterile water prior to swabbing and then transported in universal medium to the Research Laboratory at the University of Alberta by the investigator. The swabs will be plated onto blood agar aerobically and anaerobically. Significant pathogens such as *Staphyloccus aureus* and β-hemolytic *streptococci* will be identified and reported using standard methods as small, medium, and large growth. Cords that clinically appear infected will be treated as per institution protocols. A swab will be sent to the institution laboratory as well as to the research laboratory.

Internal Validity

Threats to internal validity include history, maturation, testing, instrumentation, attrition, and selection (Cook & Campbell, 1979). Each infant will only be in the study for a short time, and the pre- and post-test will be checked with the umbilical swabs. By randomizing a sufficiently large number of infants, the problem of attrition should be minimized. As each infant is in the study for only 8 to 10 days, randomization can continue until at least 100 infants have completed the protocol. Each mother will be contacted on Day 10 if she has not phoned the researcher before to ascertain if the cord has separated. As each mother and baby is discharged home early, the chance of the mothers' discovering that one or another treatment promotes faster separation will be minimized.

RELIABILITY AND VALIDITY OF MEASUREMENT

Reliability of Instrumentation

Each infant will be assessed to have had cord separation in time from delivery. This will entail an accurate time of birth, and subsequently a more accurate time of cord separation. In most institutions, a baby born after 12 noon is arbitrarily designated as day 0. Day 1 starts at 12 midnight. If this was used in the study, a baby whose cord separates on day 4 at 12 noon could be as young as 55 hours or as old as 77 hours. Cords will be assessed as separated by the principal investigator. This is important as the mother may think the cord has separated when it has shriveled and shrunk in size. The mother may not notice exactly the time the cord separates; the time will be taken from when she notices, for example, when she changes the diaper. As each infant is changed approximately 6 times in a 24-hour period, the times should be accurate enough over the whole study.

Swabs will be identified by study numbers. The research laboratory will not know if the swabs are from control or experimental infants. The results will not be made available to the principal investigator until completion of data collection. If the investigator is suspicious that an infant has an umbilical infection, a second swab will be collected and sent to the laboratory, the appropriate physician will be notified, and treatment as specified will be initiated. Swabs that are correctly collected and plated onto blood agar and placed at the correct temperature will either grow pathogens or not. The designation of small, medium, or large amount of growth is an issue for the Research Laboratory.

The principal investigator and designates will practice swabbing cords and transferring the specimens to the blood agar plates. The Clinical Microbiologist will assess the techniques. Admission to the study will not take place until the investigator's technique is established. Mothers will be questioned closely to ensure that no other lotions are placed on the umbilical cord. Infants that do receive other lotions will be excluded from the study.

Validity of Instrumentation

To ensure the validity of the medium of agar plates, the advice of the Clinical Microbiologist will be sought. The Clinical Microbiologist has indicated that blood agar plates will be sufficient for colonization studies of skin flora. The information sheet will be pilot tested on a number of mothers prior to starting the study. Face validity will be established using a panel of midwives and nurse researchers.

DATA ANALYSIS

The time in age of each infant at time of separation of the cord will be analyzed for each group using the mean, variance, and standard deviation. A t-test will be used to compare the control and experimental groups. Demographic data such as gender and type of delivery will be analyzed using percentages to describe the sample.

Colonization studies between groups will be compared using a t-test. Infants born by Lower Segment Caesarian Section will colonize later in time than the infants born vaginally. Any infants who meet admission to the study criteria who subsequently develop clinical infections will be presented separately. Post hoc chi-square may be used to analyze demographic data.

ETHICAL CONSIDERATIONS

Ethical review will be sought from the Faculty of Nursing, University of Alberta and Capital Health Authority for this study. Informed consent will be obtained by the investigator from each mother during admission, labor, or post delivery. Prospective parents will be given an information sheet by the nurse who admits the patient to the labor ward. At this time those mothers who are interested will then be seen by the investigator.

Potential Benefit to Nursing

The benefit to nursing of such a study will be monetary and timely. There has been a recognition that much of nursing practice is based on habit and is not based on theoretical knowledge. If, as is hypothesized, umbilical cords wither and separate faster when nature is left alone, then it seems reasonable to leave the cord alone. Mothers are then able to spend time learning more relevant practices such as feeding, changing, and comforting their newborn infants. The time saved by nurses who are not teaching complicated cleaning regimes will not be easily quantified; however, over a year the monetary savings by not using alcohol swabs should be realized.

Potential Risks to the Infants in the Study

Umbilical cord care around the world varies. In developing countries the practice of benign neglect appears to encourage early separation of umbilical cords in the postnatal period. During the proposed randomized experiment, each infant will have three swabs taken from the umbilical area; this is three more than would be normal in the postnatal period. Mothers and babies are discharged home, often within 48 hours of delivery, and may not be visited by a health care professional at any time in the first two weeks. Each mother and infant enrolled in the study will be visited at least once in the first few weeks and may have two visits if they go home prior to day 3. If an infant appears to be infected, or if the potential for infection is noted, the infant will be referred to the appropriate physician. The investigator is an experienced midwife with eight years experience, as well as neonatal intensive care experience, and is well qualified to assess these babies in their home environment. While no research study can guarantee that no harm will come to enrolled subjects, it is anticipated that no harm will come to these infants.

Anonymity and Confidentiality

The investigator will be the only person who knows the names, addresses, and telephone numbers of the participants. The biographical data will be kept separate from the colonization and time of separation of umbilical cord data. Parents will be assured that their names will not appear in print or be given at meetings when the results of this research project are presented. Parents will also be assured that if the information is to be used at a later date, an ethical review will be required. Parents may also receive a written report of this research if they wish. Raw data from this study will be kept in a locked container for a minimum of 5 years and may then be destroyed. The demographic data will be kept for 7 years. The data will belong to the researcher and may not be used without permission and ethical review. The informed consent form is included in Appendix B. The RightWriter assessment of the consent form is in Appendix C.

CONCLUSION

The research proposed will be a randomized study to ascertain the method of cleaning the umbilical cord of normal term infants that promotes faster separation. The control group will use alcohol swabs to clean the cord, the experimental group will use water to clean the cord. A tertiary care hospital will be used for the study in order to obtain a sample that reflects the population of infants born to women living in Edmonton, in order that the study findings can be generalized to the total population of women having babies. Colonization studies to determine the difference, if there is one, of growth of normal skin flora will be carried out at the same time.

Maintaining Catheter Patency Using Recombinant Tissue Plasminogen Activator

COLLEEN M. ASTLE, BScN
University of Alberta

Chronic renal failure is an insidious, progressive deterioration of renal function. The most common causes include diabetes mellitus, hypertension, glomerulonephritis, poly-cystic kidney disease, interstitial nephritis, obstructive disorders, vascular disease, and AIDS-related disorders (Lancaster, 1991; Central Organ Replacement Register, 1998). Chronic renal failure is described as insidious because it is usually not diagnosed until there is an approximately 75% loss of function and the patient's vaguely described symptoms become more pronounced. Even in the face of deteriorating numbers, the glomeruli adapt with hyperfiltration in order to maintain a normal homeostatic environment (Andreoli, Bennett, Carpenter, & Plum, 1997). When function has decreased to between 5 and 10%, the diagnosis of end-stage renal disease is made.

As of 1998, more than 210,000 people in the United States with end-stage renal failure were receiving treatment, the annual growth trend of the disease being 7.8%. In Canada, as of December 31, 1998, the number of patients alive on renal replacement therapy was 21,992, including 9,114 with a functioning transplant and 12,808 patients in various treatment modalities. The majority of patients were on hemodialysis (73%), and the balance was on peritoneal dialysis (27%). In 1998, there were 4,025 new patients receiving treatment, representing a rate of 132.5 patients per million population. From 1981 to 1998 the annual growth rate of the disease was 6% (Canadian Organ Replacement Register, 1998). With the increase in life expectancy in the aging population, the United States reported a 150% increase in renal failure in people over 60 years of age between 1984 and 1993. Thirty-six percent of those people were diabetics (Kinzner, 1998). These numbers reflect a growing trend in chronicity that will burden the health care system in both Canada and the United States in coming years.

The patients with end-stage renal failure require ongoing medical intervention to sustain life. The treatment options available include peritoneal dialysis, hemodialysis, or transplantation. Peritoneal dialysis involves the peritoneum as the dialyzing membrane. A sterile, physiologically prepared solution is introduced into the peritoneal cavity and by the principles of osmosis and diffusion, fluid is removed and the blood is cleansed of its toxic impurities. The patient is required to do four or five exchanges each day. In contrast to peritoneal dialysis, hemodialysis involves passing the patient's blood through an artificial kidney where diffusion and ultrafiltration remove fluid and the waste products of metabolism, normally excreted by the kidneys. This procedure averages 4 hours three times per week. Both peritoneal dialysis and hemodialysis require the use of a patent, functional access, a means with which to dialyze the patient.

The three types of vascular access used for hemodialysis include the arteriovenous (AV) fistula, the synthetic arteriovenous graft, and the central venous catheter. Since 1966, the AV fistula has been, and continues to be, the preferred form of hemodialysis access (Berkoben & Schwab, 1995; Ezzahiri, Lemson, Kitslaar, Leunissen, & Toridor, 1999; Kapoian & Sherman, 1997; Laski, Pressley, Sabatini, & Wesson, 1997; Mysliwiec, 1997; Tisher, 1999). Primary AV fistulae are typically created by an end-to-side vein–artery anastamosis of the cephalic vein and radial artery or the brachial artery and the cephalic vein in the nondominant arm. They take 2 to 6 months to mature. Once mature, they have long-term patency rates and are rarely associated with infectious complications. The fistulas can serve as a permanent hemodialysis access for 20 years. Not all people, however, are suitable for the creation of a fistula. Veins that have previously been used for infusion of medication, intravenous therapy, phlebotomy, or laboratory blood sampling are precluded from developing into a successful access. Also, because of an aging and diabetic population there is a lack of suitable blood vessels for creation of fistula access (Kapoian & Sherman, 1997; Konner, 1999; Polaschegg & Levin, 2000).

If the dialysis patient is unable to support a native fistula, an AV graft using synthetic materials such as polytetrafluoroethylene (PTFE) may be created. PTFE grafts are placed in the forearm, upper arm, or upper thigh, in either a straight (distal radial artery to basilic vein) or loop(brachial artery to basilic vein) configuration. Maturation requires 3 to 4 weeks. PTFE is a durable material and will withstand multiple thrombectomies and revisions, but it does have a finite functional life and will wear out with repeated needle puncture. The complications associated with grafts include infection, thrombosis, steal syndrome, formation of an aneurysm, and reaction to the graft material (Obialo, Robinson, & Braithwaite, 1998).

Central venous catheters are routinely used in the medical management of many types of patients (Farrell, Walshe, Gellens, & Martin, 1997). They provide access for the delivery of fluids, medications, blood products, chemotherapy, and parenteral nutrition. They are also useful for frequent blood sampling, hemodynamic monitoring, or hemodialysis. Central venous catheters are inserted into deep veins such as the subclavian, jugular, or femoral veins and are advanced into the vena cava (Brunier, 1996). They may be placed percutaneously or by using a cutdown technique. Maturation time is not required; rather they may be used immediately after placement. Associated complications include infection, thrombosis, permanent central vein stenosis, and lower blood flow rates than other accesses (Johnson, 1998).

Central venous catheter occlusion is a common complication, which can result in loss of function, delays in treatment, high costs, patient discomfort, and patient and nurse frustration. Additionally, intraluminal clotted blood and fibrin increase the risk of catheter-related sepsis (Wickham, Purl, & Welker, 1992). Thus far, various concentrations of heparin have been used to maintain the patency of the catheters. In the past, when clotting occurred in the presence of heparin as the instillation, streptokinase and then urokinase were used to lyse the clot. Presently, 2 milligrams (mg)/2 milliliters (ml) of recombinant tissue plasminogen activator (rTPA) is being used. After a specified period of time the catheter is checked for patency and if successful, dialysis is resumed. The advantage of using rTPA is that it is frequently successful in the lysis of intraluminal dialysis catheter clots. The disadvantage is the cost of the medication. For each 2-mg syringe of rTPA the cost is $54.00 for the Northern Alberta Renal Failure Program. The following questions then arise: What concentration of rTPA would be effective in the prevention of a thrombus in a hemodialysis catheter? What should the dwell time be for this concentration of solution?

CATHETER-RELATED THROMBOSIS

The use of a central venous catheter for either temporary or chronic hemodialysis has become an acceptable bridge to internal, permanent vascular accesses (Farrell et al., 1997; Brunier, 1996, Ouwendyk & Helferty, 1996; Choudhry, Ahmed, Giris, & Kronfli, 1999; Richard, 1986). It is easily inserted at the bedside by an experienced physician thereby reducing the need for expensive and often unavailable operating room time. It can provide long-term access in children, the elderly, the morbidly obese, or in diabetics whose vessels are not suitable for the creation of an internal fistula or graft. It is necessary for patients requiring emergency dialysis or patients who are described as access failures, having used up the vessels required to create a permanent access. Central venous catheters serve as a backup for the fistulas and grafts that require ligation due to high output failure states caused by their development and use. Further, these catheters are inserted as a temporary access while awaiting the development of the permanent access. The survival rates of these catheters are reported to be 75% at 1 year and 50% at 2 years thereby allowing them to become alternative forms of long-term accesses (Parker, 1998). Berkoben and Schwab (1995) reported a survival rate of 47–74% at 1 year and 41–43% at 2 years. Despite the consensus that the construction of the primary AV fistulas represents the best choice for permanent vascular access, the trend since 1980 has been a continual increase in the use of these access devices. Kapoian and Sherman (1997) reported a 5% use of central venous catheters in 1980, which increased to 30% in 1993.

Catheter-related thrombosis is the most common cause of catheter dysfunction (Barendregt, Tordoir, & Leunissen, 1999; Buturovic, Ponikvar, Boh, Klinkmann, & Ivanovich, 1998; Johnson, 1998; Mysliwiec, 1997; Northsea, 1994; Parker, 1998; Twardowski, 1998a). It can result in an impaired ability to withdraw fluid from or infuse fluids through the catheter. The literature reports an incidence of thrombosis from 55% to 85% (Daeihagh, Jordan, Chen, & Rocco, 2000; Kohler & Kirkman, 1998). This broad range reflects the lack of a standardized method for evaluating and diagnosing this complication. Further, the term catheter-related thrombosis does not appear to be well defined. It may refer to the thrombotic occlusion of the lumen of the catheter, the formation of a fibrin sheath around the catheter, the formation of thrombus at the site of catheter insertion into the vessel, or a true thrombosis within the central vein (Wickham et al., 1992).

Catheter clotting may result from either external or internal mechanical obstruction. Kinks in the external tubing or the catheter itself can reduce or totally obstruct flow through the lumen. Internal causes of catheter occlusion include internal malposition, catheter pinch-off syndrome caused by threading the subclavian catheter under the clavicle during insertion, drug precipitate, fibrin buildup, and blood clots (Kohler & Kirkman, 1998; Muhm, Sunder-Plassmann, Aspner, Kritzinger, Hiesmayr, & Druml, 1997). Clot occlusion also occurs as a result of a retrograde flow of blood into the catheter tip during fluctuations in central venous pressure, such as when a patient coughs.

There are several sites at which thrombi are likely to form: the lumen of the catheter, the site at which the catheter enters the vein, the catheter tip, and the external surface of the catheter. The types of thrombotic occlusions include intraluminal thrombus, mural thrombus, fibrin sheath, also known as fibrin sleeve, and fibrin tail, known as fibrin flap. A fibrin sheath can form along the external surface of the catheter and resembles a sock over the catheter (Kohler & Kirkman, 1998; Northsea, 1996). It may occur soon after insertion and extends from the insertion site to the catheter tip. This may develop within 48 hours after placement. Fibrin tail forms when fibrin adheres to the end of the catheter. Often it acts as a one-way valve, permitting infusion but not withdrawal of fluid from the catheter. Mural thrombus, which forms when the fibrin from a vessel wall injury binds to the fibrin covering the catheter surface, may lead to the formation of a venous thrombus (Wickman et al., 1992).

Thrombus formation may be related to a number of factors. Insertion of the catheter may cause endothelial injury of the vessel wall, triggering the release of thromboplastic substances that cause platelets to aggregate at the site. Endothelial injury may also cause formation of small or large thrombi that attach to the vessel wall. Another factor may be the large-bore catheters commonly used for dialysis, which alter the blood flow in the vein and activate the release of the thromboplastic substances and platelets, thereby producing fibrin formation (Northsea, 1996; Wickman et al., 1992).

The patients at greatest risk for the development of catheter-related thrombi are those who experience venous thrombus, enhanced blood coagulability, or trauma to the vessel wall. Venous stasis can occur when dehydration, hypotension, immobility, heart failure, or intrapulmonary/mediastinal diseases are present. Coagulability can be altered by conditions such as malignancy, sepsis, chronic renal failure, or the administration of chemotherapy (Schenk, Rosenkranz, Wolfl, Horl, & Traindl, 2000).

The vast majority of thrombi related to central venous catheters develop without symptoms. Warning signs are insidious. As the thrombus begins to form, the catheter appears problematic, causing monitoring alarms. The blood flow appears sluggish (Berkoben & Schwab, 1995; Daeihagh et al., 2000; Northsea, 1994; Twardowski, 1998a). In some instances, it is possible to infuse fluid into the catheter but the withdrawal is impaired. The diagnosis of catheter-related thrombosis may be based solely on symptoms or can be confirmed with the aid of imaging techniques. When the central venous catheter becomes occluded the goal is to restore patency in a cost-effective manner with minimal risk to the patient. Catheter salvage is preferred over catheter replacement in an effort to limit the interruption to therapy, reduce the risk of trauma to the patient, reduce the risk of complications, and decrease the costs.

One factor that has been considered in the literature concerning catheter-related thrombosis is the type of catheter used (Berkoben & Schwab, 1995; Muhm et al., 1997; Sehenk et al., 2000). In the study by Leblanc, Bosc, Vaussenant, Maurice, Leray-Moragues, and Canaud (1998), blood flow and recirculation rates were reviewed in 33 well-functioning internal jugular vein catheters. The catheters described were able to maintain adequate blood flow rates between 200 and 275 ml/min without major increments or decrements in arterial and venous pressures. The study concluded that the blood flow rates were achieved because of the type of catheters chosen. Little information was provided about the characteristics of the sample population, including age, health, comorbid conditions, or diagnosis. The concern is whether the catheter used in this study could be used for a patient whose coagulability had been altered by conditions such as sepsis or malignancy.

Muhm and colleagues (1997) reviewed the use of large-bore, dacron-cuffed catheters using the supraclavicular approach in 175 patients during an 18-month period.

Five types of large-bore catheters were reviewed. There was no clinically significant incidence of central vein thrombosis or stenosis. Intraluminal fibrinolysis occurred in three cases. The supraclavicular approach has proven to be preferable to the subclavian approach and is now an accepted practice in many dialysis units.

The lock solutions used in the central venous catheters have been extensively reviewed in the literature (Buturovic et al., 1998; Leblanc et al., 1998; Twardowski, 1998b). The purpose of the lock solutions is to fill the length of the catheter and prevent thrombosis. Heparin appears to be the standard lock solution in most hemiodialysis catheters (Barendregt et al., 1999). Heparin prevents the clotting of blood by inhibiting factors involved in the conversion of prothrombin to thrombin. Buturovic et al. (1998) compared heparin with citrate or polygeline locks and found no difference regarding catheter patency and clot volume between groups.

Schnek and colleagues (2000) were responsible for a prospective, randomized crossover study comparing heparin and rTPA as an instillation in 12 dialysis patients over a 4-month period. Blood flow rates, arterial pressure, and venous pressure were monitored at each dialysis session. rTPA proved to be superior as a lock for the central venous catheters as measured by reduced blood flow problems and clotting.

Intradialytic urokinase has been extensively used in many dialysis units to lyse catheter thrombosis. Urokinase, a thrombolytic agent derived from human kidney cells, is a protein enzyme that acts on the endogenous fibrinolytic system, converting plasminogen to plasmin. Plasmin degrades fibrin clots, fibrinogen, and other plasma properties. Northsea (1996) used urokinase to restore patency in 95 of 102 permanent or double lumen catheters. Twardowski (1998b) suggested that warfarin be used in conjunction with urokinase. Urokinase proved to be effective in restoring catheter patency but fibrin tended to reoccur without the use of warfarin. Ouwendyk and Helferty (1996) suggested the use of baby aspirin or one-half of a 325-mg tablet of aspirin daily after central venous catheter insertion and the use of aspirin and warfarin together to prevent catheter clotting.

Since the early 1990s. rTPA has been used to restore catheter patency and lyse thrombus. rTPA is a genetically engineered enzyme involved in the breakdown of blood clots. It has been used successfully in the treatment of myocardial infarction, dissolving the clot and restoring the blood supply to the heart muscle. Davis, Vermeulen, Banton, Schwartz, and Williams (2000) used rTPA starting at 0.5 mg and escalating the dose to 1 and 2 mg sequentially until 50 central venous catheters were cleared and patency was restored. In 3.4% of the catheters, rTPA was unable to clear the occlusion. In a study by Daeihagh and colleagues (2000) rTPA was used to restore the patency in 49 of 56 catheters. Two milligrams was infused into each port of the catheters. The dwell time ranged between 2 and 96 hours. The literature supports the use of rTPA for the lysis of intraluminal thrombus, but further research needs to be done with the use of rTPA in 0.5 mg concentrations. The standard concentration used in most studies is 2.0 mg/2 ml. A decreased concentration of rTPA results in the added benefit of reduced costs.

PURPOSE OF THE STUDY

The purpose of the proposed study is to test the following hypothesis: 0.5 mg of recombinant tissue plasminogen activator (rTPA) is as effective as 2.0 mg of rTPA in the prevention of thrombosis in central venous catheters in two samples of 15 long-term, maintenance, hemodialysis patients over a 2-month period. At the end of 2 months each group will cross over to the alternate group for study. A prospective, randomized, double-blind crossover study will therefore be performed.

DEFINITION OF TERMS

Central venous catheter thrombosis is the presence of a thrombus located within the lumen of the central venous catheter that is responsible for a reduction in blood flow/fluids during aspiration and instillation of the catheter. This is evidenced by blood flow less than 200 ml/min, arterial pressure less than -250 millimeters of mercury (mm Hg), and venous pressure greater than $+250$ mm Hg.

Recombinant tissue plasminogen activator (rTPA) is a recombinant drug used as a lock solution in concentrations of 0.5 mg and 2.0 mg in the central venous catheters of two groups of 15 hemodialysis patients during a 2-month period. The selection of 0.5 mg for comparison was made because the literature suggests that this is the least amount of the drug evaluated during previous studies (Davis et al., 2000). Two milligrams of rTPA is a standard concentration presently used in dialysis units.

METHODOLOGY

Research Design

A prospective, Level III, experimental design is the framework upon which this proposed study will be built. Two groups will be compared and three variables of interest will be studied. Three physiological measures and specific laboratory values concerned with clotting will be monitored during the study. The two randomized, double-blinded groups will be used to compare 0.5 mg and 2.0 mg of rTPA as a lock solution in the central venous catheters of hemodialysis patients. The formation of thrombus, as determined by catheter function, is the dependent variable, and the use of rTPA and its effect on clotting constitute the independent variable. Each sample group will consist of 15 randomly selected patients with end-stage renal failure. The physiological measures that determine catheter performance, indicating clotting, are arterial pressure, venous pressure, and blood flow, because, as the thrombus forms, the catheter appears problematic causing monitoring alarms (Daeihagh et al., 2000; Northsea, 1996; Berkoben & Schwab, 1995; Twardowski, 1998a). The laboratory tests used to determine anticoagulation such as hematocrit, platelet count, prothrombin time, activated partial thromboplastin time, and fibrinogen will also be examined. Interval data will be collected from the above mentioned tests and measures for use in the data analysis.

Sample/Setting

The representative sample to be chosen for the study will include persons with end-stage renal disease who are treated with hemodialysis, and are followed by the Northern Alberta Renal Failure Program in northern Alberta, Canada. The actual field setting will be the incenter hemodialysis unit located in a large urban hospital. The patients, including both men and women, will be from various backgrounds, ethnic groups, and ages, and have various diseases. An attempt to control for extraneous variables will be possible through randomization of this convenience sample. All patients will have progressed to end-stage renal failure, thereby necessitating treatment for survival. All members of the sample will have a central venous catheter (CVC) as their dialyzing access. The catheters will be inserted using the same method of insertion by one of four experienced nephrologists. The catheters will be soft, dacron-cuffed, dual-lumen catheters used for long-term maintenance hemodialysis. The sample patients will be approached about consent for the study within 3 weeks of starting treatment, when it is recognized that the patients are receiving optimum treatment with maximum blood flow rates. Table 1 includes the demographic and relevant information required for initiation in the study.

The convenience sample population will be randomized by the hospital's pharmacist using a statistical program responsible for generating a set of random numbers to determine the two groups within the study (Appendix A). The patients to be excluded from the study are those who are not of legal age for consent, those with a current infective process, those with bleeding disorders that may affect patient welfare, and those with cancer in whom coagulability is altered by the nature of the disease (Schenk et al., 2000). Children will not be included in the study as they are not representative of a hemodialysis population that is usually comprised of adults. Rather, children are often redirected to the less invasive treatment and more tolerable modality of peritoneal dialysis.

TABLE 1	*Patient Demographics and Relevant Central Venous Catheter Information: Group A/Group B*						
Patient No.	Sex/Age	Causes of Renal Failure	Duration of Dialysis (days)	Dialysis Membrane	Dialysis Regimen	Duration of CVC (days)	CVC Site
1							
2							
3							
4							
5							
6							
7							
8							
9							
10							
11							
12							
13							
14							
15							

Sample size will be calculated using a confidence interval of 95%, a power of 0.8, and calculated variability of 18 and difference between the means of the groups (10). The calculated variability is the standard deviation of the means of two hemodialysis samples comparing blood pump speed known as the effect size. A two-tailed test will be used because the two representative samples are hypothesized to be equal. The following formula was used in the calculations for size of the groups:

$$\text{Sample} \quad \frac{(Z\alpha + z\beta)}{d} = \frac{(1.96 + 0.8)}{10} \times 18 = 25. \qquad \begin{aligned} Z\alpha &= \text{confidence interval} \\ z\beta &= \text{power} \\ d &= \text{effect size} \end{aligned}$$

The sample size will be 25 with an additional 5 for drop out (Senn, 1993). The total sample will consist of 30 hemodialysis patients, with 15 per group.

Methods

Approximately 3 weeks from the time of insertion of the central venous catheters, when maximum blood pump speeds are achieved, individual patients will be approached and asked to participate in the proposed study. An informed and witnessed consent will be obtained. The researcher conducting the study will fill out a demographic information sheet. Prior to the initiation of each dialysis treatment thereafter, as per unit protocol, the locking solution will be aspirated from the central venous catheter. Dialysis will commence and the patient will be monitored at least hourly for vital signs, blood flow rates, and arterial and venous pressures. This data will aid in the determination of catheter function. Blood flow rates below 200 ml/min, arterial pressures less than −250 mm Hg, and venous pressures of greater than +250 mm Hg reflect the presence of a thrombus. The blood flow rate or pump speed is a measure of how fast the pump is able to rotate based on catheter performance. Arterial pressure reflects the ease of removing the blood from the patient through the access for dialysis. The blood that is being withdrawn from the patient creates a negative or minus reading. Venous pressure is a measure of the ease of returning the patients blood once it has gone through the artificial kidney. This pressure is interpreted as a plus value because it reflects a positive force. Systemic heparin will be administered according to individual patient clotting times to prevent clotting of the extracoporeal system and to allow patients to be monitored for bleeding. Measuring hematocrit, platelet count, prothrombin time (PT), activated thromboplastin time (APTT), and fibrinogen each month will enable patients to be monitored for anticoagulation. The same dialysis machines and bloodlines will be used for each treatment. At the completion of dialysis, the patient's blood will be returned to the patient and the catheter will be flushed with 10 ml of normal saline to remove residual red blood cells. rTPA, prepared by the hospitals' pharmacy department, will be instilled into the lumen of the central venous catheter. rTPA will dwell in the catheter until the patient returns for his or her thrice-weekly treatment. Refer to Appendix B for the unit protocol concerning catheter instillation.

Data collection will include recording interval values for blood flow rates, arterial pressure, and venous pressure per patient to monitor catheter performance and thrombosis, and anticoagulation to monitor for potential clotting. The incidence of complications such as bleeding, sepsis, and clotting will be recorded and rated according to the frequency of the event. The study is divided into two stages for each of the two groups. Each stage will include the data collected for 1 month. At the end of 2 months the groups will cross over into the alternate group. Though the literature indicates that thrombus may form from catheter insertion by disruption of the integrity of vessel walls or from the material in the catheters, the incidence of thrombosis may occur at any time within the first month after insertion. A span of 2 to 4 months is optimal to determine the effects of rTPA on clotting as determined by the literature (Daeihagh et al., 2000; Schenk et al., 2000).

Data Analysis

The statistical analysis will use repeated-measures ANOVA to analyze and compare the data. This specific statistical test is used to compare the means of two groups using three or more variables when repeated measures are taken on each subject (Norman & Streiner, 1999). The three variables of interest are treatment, sequence of time, and period of time. The treatment variable will compare the means of the two concentrations of rTPA. The sequence of time variable will compare the measurements recorded in four separate 1-month intervals. The period of time effect will include data on the specific patients within their randomized groups in one period of time such as the first month versus the second month (Table 2). The repeated-measures ANOVA will also be used to compare treatment, period, and sequence for hematocrit, platelet count, PT, APTT, and fibrinogen. Refer to Table 3 for comparison of the two concentrations of rTPA and the statistical analysis of ANOVA comparing the three variables in Table 4.

Reliability and Validity

Control has been described as the key concept in experimental designs. Randomization is one method for controlling all possible extraneous variables in a Level III design (Brink & Wood, 1988). In this proposed study, the sample described will be a convenience sample, selected because the patients are in end-stage renal failure, have central venous catheters, and are receiving long-term, maintenance hemodialysis. The patients will be of different ages, races, and sexes, and will have different diseases. They may not be representative of all hemodialysis patients because of the method of selection. The results, therefore, cannot be generalized to all hemodialysis patients. Once these patients are

TABLE 2	*p Value from the Analysis of Variance of Central Venous Catheter Flow and Pressure Performance*			
	Treatment	*Time*	*Period*	*Sequence*
Blood flow (ml/min)				
Venous pressure (mm Hg)				
Arterial pressure (mm Hg)				

TABLE 3		Anticoagulation for Dialysis, Mean Values for Hematocrit (Hct), Platelet Count (Plt C), PT, APTT, and Fibrinogen Comparing Two Concentrations of TPA: Groups A/B (1–30 patients)								
		Hct (%)	Hct (%)	Plt C	Plt C	PT	PT	APTT	APTT	Fibrinogen	
Pt no.	Heparin	rTPA 0.5	rTPA 2.0	rTPA 0.5	rTPA 2.0	rTPA 0.5	rTPA 2.0	rTPA 0.5	rTPA 2.0	rTPA 2.0	TPA 0.5
1											
2											
3											
4											
5											
6											
7											
8											
9											
10											
11											
12											
13											
14											
15											

selected they will be randomized as described previously. Randomization, a control for internal validity, helps to eliminate bias by spreading variability equally across the groups.

Similar to the control achieved by randomization, incorporating a double-blind, crossover method into the study will enhance control. The use of the double-blind method eliminates bias. Neither the patient nor the researcher will be able to positively identify which patient will receive either concentration of the drug. The use of the crossover method will allow the patient to serve as his or her own control, thereby accounting for variability among the subjects and increasing equivalence between groups.

The parametric test of ANOVA will also increase control for the experimental design. This proposed study will use the repeated-measures ANOVA, which will adjust for differences between two groups and for correlation between the means (Brink & Wood, 1998). Further, because the study will be a double-blind crossover experiment, the patients will serve as their own controls for the comparison between the two concentrations of drugs to be used.

Control of experimental conditions will be enhanced by keeping procedures and equipment constant. Though four different nephrologists will perform the procedure for

TABLE 4	*p Value from the Analysis of Variance of Hematocrit and Coagulation Parameters*		
	Treatment	*Period*	*Sequence*
Hematocrit (%)			
Platelet count			
PT			
APTT			
Fibrinogen (mg/dl)			

line insertion, the technique and actual procedure used will be the same. The type of catheter used for long-term, maintenance hemodialysis will be the same, a dacron, dual-lumen catheter. The nursing staff in the dialysis unit will be responsible for consistently performing the instillation procedure for locking the catheters. This procedure was developed and taught to all nursing staff by one clinical nurse educator, approved by the policy and procedure committee within the hemodialysis program, and reviewed on a yearly basis. The machines and bloodlines used for the dialysis procedure will be the same. This equipment will be calibrated as per the manufacturer's specifications and verified by an external pressure meter and by a qualified biomedical technician for accuracy. The degree of error as specified by the manufacturer of the dialysis machine will allow a 10% variation in the blood pump speed and a 3% variation in the pressure readings. This will permit the measures for blood flow rates, arterial pressure, and venous pressure to be reliably tested and retested. Validity concerning anticoagulation will be addressed through specific laboratory tests well utilized in the health sciences field for the determination of clotting. The quality improvement program utilized within the clinical laboratory setting is reported to regularly verify the accuracy of results. The specificity, sensitivity, and positive predictive value of the coulter hematology analyzer responsible for generating the results of the hematologic tests are reported to be 97%, 89%, and 93.5%, respectively (personal communication, level III technician, University of Alberta Hospitals, November 24, 2000). The data to be observed and recorded, measuring the function of the catheters, will be documented by one interrater observer with hemodialysis experience, enhancing the reliability of data collection.

The concern for carryover effect of the different concentrations of rTPA within the catheter will be addressed by aspirating the catheter and then flushing with 10 ml of normal saline prior to the initiation of dialysis. A clotting time can be performed to ensure no residual rTPA was left in the catheter. The catheter will then be instilled with the new solution at the end of the treatment. A 2-day span of time between treatments will also eliminate any carryover of the medication.

A pilot study is an ideal way to address some of the concerns identified in this experimental design. It could be used to identify problems in the design, refine the data collection and analysis, establish the reliability and validity of the instruments used, establish the competence of the investigator, and strengthen the case for the study being proposed. It has been calculated that a sample of 30 patients will be necessary for this study. A pilot study would require three patients or 10% of the sample population (Brink

& Wood, 1998). Though the pilot study would increase efforts related to time, energy, and expenses, the knowledge gained could prove invaluable in many aspects of the finished product.

Ethical Considerations

Prior to the initiation of the study, the Health Research Ethics Board will be approached with a request for ethical review of the proposed study. Upon introduction to the study, the participants will be informed of the purpose of the study, procedures involved, risks, benefits, voluntary participation, compensation, and confidentiality. It will be stressed that the patient is under no obligation to participate and may withdraw from the study at any time, and that withdrawal from the study will not influence care given. An information sheet will be provided outlining the above-mentioned information (see Appendix C). A consent to participate form will be signed by the participants prior to the initiation of the study and will be obtained and witnessed by a hemodialysis professional who is not involved in the study.

The risk associated with an instillation of rTPA is bleeding. Paulson, Reisoether, Aasen, and Fauchald (1993), reported rTPA dissolves clot formation efficiently and safely, citing an 11% incidence of minor bleeding with its use. A small pilot study by Atkinson, Bagnall, and Gomperts (1990) and a prospective, double-blind study by Haire, Atkinson, Stephens, and Kotulak (1994) stated there was no incidence of bleeding while using rTPA. Though the literature appears to suggest there is minimal risk associated with the use of this drug, the patient must be made aware of the potential for bleeding.

Significance of the Study

One of the limitations of this proposed study is the concern with lack of external validity or generalizability of results related to the type of sample selected. The sample will be a convenience sample, not a true representation of all hemodialysis patients with end-stage renal failure. To ensure generalizability, this type of study could be undertaken in other renal units during a multicenter trial.

The issue of cost was not addressed in this proposed study. It is well recognized that rTPA is an expensive medication, hence it is selectively used. A cost comparison concerning catheter replacement, physician time, nursing time, and radiological verification versus the use of rTPA would prove informative and may demonstrate support for more widespread use of this drug.

The insertion and removal of central venous catheters in the hemodialysis population are the responsibility of the nephrologist. The care of these catheters is the responsibility of the dialysis nurse. A high incidence of thrombosis is a well-documented complication associated with this type of vascular access. Caring for these catheters requires technical skill, problem-solving abilities, and an understanding of anatomy and catheter performance. Even for nurses armed with experience and skill, the care of central venous catheters can be a trying experience. It is understandable, therefore, that there is a search for a drug, skill, or technique that will improve catheter performance and decrease nurse frustration and patient anxiety. rTPA has proven to be effective in the dissolution of clots within the catheters. The one deterrent to its widespread use is cost. If it can be demonstrated that a decreased concentration of rTPA, such as 0.5 mg, is as effective as the standard 2.0 mg, then more of it could be used, thereby improving nursing care and practice for patients in end-stage renal failure.

REFERENCES

Andreoli, T., Bennett, J. C., Carpenter, C. C., & Plum, F. (1997). *Cecil essentials of medicine* (4th ed.). Toronto: W. B. Saunders.

Atkinson, J. B., Bagnall, H. A., & Gomperts, E. (1990). Investigational use of tissue plasminogen activator for occluded central venous catheters. *Journal of Parenteral Enteral Nutrition, 14,* 310–311.

Barendregt, J. N., Tordoir, J. H., & Leunissen, K. M. (1999). Antithrombotic measures for indwelling intravenous hemodialysis catheters—Columbus' egg yet to be found. *Nephrology Dialysis & Transplantation, 14,* 1834–1835.

Berkoben, M., & Schwab, S. (1995). Maintenance of permanent hemodialysis vascular access patency. *American Nephrology Nurses' Association, 22(1),* 17–23.

Brink, P. J., & Wood, M. J. (1984). *Basic steps in planning nursing research: From question to proposal* (4th ed.). Boston: Jones and Bartlett.

Brink, P. J., & Wood, M. J. (1998). *Advanced design in nursing research* (2nd ed.). Thousand Oaks: Sage.

Brunier, G. (1996). Care of the hemodialysis patient with a new permanent vascular access: Review of the assessment and teaching. *American Nephrology Nurses' Association, 23(6),* 547–556.

Buturovic, J., Ponikvar, R., Boh, M., Klinkmann, J., & Ivanovich, P. (1998). Filling hemodialysis catheters in the interdialytic period: Heparin versus citrate versus polygeline: A prospective randomized study. *Artificial Organs, 22(11),* 945–947.

Central Organ Replacement Register. (1998). *Canadian organ replacement register, 1997 annual report.* Don Mills, Ontario: Hospital Medical Records Institute.

Choudhry, D., Ahmed, Z., Giris, H., & Kronfli, S. (1999). Percutaneous cuffed catheter insertion by nephrologists. *American Journal of Nephrology, 19,* 51–54.

Daeihagh, P., Jordan, J., Chen, G. J., & Rocco, M. (2000). Efficacy of tissue plasminogen activator administration on patency of hemodialysis access catheters. *American Journal of Kidney Diseases, 36(1),* 75–79.

Davis, S., Vermeulen, L., Banton, J., Schwartz, B., & Williams, E. (2000). Activity and dosage of alteplase dilution for clearing occlusions of venous-access devices. *American Journal of Health-System Pharmacy, 57(11),* 1039–1045.

Ezzahiri, R., Lemson, S., Kitslaar, P., Leunissen, K., & Toridor, K. (1999). Hemodialysis vascular access and fistula surveillance methods in the Netherlands. *Nephrology Dialysis & Transplantation, 14,* 2110–2115.

Farrell, J., Walshe, J., Gellens, M., & Martin, K. (1997). Complications associated with insertion of jugular venous catheters for hemodialysis: The value of post procedural radiograph. *American Journal of Kidney Diseases, 30(5),* 690–692.

Haire, W. D., Atkinson, J. B., Stephens, L. C., & Kotulak, G. D. (1994). Urokinase versus recombinant tissue plasminogen activator in thrombosed central venous catheter: A double-blind, randomized trial. *Thrombosis and Haemostasis, 72,* 543–547.

Johnson, M. (1998). Catheter access for hemodialysis. *Seminars in Dialysis, 11(6),* 326–330.

Kapoian, T., & Sherman, R. A. (1997). A brief history of vascular access for hemodialysis: An unfinished story. *Seminars in Nephrology, 17(3),* 239–243.

Kinzer, C. (1998). Warfarin sodium (coumadin) anticoagulant therapy for vascular access patency. *American Nephrology Nurses' Association, 25(2),* 195–203.

Kohler, T., & Kirkman, T. (1998). Central venous catheter failure is induced by injury and can be prevented by stabilizing the catheter tip. *The Society of Vascular Surgery, 28(1),* 59–65.

Konner, K. (1999). A primer on the av fistula—achilles' heel, but also the cinderella of hemodialysis. *Nephrology Dialysis & Transplantation, 14*, 2094–2098.

Lancaster, L. E. (Ed.) (1991). *Core curriculum for nephrology nursing*. Pitman, New Jersey: Anthony J. Jannetti.

Leblanc, M., Bosc, J., Vaussenant, F., Maurice, F., Moragues, H., & Canaud, B. (1998). Effective blood flow and recirculation rates in internal jugular vein twin catheters. Measured by ultrasound velocity dilution. *American Journal of Kidney Diseases, 31(1)*, 87–92.

Laski, M. E., Pressley, T. A., Sabatini, S., & Wesson, D. E. (1997). National Kidney Foundation: Dialysis Outcomes Quality Initiative (DOQI): Clinical Practice Guidelines. *American Journal of Kidney Diseases, 30(4)*, S138–S237.

Muhm, M., Sunder-Plassmann, G., Aspner, R., Kritzinger, M., Heismayr, M., & Druml, W. (1997). Supracalvicular approach to the subclavian/innominate vein for large-bore central venous catheters. *American Journal of Kidney Diseases, 30(6)*, 802–808.

Mysliwiec, M. (1997). Vascular access thrombosis—what are the possibilities of intervention? *Nephrology Dialysis & Transplantation, 12*, 876–878.

Norman, G. R., & Streiner, D. L. (1999). *PDQ statistics* (2nd ed.). Hamilton: B. C. Decker.

Northsea, C. (1996). Continuous quality improvement: Improving catheter patency using urokinase. *American Nephrology Nurses' Association, 23(6)*, 567–571.

Obialo, C. I., Robinson, T., & Braithwaite, M. (1998). Hemodialysis vascular access: Variable thrombis-free survival in three subpopulations of black patients. *American Journal of Kidney Diseases, 31(2)*, 250–256.

Ouwendyk, M., & Helferty, M. (1996). Central venous catheter management: How to prevent complications. *American Nephrology Nurses' Association, 23(6)*, 572–577.

Parker, J. (Ed.) (1998). *Contemporary nephrology nursing*. Pitman, New Jersey: Anthony J. Jannetti.

Paulsen, D., Reisoether, A., Aasen, M., & Fauchald, P. (1993). Use of tissue plasminogen activator for reopening of clotted dialysis catheters. *Nephron, 64*, 468–470.

Polaschegg, H., & Levin, N. (2000). Challenges for chronic dialysis in the new millennium. *Seminars in Nephrology, 20(1)*, 60–70.

Richard, C. J. (1986). *Comprehensive nephrology nursing*. Toronto: Little, Brown.

Senn, S. (1993). *Crossover trials in clinical research*. Chichester, England: Wiley.

Schenk, P., Rosenkranz, A., Wolfl, G., Horl, W., & Traindl, O. (2000). Recombinant tissue plasminogen activator is a useful alternative to heparin in priming Quinton Permcath. *American Journal of Kidney Diseases, 35(1)*, 130–136.

Tisher, C. C. (Ed.). (1999). Clinical Practice Guidelines of the Canadian Society of Nephrology for treatment of patients with chronic renal failure. *Journal of the American Society of Nephrology, 10(13)*, S287–S321.

Twardowski, Z. J. (1998a). The clotted central vein catheter for hemodialysis. *Nephrology Dialysis and Transplantation, 13*, 2203–2206.

Twardowski, Z. J. (1998b). High-dose intradialytic urokinase to restore the patency of permanent central vein hemodialysis catheters. *American Journal of Kidney Diseases, 31(5)*, 841–847.

Wickman, R., Purl, S., & Welker, D. (1992). Long-term central venous catheters: Issues for care. *Seminars in Oncology Nursing, 8(2)*, 133–147.

APPENDIX A

Example of a Computerized Method for Randomizing Numbers

To generate a set of random numbers, enter the selections (integer values only):

How many sets of numbers do you want to generate?   Value—2

How many numbers per set?   Value—15

Number range   Value 1–30

Do you wish each number in the set to remain unique?	Yes
Do you wish to sort your outputted numbers?	Yes
How do you wish to view your outputted numbers?	Place markers within

Randomized Results:

Group A   p1 = 3, p2 = 5, p3 = 10, p4 = 12, p5 = 13, p6 = 14, p7 = 16, p8 = 17, p9 = 18, p10 = 20, p11 = 21, p12 = 22, p13 = 25, p14 = 26, p15 = 29

Group B   p1 = 1, p2 = 2, p3 = 4, p4 = 6, p5 = 7, p6 = 8, p7 = 9, p8 = 11, p9 = 15, p10 = 19, p11 = 23, p12 = 24, p13 = 27, p14 = 28, p15 = 30

APPENDIX B

Procedure

Title: Instillation of rTPA in a Central Venous Catheter

Issue Date:

Level: Departmental

Supplies: Hemodialysis tray
Tray with compartment
2 kelly forceps
3 towels and 1 fenestrated towel
1 package povodine iodine (Betadine) solution
1 transfer forceps
Mask
2 catheter caps
2 18-gauge needles
1-in. Dermiclear (bridging) tape
rTPA (prepared by pharmacy)
Normal saline vials × 2 if normal saline not available
Sterile gloves
4 3-ml syringes
2 10- ml syringes
label

Procedures:

1.0   Mask for patient and nurse.

2.0   Wash hands.

3.0   Remove bridging tape.

4.0   Open hemodialysis tray.

5.0   Use transfer forceps on outer wrap of hemodialysis tray to pick up towels, Betadine solution, kelly forceps, and place beside the tray.

6.0   Using intravenous saline from dialyzer setup, run some saline into a compartment of the tray.

OR

Twist open 2 normal saline vials and pour into a compartment of the tray.

7.0   Add 4 3-ml syringes, 2 10-ml syringes, 2 18-gauge needles, and 2 catheter caps onto sterile field.

8.0 Place prepared rTPA syringes near tray.

9.0 Glove.

10.0 Pour Betadine solution into the second compartment of the tray.

11.0 Soak 2 4 × 4 gauze with betadine solution.

12.0 Prepare 2 10-ml syringes with normal saline by drawing up from saline compartment.

13.0 While holding a catheter with a 4 × 4 gauze, position towels above and below catheter area.

14.0 Wrap the catheter with a Betadine-soaked 4 × 4 gauze for 4 minutes.

15.0 With catheter clamps closed, remove and discard caps.

16.0 While holding the wrapped catheter, lay the fenestrated towel underneath the Betadine-wrapped catheter.

17.0 Remove betadine-soaked 4 × 4 gauze on catheter and attach a 3-ml syringe to each catheter extension.

18.0 Withdraw 3 ml from each unclamped extension of the catheter.

19.0 Clamp both extensions.

20.0 Discard the withdrawn blood onto a 4 × 4 gauze to check for clots.

21.0 Attach a saline-filled 10-ml syringe to each extension.

22.0 Unclamp and flush each extension alternately with 10 ml normal saline and clamp while instilling to remove all traces of blood.

23.0 Wrapping a sterile 4 × 4 gauze around the rTPA-filled syringe, instill in one continuous motion.

24.0 Attach new caps to leur lock connectors on clamped catheter connections.

25.0 Apply bridging tapes on both catheter connections.

26.0 Attach a label over bridging tape indicating the presence of rTPA.

27.0 Wrap a 4 × 4 gauze around catheter extensions and secure with tape.

APPENDIX C

Tissue Plaminogen Activator Research Study Patient Information Sheet

Project Title: Maintaining Catheter Patency Using Recombinant Plasminogen Activator
Principal Investigator:
Colleen M. Astle, R.N. M.N. Candidate
Co-investigators:
Dr. R. Ulan, Nephrologist and Associate Professor, University of Alberta

Purpose of the study: Hemodialysis is a treatment that is available to you when your kidneys have stopped working. It will replace some of the functions normally carried out by your own kidneys such as cleaning the blood of waste products and excess fluids. To perform this procedure it is necessary to gain access to your blood. This is possible with the use of a catheter. The catheter is kept open and working by using a drug called tissue plasminogen activator. The reason for doing the study is to compare two different amounts of this drug to see which is more effective in keeping the catheter open for use.

Study procedures: Central venous catheters are a common access used for dialysis. You will have a catheter in place when this study is started. If you agree to take part in the study, an unknown concentration of the study drug will be put into the catheter to keep it open. At the end of 2 months you will move to the second group to use the other concentration of the drug. Neither you nor your study investigator will know which drug concentration is being used in either stage of the study.

Risks: There is a small risk of bleeding associated with the use of this medication and one of the drugs may be less effective in preventing the catheter from clotting. You will be kept informed if any problems develop with the catheter.

Benefits: You personally may not benefit from this study at this time, however the information gained in doing the study may help improve the care of these catheters in the future.

Voluntary participation: Taking part in the study is voluntary. Deciding not to take part will not affect the care you receive. If you decide to stop after the study has begun your care will not be affected.

Compensation: There will be no financial cost to you for taking part in the study. You will not be charged for using the drug in your catheter or for any of the procedures. By signing the consent form you are not releasing the investigator, institution, or sponsor from their legal and professional responsibilities.

Confidentiality: The information collected for this study will be kept private. Your name will not be used. Your chart will be used to collect information for the study. If you have any questions about the study please do not hesitate to call the Program Director. If you have any concerns about any aspect of this study, you may contact the Capital Health Authority patient care representative. This office has no affiliation with the study or its investigators.

Index

Note: Page numbers followed by t refer to tables.